[335 -30]

December! Well, I don't much regret the end of _this year_
for the trouble we have gone through it something dreadful—
Of course there _have_ been pleasant days but they have
been the exception rather than the rule—Uncle & Aunt are
not all-x; I took A. to the omnibus, then practised & talked
to M. who is rather incensed agnst Gemma, who said that if
she did not improve she wod. never be poor dear little M.
agn.—It was an unkind thing to say, & what does not
mend matters, it was said before Mrs Stretton! I met Mr W.
as I came home this x, he looked as "jolly" as ever, & removed
his hat with a flourish. P. has a ticket for the private view of
Holman Hunt's new picture "The shadow of Death", but unfortunate-
-ly it was sent too late on Saturday for him to go. Mr.
-tt told Uncle he shd. so much like to go to P.'s lecture at the
Academy (tonight), so P. has sent him a ticket. I am very
glad. It does not seem as if he did. call there in a hurry—
I bound a bracket with green silk, which looks very
pretty indeed, & have cost next to nothing, as I used
up odds & ends I had. Aunt intends to "return by
the mail-train tonight," having seen all she wanted,
& Uncle goes back tomorrow x. . P. gave his lecture, but
felt dreadfully nervous at the idea. Uncle & J. went
with him. It was very full, & went off very well, so
everyone said. Aunt said goodbye, & went off to St.
Pancras, & — returned! having missed the train!—
So, she will go with Uncle. I slept upstairs for the
last time for some time I hope; I like my own room.
Aunt does not intend to have the old people to her
party this year; I am so pleased! Then Stella & Leonie
are up a list of the invites, a proposition I made

THE PRECARIOUSLY
PRIVILEGED

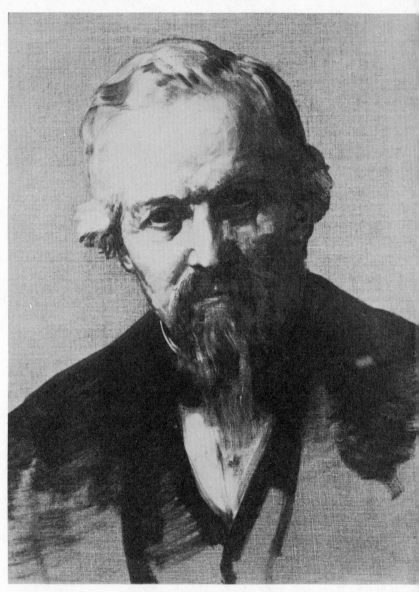

JOHN MARSHALL, FRS

Alphonse Legros, 1837–1911, Slade Professor of Fine Arts at University College, London, painted this portrait in 1879, and presented it to the South Kensington Museum in 1880. When it was exhibited at the Grosvenor Gallery in May 1880, the sitter's daughter commented: 'Legros' portrait of P. is atrocious, much too dark, with a forbidding expression, & a crooked look wh. is quite distressing to contemplate.'

THE
PRECARIOUSLY
PRIVILEGED

*A Professional Family
in Victorian London*

Zuzanna Shonfield

Oxford   New York

OXFORD UNIVERSITY PRESS

1987

Oxford University Press, Walton Street, Oxford OX2 6DP

Oxford New York Toronto
Delhi Bombay Calcutta Madras Karachi
Petaling Jaya Singapore Hong Kong Tokyo
Nairobi Dar es Salaam Cape Town
Melbourne Auckland

and associated companies in
Beirut Berlin Ibadan Nicosia

Oxford is a trade mark of Oxford University Press

British Library Cataloguing in Publication Data

Shonfield, Zuzanna
The precariously privileged: a professional family in Victorian London.
1. Middle classes—England—London—History—19th century 2. London (England)
—Social life and customs—19th century
I. Title
942.1081'0880622   HT690.G7

ISBN 0-19-212265-7

Library of Congress Cataloging in Publication Data

Shonfield, Zuzanna.
The precariously privileged.
Includes index.
1. London (England)—Biography. 2. Marshall family. 3. Middle classes—England
—London—History—19th century. 4. London (England)—Social life and customs
—19th century. 5. Physicians—England—London—Family relationships—History
—19th century.   I. Title.
DA676.8.A1S56 1987   942.1'081'0922 [B]   86-12801

ISBN 0-19-212265-7

Printed in Great Britain by
Butler & Tanner Ltd.
Frome, Somerset

FOREWORD

THIS book is focused on the Marshalls of Savile Row, one of the many recent arrivals who rose to the top of the establishment at the time of the great surge of middle-class growth in nineteenth-century London. Migrating from the provinces (or, in a few instances, from abroad), they swelled the professional and artistic élite which serviced this new class and provided it with an intellectual core. Being recently uprooted, they were prone to the special problems which make immigrant communities vulnerable and unstable. London offered special opportunities, first-class educational facilities, the feeling of being at the centre of things, the freedom to defy convention without exciting comment. But it also took the toll charged by every great city: it made the newcomers feel isolated and defenceless. Much of this had to do with an uncertainty as to where they belonged. They found it difficult to place people whom they met in their new circumstances, and this contributed to an awkwardness and lack of spontaneity in all their relationships. What suffered most was the process of forming the alliances of friendship and marriage.

Casual evidence of social mobility abounds in the autobiographies and biographies of nineteenth-century professionals, but it is only continuous records over long spans of years, such as are found in diaries, that show how sequences of almost imperceptible adjustments eventually add up to massive shifts in status. The history of the Marshalls is a good instance of such movement up and then downwards, and also laterally, out of the professional sphere. The very sequence of the family's London residences, the shift westwards and to the south-west, illustrates how the metropolis rewarded the rise or the decline of privilege.

John Marshall (1818–91), the head of the family, came from Ely. His career as surgeon and anatomist is a model of the success of a hard-working and ambitious Victorian migrant from the provinces. Helped by the propitious environment of the fast-growing capital he rose from the anonymity of the new settler, with few means and even less patronage, to the summit of the medical profession. His wife and children were also hoisted for a time out of a humdrum middle-class existence on to the upper stratum of the professional élite. This elevation made one or two of them open to innovatory, even radical notions and sentiments. But the accent here is on the conventional, delineating its limits and aiming to show the process by which it became eroded by contact with the unconventional and by the wear and tear of family life.

When Marshall reached the peak of his profession, he brought home, in terms of today's buying-power, over £100,000 net a year, yet he left no great fortune. As in the case of many other professional families, a son who had to be maintained through a slow educational process, and daughters who never became entirely self-supporting, made both the savings and status that had been the reward of his life's effort too insubstantial to meet the needs of his ultimate heirs. There is a great deal of evidence to show that the elevated situation in which the successful new professionals found themselves in the latter part of the nineteenth century was decidedly precarious. One is led to speculate that it was the insecurity of their standing and of their standard of living that made the daughters of these new top professionals a drag on the marriage market.

Getting married was the chief preoccupation of the twenties and early thirties of John Marshall's elder daughter, Jeannette, the diarist on whose records the bulk of this book is based. In the 1870s and '80s it was still the rule to aspire no further than to a few years of glorious fun at balls and garden parties, followed by a suitable match and then, after the honeymoon, a succession of more staid convivial occasions. Enterprising, ambitious or public-spirited women who went in for serious-minded pursuits (or those who flouted convention for the sake of frivolous gratification) were still the exception.

In girlhood and early womanhood Jeannette Marshall had seen herself as one of the fortunates. Good-looking, worldly, clever, and in all obvious ways thoroughly eligible, she thought she could pick and choose the man on whom to bestow her favours. But by the age of thirty-five, in 1890, after some seventeen or eighteen years of fleeting flirtations and near-offers, and mid-way through yet another unsatisfactory affair of the heart, she was forced to reflect: 'somehow my matrimonial hand-mark does not seem to be a true one.' Four out of her five aunts (and of course her mother) had married; the exception

had been her mother's blind sister Eliza, whose infirmity was a sufficient explanation for her celibacy. To remain on the shelf was a new
experience in Jeannette's family—though shared with a good many
Victorian middle- and professional-class women.[1] Not only she and
her sister Ada, but fifteen out of twenty of her adult girl cousins were
in 1890 still unmarried. Eventually a few would find husbands, but
even so, the proportion of single to married women in Jeannette
Marshall's own circle would remain far greater than in her mother's
generation.

At fifteen, she had declared that in literature she preferred the 'école
realiste' to the 'école romantique'. And she herself exemplified what,
in fiction at least, was a return to realism, to the unembellished
portrayals for which Jane Austen provided memorable prototypes. In
writing of herself she was reticent, and made no attempt to unveil her
personality nor examine her purpose in life. But in a daily record of
nearly eight thousand closely written pages much that is intimate
naturally seeps out. For one thing, the pattern which is revealed as the
diarist records fragments of family conflicts illustrates, with uncon-
scious frankness and some subtlety, the pressures of Victorian home
life.

She chose to write, in the curiously debunking tone which was
fashionable among the bright young women of the period, of doings
and comings and goings, with no thought for the inner layers of
connecting causes and effects, of motives and fulfilments and disap-
pointments. Medicals, politicians, men of letters, artists (with the Pre-
Raphaelite friends of her father's youth to the fore), foreign patrons
and indigenous eccentrics—she scoffed at them and gossiped about
them without a shade of deference. It took reversals of fortune and
the prospect of permanent spinsterhood to rub down some of Miss
Marshall's smug self-satisfaction, reveal resources of stoicism and
courage, and show that she knew how to bend and adjust to achieve
her objectives.

[1] On the basis of 1851 census figures it is estimated that 30 per cent of all women
between the ages of 20 and 40 were single (Janet H. Murray, *Strong-minded Women,
and other lost voices from nineteenth-century England*, Harmondsworth, 1984, p. 48). The
problem was especially marked in London and most acute among daughters of upper
middle-class families. In their case, marriage was the exception rather than the rule (see
Dorothy Crowther, 'Kinship and Occupational Succession', *Sociological Review*,
n.s. xiii.1 (1965), p. 18). John Burnett, in *Plenty and Want* (Harmondsworth, 1968),
p. 234, even comes to the extravagant conclusion that in the 1870s 'the greatest
feminine problem' was the 'scarcity of husbands for middle-class girls'.

Jeannette Marshall left twenty-two volumes of diaries, covering the years 1870 to 1892 (1890 and 1891 are under one cover). She wrote them almost invariably in Pettitt's Octavo Diaries, elegant volumes bound in olive-green, gold-embossed cloth.[2] The daily entries, rarely less than three hundred words long, were jotted down for the most part before she retired to bed. In the process of summarizing the screeds of detail some of what interested her most—clothes, entertainment, music, travel—has been foreshortened to make way for the wider perspective in which her existence and those of her relatives were set. Jeannette's spelling and punctuation have been preserved, except in a relatively small number of cases where substituting conventional orthography or punctuation clarifies the meaning.

What came before 1870, her family's antecedents, her father's career and her own childhood, is outlined under the heading 'Points of Departure', and stems in the main from the account of her childhood which Jeannette wrote at eighteen, backed by genealogical material from her Commonplace Book and the usual gleanings from archives, directories, parish records and gravestones. In a final section, entitled 'Aftermath', the post-1892 fortunes of the descendants of John Marshall the surgeon are encapsulated from fragmentary memoirs Jeannette wrote in her fifties, supplemented by family letters and photographs, and also by the relevant portions of the journals another compulsive diarist, Rosalind Seaton, wrote in five volumes through the years 1916 to 1940. Some of the protagonists and events of this relatively recent phase are of course still remembered by people now living; their eye-witness accounts round off the history of the Marshall family.

I owe to Caroline Miles the privilege of gaining the permission of her mother Rosalind Leslie to use the Marshall papers for this book. It was Mrs Miles who saw the relevance of these records to a task which I had set myself, that of studying the life of professionals in late-Victorian London, and with great tact and good humour she allowed me to range freely in the histories of her ancestors and to interpret them without undue reverence.

I would like to thank Janet Percival, the Archivist of University

---

[2] They cost 4s. 6d. each, about £6.50 in today's terms. Throughout this book a factor of c.30 has been used to convert late Victorian values into present-day ones. An explanatory note to the facsimile edition of the 1886 Statistical Abstract of the UK (HMSO, 1986) reckons that 'in 1986 one would need more than £32 to buy what could be bought for £1 in 1886'.

College, London, for several fruitful explorations of the records of University College Hospital, and also the staff of the library at the European University Institute in Florence, who for several years tolerated an unscheduled researcher. C. R. Jakes of the Local Studies department of the Cambridgeshire Libraries and Information Service has helpfully located elusive facts about the poet William Harrison. Reginald Holmes, a historian and lover of Ely, told me a great deal about the town and its past inhabitants.

Few of my friends and relatives escaped the chore of helping with the design of the book and advising on its contents, but some contributions have been so specific that those who made them must be singled out by name. Bonnie Bonis in Florence and Alison Richmond in London learnt to decipher my scrawl and induced me to clarify my sentences. Leslie Dick made order out of chaos; above all, she acted as touchstone for my tentative attempts to interpret the diarist's character. Linda Levy Peck's reading of some of the early draft set me a historian's professional standard. Jeremy Schonfield's special contribution has been to make me take heed of editorial requirements.

To Dharma Kumar, Pauline Pinder and Irena Szymańska I am specially indebted. Each of them put in long hours of creative and clear thinking about what I was trying to convey, and then advised me how to improve my rough-hewn texts. Irena Szymańska also took on the task of inspiriting me whenever the courage to continue with the venture was about to desert me.

Several people died before I had a chance to thank them for their help. To my mother, Stefania Holt, I owe all I know about costume. Pym (K. P.) Mannock enthusiastically searched for elusive information on the ancestry of the Marshall, Walton and Williams families. My husband died in 1981, but there is little in the book that was not thrashed out in conversation with him, and it was he who gave the undertaking its initial spurt.

Our children took over many of the functions that would have been their father's. Katherine has set me an example of single-mindedness over a self-imposed task; David explored and guessed and interpreted my often arcane ideas. My thanks go to them and also to Pat for bearing with my obsession and sharing me with a nineteenth-century, surrogate, family.

S. Leolino–London
1986

CONTENTS

LIST OF ILLUSTRATIONS

John Marshall, FRS   *Frontispiece*

Note: Quotations in captions are from Jeannette Marshall's diaries and other writings. The author wishes to acknowledge the following photographs: *Frontispiece*: by courtesy of the Board of Trustees, Victoria and Albert Museum; Pl. 1 (*a*) by kind permission of Sir John Summerson; Pl. 1 (*b*) by kind permission of Henry Poole & Co.; Pl. 1 (*c*) copyright B. T. Batsford Ltd.; Pl. 13 copyright Photographic Unit, Department of Architecture & Civic Design, Greater London Council; the remaining photographs are reproduced by kind permission of Mrs Caroline Miles.

THE MARSHALLS

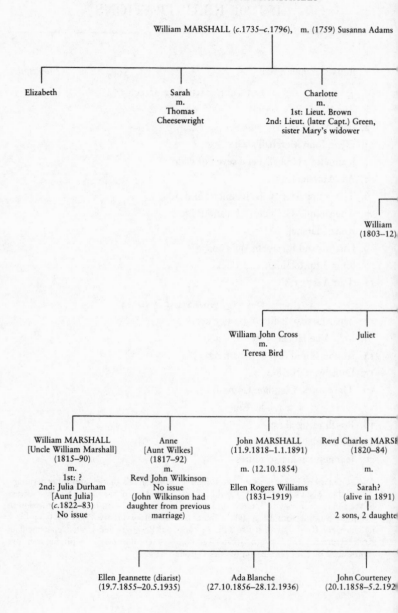

William MARSHALL (*c*.1735–*c*.1796), m. (1759) Susanna Adams

Elizabeth

Sarah
m.
Thomas
Cheesewright

Charlotte
m.
1st: Lieut. Brown
2nd: Lieut. (later Capt.) Green,
sister Mary's widower

William
(1803–12)

William John Cross
m.
Teresa Bird

Juliet

William MARSHALL
[Uncle William Marshall]
(1815–90)
m.
1st: ?
2nd: Julia Durham
[Aunt Julia]
(*c*.1822–83)
No issue

Anne
[Aunt Wilkes]
(1817–92)
m.
Revd John Wilkinson
No issue
(John Wilkinson had
daughter from previous
marriage)

John MARSHALL
(11.9.1818–1.1.1891)

m. (12.10.1854)

Ellen Rogers Williams
(1831–1919)

Revd Charles MARSH
(1820–84)

m.

Sarah?
(alive in 1891)

2 sons, 2 daughte

Ellen Jeannette (diarist)
(19.7.1855–20.5.1935)

Ada Blanche
(27.10.1856–28.12.1936)

John Courteney
(20.1.1858–5.2.192

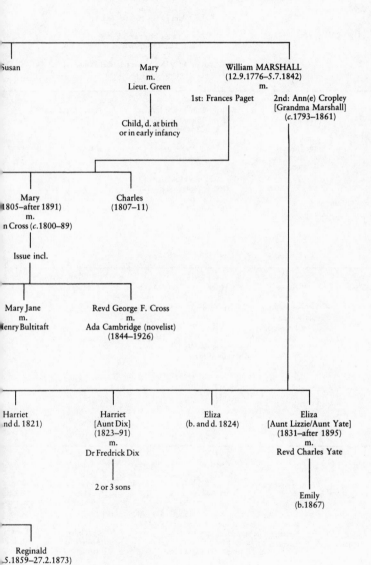

THE WILLIAMS FAMILY

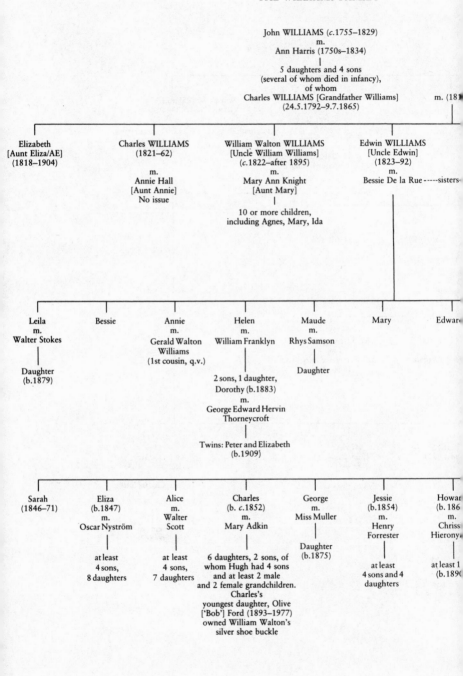

John WILLIAMS (c.1755–1829)
m.
Ann Harris (1750s–1834)

5 daughters and 4 sons
(several of whom died in infancy),
of whom
Charles WILLIAMS [Grandfather Williams]   m. (18▊
(24.5.1792–9.7.1865)

Elizabeth
[Aunt Eliza/AE]
(1818–1904)

Charles WILLIAMS
(1821–62)
m.
Annie Hall
[Aunt Annie]
No issue

William Walton
WILLIAMS
[Uncle William Williams]
(c.1822–after 1895)
m.
Mary Ann Knight
[Aunt Mary]

10 or more children,
including Agnes, Mary, Ida

Edwin WILLIAMS
[Uncle Edwin]
(1823–92)
m.
Bessie De la Rue ----sisters-

Leila
m.
Walter Stokes

Daughter
(b.1879)

Bessie

Annie
m.
Gerald Walton
Williams
(1st cousin, q.v.)

Helen
m.
William Franklyn

2 sons, 1 daughter,
Dorothy (b.1883)
m.
George Edward Hervin
Thorneycroft

Twins: Peter and Elizabeth
(b.1909)

Maude
m.
Rhys Samson

Daughter

Mary

Edwar▊

Sarah
(1846–71)

Eliza
(b.1847)
m.
Oscar Nyström

at least
4 sons,
8 daughters

Alice
m.
Walter
Scott

at least
4 sons,
7 daughters

Charles
(b. c.1852)
m.
Mary Adkin

6 daughters, 2 sons, of
whom Hugh had 4 sons
and at least 2 male
and 2 female grandchildren.
Charles's
youngest daughter, Olive
['Bob'] Ford (1893–1977)
owned William Walton's
silver shoe buckle

George
m.
Miss Muller

Daughter
(b.1875)

Jessie
(b.1854)
m.
Henry
Forrester

at least
4 sons and 4
daughters

Howar▊
(b.186▊
m.
Chriss▊
Hierony▊

at least 1
(b.189▊

William Walton (*c.*1750–1806)
m.
1st: ?Elizabeth—no surviving issue
2nd: Sarah Bean (1764–1834)
|
2 sons who did not survive early
childhood and 1 daughter,
Elizabeth [Grandmother Williams]
(7.1.1797–24.10.1876)

John WILLIAMS
[Uncle John]
(1824–after 1895)

m. 1st:
ry De la Rue
|
ns* of whom
rald Walton
m.
h Kent (d. 1890)
sue: 3 or 4
Annie Williams
cousin, q.v.)
|
Anthony Walton
(b. 1893)

m. 2nd:
Elizabeth 'Liz' Gray,
née Abrahams
(4 or 5 daughters* and
several sons from
previous marriages)

Sarah Walton
[Aunt Startin]
(1827–92)
m.
George Startin
[Uncle Startin]
(1808–85)

Anna Maria
(1828–31)

Ellen Rogers
(9.5.1831–5.4.1919)
m. (12.10.1854)
John Marshall

*see Marshall
family tree*

16 children, of whom
3 died in infancy.
The surviving ones
were:

ard   Constance   Kitty   Helen   Fanny   Walter William
92)   m.   (1871–83)
                       Charles Cassidy
                             |
                          at least
                       1 son (b. 1894)

* Two of John Williams's sons married their stepmother's daughters by a previous marriage.

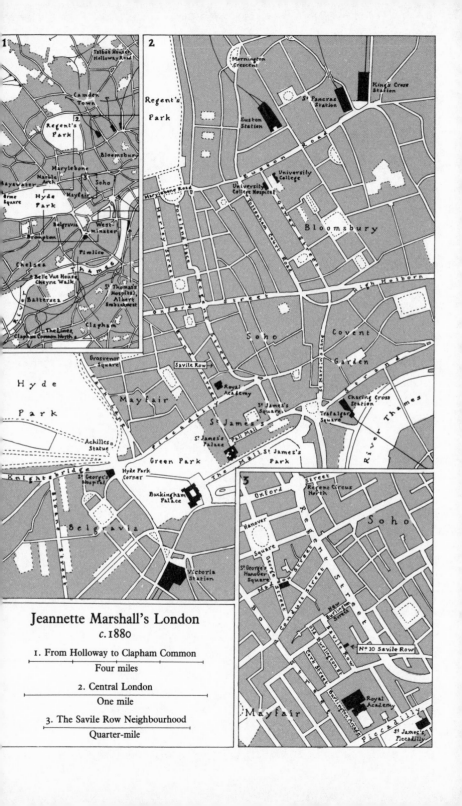

1

Talbot House
Holloway Road

Camden
Town

Regent's
Park

2

Regent's
Park

Bloomsbury

Marylebone

Marble
Arch

Bayswater

3

Soho

Orme
Square

Mayfair

Hyde
Park

Belgravia

West-
minster

Brompton

Pimlico

Chelsea

Thames

Belle Vue House
Cheyne Walk

St Thomas's
Hospital,
Albert Embankment

Battersea

Clapham

The Limes
Clapham Common North

2

Mornington
Crescent

King's Cross
Station

St Pancras
Station

Euston
Station

University
College

University
College Hospital

Marylebone Road

Bloomsbury

Euston Road

Tottenham Court Road

Gower Street

High Holborn

Oxford Street

Soho

Covent
Garden

Savile Row

Royal
Academy

St James's
Square

St Martin's Lane

Strand

Charing Cross
Station

Trafalgar
Square

Hyde
Park

Grosvenor
Square

Mayfair

Piccadilly

St James's

Pall Mall

St James's
Palace

The Mall

St James's
Park

River Thames

Achilles
Statue

Green Park

Knightsbridge

Hyde Park
Corner

St George's
Hospital

Buckingham
Palace

Belgravia

Victoria
Station

3

Street

Oxford

Regent Circus
North

Soho

Hanover
Square

Regent Street

St George's
Hanover Square

George Street

Conduit Street

New
Burlington Street

Bond Street

Old Burlington Street

Savile Row

Nº 10 Savile Row

Mill Street

Maddox Street

Cork Street

Clifford Street

Burlington Arcade

Royal
Academy

Mayfair

Piccadilly

St James's
Piccadilly

Jeannette Marshall's London
c. 1880

1. From Holloway to Clapham Common

Four miles

2. Central London

One mile

3. The Savile Row Neighbourhood

Quarter-mile

POINTS OF DEPARTURE

EARLY in December 1854 the painter Ford Madox Brown called on his friend John Marshall at 10 Savile Row and found the surgeon and his wife 'in a splendid room without fire—both look starved & pinched'.[1]

John and Ellen Marshall had married on 12 October and at the time of Brown's visit Ellen was some eight weeks pregnant. The comfortless room in which she, her husband and their guest shivered with cold was no doubt the first-floor front drawing-room. With its tall windows, elegant panelling and finely carved cornice, this was indeed impressive. So was the whole house, a fit domicile for the top professional Marshall hoped to become. Throughout the nineteenth century, the Savile Row area, as well as Wimpole Street and Harley Street, housed the pick of London's physicians and surgeons.

By now in his middle thirties, Marshall was relatively behind in the race to the summit.[2] He had come to London from Ely, then as now a small, cathedral-dominated place, in 1838 or 1839 and had worked his way up to the position of assistant surgeon at University College Hospital. This appointment had come to him when he was thirty, well within the usual age norm, but since then his progress had slowed. Some of this had to do with the limits of his expertise and also with the vacancies within the College and its Hospital. Even so, much of the handicap was of his own making. The exhilarating sense of freedom imparted by the move to London had impelled him at fortuitous tangents away from the obvious path to professional heights.

Ely had been the home of his ancestors for as long as family memory went back. The pre-Victorian Marshalls are remembered there, first

---

[1] Most of the material on the relationship between John Marshall and the young Pre-Raphaelites stems from *The Diary of Ford Madox Brown*, Virginia Surtees ed. (New Haven, 1981), and William Michael Rossetti's *Some Reminiscences* (London, 1906).

[2] M. Jeanne Peterson, *The Medical Profession in Mid-Victorian London* (London, 1978) has been used for comparisons of Marshall's career with those of his contemporaries.

among the respectable tradesmen and then, by the second half of the eighteenth century, as attorneys and auctioneers, a line of business which earned them their living until the death of the last of the Ely tribe in 1890. Although these forebears appear from a distance as immutable as the Cathedral or the Ely Porta, a degree of change came in the last quarter of the eighteenth century. John Marshall's father, William (1776–1842), had been articled to a Cambridge solicitor and finished his legal studies in London, where he found his first wife. But being an only son, he returned to the fold and was reabsorbed into Ely. A local girl, Ann Cropley, became his second wife.

Their first child, also William (1815–90), born a few weeks before the battle of Waterloo, in time took over his father's legal practice. According to the custom prevailing among provincial professionals, the next son, John (1818–91), was directed into medicine. In the first three decades of the century four out of every five top physicians—those who became Fellows of the Royal College of Physicians—had been funded at considerable expense through Oxford or Cambridge. Though less prestigious, surgery was the only realistic specialization for the ambitious son of a relatively impecunious small-town lawyer, and a provincial apprenticeship was the obvious first step into surgery. Accordingly, on leaving school John was apprenticed to Messrs Wales, who combined the functions of surgeons and general practitioners in nearby Wisbech.

A bare five years later, in 1837 or 1838, young Marshall, probably not yet twenty, inscribed himself at University College, London. The College was new (its charter dated from 1828) and non-sectarian, which earned it the label of the Godless College in Gower Street. It attracted a heterogeneous mix of lively students and unconventional, enthusiastic teachers. Marshall, a 'most industrious and intelligent student',[3] distinguished himself as early as 1840 by winning an essay prize founded by William Sharpey, his physiology teacher. The award, and especially the gold medal that went with it, brought a student to the special notice of appointment committees and the medical press; to Marshall, with no family connections or other private patronage to back him, such distinction must have been particularly useful.

<hr>

[3] Reports of the University College sub-committees on applicants for academic and hospital positions and W. R. Merrington, *University College Hospital and its Medical School: a History* (London, 1976) are the chief sources for Marshall's early career at UC and UCH.

The first fruits of the 1840 honour and of his hard work came in 1842 with his appointment to the curatorship of the College's Anatomy Museum. At a modest annual stipend of £75 for some thirty-five hours a week, it was no sinecure. But, like his father and his elder brother William, John Marshall had an aptitude for accurate observation of physical phenomena and was moreover a fine draughtsman; both gifts attracted him to the field of anatomy. His time at Wisbech had taught him some straightforward skills such as the preparation of simple remedies; but as far as surgery proper was concerned, the emphasis had been on passive learning, through 'considerable opportunities of witnessing surgical practice', of which he had 'availed himself . . . with great assiduity'. The surgeons who taught him at University College Hospital had more to offer. In 1844 Marshall became personal assistant to Robert Liston, whose dexterity and exploits in lightning surgery had won him the reputation of an ace. His uncouth exuberance was legendary. 'Time me, gentlemen, time me!' he would call to his students as the scalpel drew blood. In contrast to Liston, Richard Quain, for whom Marshall worked as an assistant demonstrator in the mid-forties, was a cautious, unhistrionic surgeon and a sensible painstaking teacher. However, neither the example of Liston nor that of Quain overcame Marshall's lack of 'special surgical aptitude'; his operating techniques remained 'slow and the reverse of brilliant'.[4] He called himself surgeon and would eventually earn a good living by an amalgam of surgery and general practice. But anatomy moulded important parts of his career and it was as anatomist that he made his scientific mark.[5]

Anatomy also opened the way to unorthodox friendships. Back in 1844 Marshall, newly qualified and in the throes of coping with the demands of Liston, set up in private practice. The location he chose, Crescent Place, Mornington Crescent, was only a few minutes' walking distance from his hospital. Here rents were low; here the untried practitioner, who charged no more than 1s. or 1s. 6d. per consultation, would find patients tolerant of his provincial ways. Some of his neighbours he would soon be treating for free.

---

[4] *Plarr's Lives of the Fellows of the Royal College of Surgeons of England*, revised by Sir D'Arcy Power with W. G. Spencer and G. E. Gask (Bristol, 1930), and Sir Edward Sharpey Schafer, 'Surgery and Physiology', *Lancet*, 27 October 1923, p. 921.

[5] His major contribution to anatomical literature was the *Anatomy for Artists* (London, 1878), which went into several editions. His name is attached to the oblique vein on the posterior wall of the left atrium.

Round the corner from Crescent Place, at the point where Arlington Road runs northwards out of Mornington Crescent, stood Tudor Lodge, a cluster of artists' studios in one of which Ford Madox Brown had stayed briefly in 1844. On returning from abroad after the death of his first wife, the painter found work space of a less transient kind within easy walking distance of Arlington Road. For some years he and his Pre-Raphaelite coterie continued to haunt Tudor Lodge. He and several of his friends, such as Charles Lucy, Walter Deverell and the Rossetti brothers, Gabriel and William Michael, availed themselves of Marshall's professional services. Their acquaintance with Marshall, at first that of patients and medical adviser, soon grew into something close to an intimacy. Brown, like Marshall, was a newcomer to London, having lived and studied in France and Belgium. A hypochondriac, with a medical grandfather and a surgeon for father-in-law, he may have found Marshall's company congenial and reassuring. The relations between the two young men, Marshall thirty or so, Brown twenty-seven, were familiar and relaxed: 'John Marshall came in, went out with him . . . came in, stopped till ten . . . Thomas and John Marshall came in. I did no more work . . . called on Marshall . . . walked all the way to my study with me at 2 in the morning . . . called in: talked a great deal about the approaching revolution; what is to be the upshot of it?'[6] As a mark of acceptance into the Pre-Raphaelite set, Brown perpetuated the surgeon's features in the huge canvas of Chaucer at the Court of Edward III. John Marshall, fair, snub-nosed and as yet beardless, is there as the Jester, 'so absorbed in Chaucer's tale as to have forgotten his calling', an insight perhaps into the young provincial's fascination with the life of the artists.

Certainly, for Marshall the easy, informal relationships among these bohemians supplied some of the heady excitement which other young medicals got through foreign travel, service in the navy or in the colonial army and spells of practice in hospitals abroad. What he had to offer in return, beside free care in sickness,[7] were a few contacts with

[6] Entries in Brown's diary, op. cit., for 8 September and 1 November 1847, and for 11 January, 4 February and 7 April 1848. Thomas was almost certainly William Cave Thomas, an intimate of Brown's. The subject of Brown's and Marshall's political discussion may have been the contemporary republican revolution in Paris, or, more likely, the aftermath of the Chartist riots.

[7] S. C. Dyke, 'Some Medical Aspects of the Life of Dante Gabriel Rossetti', *Proceedings of the Royal Society of Medicine*, lvi, December 1963, writes that Marshall 'attended all the Pre-Raphaelite Brethren in the early days of the movement, apparently free of charge'. Brown, for one, discharged his debt in kind, by presenting the surgeon

the University College establishment, paving the way to academic commissions and best of all, access to the dissecting rooms at his hospital, with corpses for anatomical study. The reforming measures introduced way back in 1830 to stop the scandalous abuses of the trade in bodies for dissection had forced the merger of two of London's largest independent schools of anatomy with St George's and St Thomas's hospitals and the closure of most of the smaller schools.[8] Deprived of these private schools, artists had nowhere to gain practical knowledge of anatomy through dissection, unless a well-disposed surgeon smuggled them into a hospital dissecting room. Marshall did just that, at least for Ford Madox Brown; the painter was amused, if somewhat squeamish:

. . . to University Hospital to ask John Marshall about a dead boddy. He got the one that will just do. It was in the vaults under the dissecting room. When I saw it first, what with the dim light, the brown & parchment like appearance of it & the shaven head, I took it for a wooden imulation of the thing. Often as I have seen horrors I really did not remember how hideous the shell of a poor creature may remain when the substance contained is fled. Yet we both in our joy at the obtainment of what we sought declared it to be lovely & a splendid corps. Marshall evidently loves a thing of the kind . . .

. . . to the University by $\frac{1}{2}$ past 10. Drew the corps till $\frac{1}{2}$ past 2. Got on quite merrily & finished it 2 hours sooner than was obligate on me. As I was going met Marshall who could not keep away from the sweets of the charnel house.

These entries from Brown's diaries referred to 13 and 14 March 1856. On the second occasion, the painter added: 'I went home with him, he talking away as ever. He has lots of work on hand. I saw his little girl, very nice.' The child was Marshall's first-born, Jeannette, then eight months old.

Unlike her husband, Ellen Marshall, the new baby's mother, was a Londoner, born and brought up in Holloway. Her paternal grand-father John Williams had come to the capital from South Wales in the 1770s or '80s and founded a successful family business which lasted a hundred years or so. By the second half of the nineteenth century the

with at least two examples of his work, a sketch for *Chaucer*, 'The Seeds and Fruits of English Poetry' (plate 6 in the 1984 catalogue of the Tate Gallery's Pre-Raphaelite exhibition) and a coloured lithograph of Lake Windermere (ibid., pp. 60–1).

[8] See M. J. Durey, 'Bodysnatchers and Benthamites: the Implications of the Dead Body Bill for the London Schools of Anatomy, 1820–42', *The London Journal*, ii.2 (1976).

prejudice against manufacturing and trade had crystallized sufficiently for his descendants to suppress the nature of the industry on which the family's fortunes depended. Jeannette wrote vaguely that her great-grandfather Williams on coming to London 'went into business, "something in the City" ', though his sarcophagus, still in the church-yard of St Mary Magdalene's, Holloway, clearly identifies itself as the 'Family Vault of Mr John Williams of this Parish and of St. James's Clerkenwell—Soap Manufacturer'.[9]

There was no such ambiguity about the career of Jeannette's other maternal great-grandfather, William Walton, who had for thirty-eight years been in the employ of the Bank of England; for the last six years before his death (in 1806) he occupied one of the three most esteemed positions on its staff, that of Chief Accountant. According to family tradition it was while accompanying his widowed mother on a walk through a City churchyard that he 'saw a tombstone dedicated to the memory of . . . Chief Accountant of the Bank of England, and remarked "That's what I should like to be", and sure enough it was what he became'; a very Victorian vignette, designed to satisfy the progeny rather than to convince the unbiased outsider. Report also had it that his mother's means had been very modest and that William was her only child; in reality he had a sister, a spinster who survived at least until 1802, when she was remembered in Walton's will.

To his descendants Walton was the only forebear of importance, ennobled—in their eyes—by his contact with the august institution for which he worked throughout his adult years. To them there was a whiff of refinement about the few relics that came down from him: a watch, a silver shoe-buckle and a scrap of an engraving of a coat of arms, three boars surmounted by a boar's head with the motto *Semper pro Patria* on a scroll underneath, seemingly a book-plate. Walton's descendants put the buckle and watch on the scales of gentility to counterweigh the soap manufactured by the Williams family, yet both the silver buckle and the silver watch would not have been out of place

---

[9] Jeannette Marshall's diaries are also reticent on how other maternal relatives earned their living. A few oblique references to the ups and downs of their business, coupled with evidence from directories, bear witness that two of John Williams's grandsons, Edwin and John, were importers of sugar and other colonial commodities such as indigo, with offices in the City. Their brother-in-law George Startin (Jeannette's uncle by marriage) also imported sugar, besides being a wholesale grocer. The soap business had been carried on, in Clerkenwell and later in Hoxton, by Charles Williams, Jeannette's grandfather, and by his eldest son (who predeceased him); it was eventually taken on by another of Charles's sons, William Walton Williams.

among the possessions of any moderately successful eighteenth-century artisan or even labourer.[10] More to the point, Walton died a wealthy man. His top salary at the Bank was £500 a year, a comfortable income, but not one which would allow savings sufficiently high to found a large fortune. However, working for the Bank opened other ways of amassing wealth. Walton's colleague, the Chief Cashier Abraham Newland, who up to the age of eighteen had helped his father bake bread in the family business, died a very rich man. Estimates of what he left topped £200,000, with a great deal of scandal attaching to the method of accumulating so vast an amount. Walton's gleanings were less spectacular; even so his only surviving child and residual heiress, Elizabeth, the wife of Charles Williams and the mother of Ellen Marshall, eventually inherited something of the order of £30,000.

John and Ellen Marshall may have married for love; years later Jeannette wrote of a 'desk-full of love letters' sent by her father during his courtship. He was thirty-six to his bride's twenty-three at the time of their marriage. His earnings had only just begun to rise. It must have been comforting to know that Ellen could confidently expect sizeable inheritances from both her father's and her mother's side. In the meantime the dowry which Charles Williams no doubt provided for his daughter helped the newly weds into the Savile Row house and bought some of the trimmings indispensable for life at a fashionable medical man's address.[11]

After Jeannette, Ellen gave birth to three more children, Ada, John and Reginald; they came at almost regular intervals of fifteen or sixteen months, four children altogether, all born within the first five years of marriage. In the 1850s four made a small family, two less than the

[10] See M. Dorothy George, *London Life in the Eighteenth Century* (Harmondsworth, 1965), p.173.

[11] A hint of what Ellen might have brought John Marshall on marriage is in Charles Williams's will, dated in the early 1860s. There a special extra share, £2,000, was earmarked out of trust funds for the one unmarried daughter, Eliza. Assuming that the father intended to make equal provision for his three daughters, Ellen and her sister Sarah would each have had dowries of £2,000 or the income from it. It is of course possible that the £2,000 was left to the blind Eliza precisely because she had not married.

Ellen's long-term expectations were on a more generous scale. The income which eventually accrued to her was in the range of £200–£400 a year, implying a capital of some £4,000–£8,000 as her share of a substantial fortune.

middle-class average.[12] It was indeed not up to Williams standards: Ellen's elder sister Sarah Startin was to give birth to sixteen (three of whom died in infancy), and the two most prolific Williams sisters-in-law, Mrs William and Mrs Edwin, ended up with families of some ten and eight apiece.

Ada was a pretty but unassertive child. John, the first boy, had a muscular or bone defect in his legs, which had eventually to be corrected by a period in leg-irons: he was less than perfect. Not until the birth of Reggie was Jeannette's advantage as first-born challenged. The nurses—there were two of them for a time, one to look after the three older children, the other devoted to the new arrival—'used rather to "put upon" me, I being the eldest of the four, and very tall for my age.' Her ready smile won her the nickname Sunshine: 'very sharp-looking with black eyes & a snub nose, with very beautiful golden hair' is how she described her childhood self. On the earliest surviving photograph, aged no more than eight, she looks a fine figure of a girl, with delicate features, her hair in tight plaits round the shapely head, gazing at the world confidently and urbanely, if a little smugly. She wrote of toys as if they were financial assets. The two or three dolls she mentioned in passing lack charm and individuality; they were remembered chiefly as gifts from unexpected donors on unexpected occasions and did not acquire names of their own.

It may have been the responsibilities of the eldest that, years later, prompted her to describe herself in an excess of adolescent self-dramatization as 'never young'. And yet she and the other children of Ellen and John Marshall grew up in a seemingly idyllic environment; today it would be called 'child-centred'. Even the nursery, in an extension across the yard where the children could romp without disturbing their father's patients, was comfortably adapted to the needs of the young:

It was a large room, with a high fireguard round the grate, and two little chairs, my sister's and mine, one on each side of the fire-place. I can also remember a cupboard with some fluffy mats with cups & saucers arranged on them on the top; & a low washing-stand with a large white bason, in which we used to be

[12] The average number of children in 'families of gentlemen with private means' for marriages contracted between 1851 and 1860 was 6.01. See J. A. Banks, 'The Way They Lived Then', *Victorian Studies* (Bloomington, Indiana), xii.2 (December 1968), p. 200, quoting the 1911 Census of Population.

placed, bodily, for cleansing purposes. There was a table in the middle of the room, and a high chair with a rest for the feet, and a bar to fasten the small occupant in.

Soon after the birth of their fourth child, as if to mark that the family was now complete, John and Ellen rented a suburban villa in Kentish Town (close to the Williams' grandparents' Talbot House) so that the children might have better air and more freedom than at Savile Row. No. 19 Roseberry Villas, York Road, looked over a vast expanse of greenery towards Holloway. At the back there was a view of a cricket ground and open fields. Including the nurses and servants, six adults plus four children squeezed into one small, though detached, house. Marshall, at some inconvenience to himself, went backwards and forwards to and from Gower Street and the West End, with 10 Savile Row part sub-let and part consulting rooms. It cannot have been a comfortable life for him, always on the go and without much money to spare when the expenses of two homes had been met. The arrangement continued till Jeannette was nearly nine, in 1864; when six years later Marshall suggested that the experiment be repeated, this time at Wood Green, where he had professional engagements, his wife and adolescent daughters jointly defeated the proposal. Unlike himself, the three of them were London-born and not to be palmed off with an outer suburb.

On her wedding likeness and in photographs taken later in life Ellen Marshall looked handsome, if slightly forbidding—like a staid French matron, with a rounded baby's forehead above an aquiline nose. Some youthful charm or indeed magnetism there might have been; if so, these qualities did not survive marriage and motherhood. Perhaps as the result of some childhood infection, she was from early on rather deaf, extremely short-sighted and also somewhat bald. What had been in her youth an interestingly high hair-line required from her forties onwards the camouflage of a clever toupee:

P. went to Truefitts to get his hair cut, M & I were to follow in order to discuss the weighty matter of some false hair for M. We walked upstairs wh. P. soon joined us. There ensued a fearful consultation on 'Universals', 'Cache follets', false hair of all descriptions. Mr Truefitt was called to give an opinion as to whether M's hair would ever grow agn, the foreman of the wig department to give _his_ opinion as to what style of hair would suit M.; besides these 2 great guns there was a woman & P.; I held my peace . . .

The disabilities, though minor, made Ellen uncertain in social situations. Moreover, she suffered from prostrating migraines and, like so many other migraine sufferers, allowed her indispositions to dominate the life of her closest family.

Jeannette learnt to accept the ups and downs of her mother's constitution and the moodiness arising from them with equanimity. She noted physical and emotional symptoms alike with detached objectivity. 'M. has days when she is dreadfully deaf' she wrote, and a few days later, in an amused (though cryptic) aside, remarked that Ellen had a list of 'devils': 'Ten males, 54 females!!!'; just before a major fracas she described her mother as 'very tired, & (à vrai dire) very cross likewise!' On occasion, indeed, it came to a full-size scene between mother and daughter. Ellen would then sulk and withdraw from all intercourse, not only with the culprit who had defied her authority but also with the rest of the family, till at last a *démarche* by Marshall himself brought a token apology from the offending party and peace was restored. None too soon: in 1871 one such crisis—over a 'hideous' hat which Jeannette refused to wear in defiance of her mother's wishes—lasted a full three days.

Because of all this, 10 Savile Row was, in Jeannette's girlhood, a rather inhospitable place, Ellen's farouche edginess prevailing over Marshall's social ease. She treated the whole elaborate ceremonial of reciprocal visiting as a chore. Even casual calls by members of her own family were tolerated rather than encouraged. This goes some way to explain why the young Marshalls, and especially the two girls who, unlike their brothers, received their schooling at home, had very little regular contact with other children. Once when Jeannette was already in late adolescence she was sent to Aunt Sarah Startin to convalesce after rheumatic fever. The Startins and nine of their surviving twelve children lived in a recently built house, 13 Thurlow Road, off Fitzjohn's Avenue in Hampstead, where the air was purer than in central London. Aunt Startin cosseted her niece and served up delicacies to tempt the convalescent's palate. The cousins romped, teased and made practical jokes. For Jeannette it was a welcome return to carefree nursery days. Cousin Jessie became something of a friend: 'I suit her better than Ada, being more lively, & more conversationally inclined . . . Jessie's room is a very pretty one, & now I have got used to dressing & undressing before my dear Cousin, I like staying here very much indeed.'

But five days were too short to consolidate the friendship and the stay at Hampstead remained an isolated event. Festive occasions when the entire Williams clan gathered at Holloway were also too infrequent to forge lasting friendships. In a family in which there were, in London alone, some thirty or forty first cousins from which to choose play-mates, Jeannette and Ada, John and Reggie, relied almost entirely on one another's company. For adolescents, curious of what the world had to offer and eager for its approval, such isolation was hard to bear. No wonder that to Jeannette confiding in a diary proved a solace. Within months of beginning her daily record she wrote: 'Whatever should I do without it? It is really part of my life, almost. I love it so much.'

CHAPTER I

'UNE DEMOISELLE FAITE'

IN the middle of the first page of the first volume of the diary, in a space which Jeannette on New Year's Day 1870 providently reserved for the end-of-1870 summing-up, she wrote under the date of 31 December:

I have now tried keeping a diary for a year, during which time I have not missed a single day. The best recommendation I can give is that I have already invested in a larger Diary, ready to commence 1871, & all I can say is that I shall write it regularly. This year has been, on the whole, a very happy one for me, although many poor people have had their homes devastated; & their nearest and dearest gone away to fight for their country. For my part, I am sick of patriotism! Ce n'est que le 'sentiment'!—I think I have learned a good deal during this year ... 1½ years more lessons, & then I shall be, if I live, 'une demoiselle faite', so I have not much time to lose. I am sorry that I cannot sit up to see my poor old friend go out & become a thing of the past. Poor 1870!

'Une demoiselle faite', a fully-fledged young lady, is how she appeared to herself by her mid-teens. In the early months of the 1870 record, before her fifteenth birthday, there were several signs of her regarding herself, and being treated, as a near-adult. The time (and diary space) devoted to her wardrobe, the lengthening of skirts, the constant experimentation with new hair-styles were some of them; so too was the decision to embark on a regular journal. At fifteen or so she claimed to have stopped growing, although in fact she continued till around 1874, when she measured five foot six-and-a-half inches in her stockinged feet. She was slim for her height, with a twenty-two inch waist of which she was, and remained, proud. Her hair was beginning to darken from the golden tint of her first childhood, and had reddish gleams. She wore it now in fluffs, now soft and frizzy, or brushed back high over the forehead. She still smiled a great deal; her expression was pleasant, but round the chin were beginning to show signs of the determination which would in adulthood make her face handsome rather than attractive. This expression corresponded to moods which showed her to be obsessed with herself though by no means inward-looking or anxious.

The particular forms of this obsessiveness connected with orderliness were already a trait so marked that she herself saw them as oldmaidish, commenting in an access of rare introspection: 'I do so rejoice in seeing things perfectly neat.' Her adolescent poise verged on complacency. She described her looks as 'moderate generally & sometimes pretty good. That is the truth, with no vanity or false modesty.' 'When I make up my mind that anyone shall like me, I generally succeed' she boasted. A happy character on the whole, but also one with little of the genuine spontaneity of adolescence. Apart from an occasional hyperbole about an 'angelic party' and a very few passionate outbursts of frustration or anger, she continued to emphasize her self-image of someone 'never young'.

While many professionals of Marshall's rank sent their sons to Rugby and similar modernized or recently established public schools where they mixed with the sons of the aristocracy and gentry, the two Marshall boys attended University College School in Gower Street, an unpretentious, non-sectarian and progressive place, chosen most probably for precisely those qualities. To Marshall's way of thinking, his girls deserved an education on much the same lines as that of their brothers, but Jeannette and Ada completed their schooling at home, as did scores of daughters of other men of their father's standing.[1] What in the end weighed the scales down on the side of home tutoring was that while boys were regarded as capable of remaining on the social heights reached by their professional fathers, it was thought that girls had to be protected from the dangers of indiscriminate associations with schoolfriends of the wrong sort.

And so Jeannette, and Ada too, grew up in a secluded schoolroom

---

[1] The daughters of Marshall's fellow medical men James and George Paget were among the girls educated at home. Marshall's acquaintance George Buchanan sent his three eldest daughters to Octavia Hill's establishment in Nottingham Place; one of them eventually boarded at Cheltenham Ladies' College (see M. Jeanne Peterson, 'Myth and Reality in a Victorian Family: The Pagets as a Case Study', paper presented at Anglo-American Conference, University of Indiana, 1982, and Lilian Adam Smith, *Recollections of a Grandmother*, ed. Janet Adam Smith, privately circulated, 1977). Of the day schools easily accessible from Savile Row, the Nottingham Place institution would have been the obvious choice for the Marshall girls if sending them to day school had been considered. Nottingham Place and Miss Buss's North London Collegiate School for Ladies in Camden Street were nearest in spirit to University College School, where the ideas included flexible time-tabling and novel disciplinary methods, with no recourse to corporal punishment or 'lines'.

without the companionship of other girls, and also without the urge to emulate or the need to defend one's position. In terms of formal knowledge, they probably picked up more, and less painfully, from their teachers at home than they would have learnt at school. But the lack of practice in the making of friends, in living a communal life not just with intimates but with people at large, was a handicap that would dog them for life.

By the time Jeannette reached early adolescence a succession of governesses had moved through the Marshalls' schoolroom. With the exception of a short interregnum when a spinster friend of Grandmother Williams was in charge, all of them were continental Europeans, teaching Jeannette and Ada fluent French and German, as well as the rudiments of other subjects.

The tutors who succeeded them were of an altogether different quality. Occasionally a woman of independent spirit and inquiring mind would be propelled by personal circumstances into the unenviable role of private tutor, only to find in it a genuine vocation. Jeannette had the good fortune to be taught in adolescence by three such women. The one who came first, between Jeannette's eleventh and fourteenth birthday, was a highly qualified schoolteacher, Jane Agnes Chessar. Marshall had known Miss Chessar ever since, in her middle twenties, she had been his student at a special course in physiology for women which he ran at University College in 1861. She had come to London from her birthplace, Edinburgh, at the age of sixteen and after only a year's training, took over a class at the Home and Colonial Training College and School in Gray's Inn Road, a progressive institution run on Pestalozzi lines. According to the *Dictionary of National Biography*, she 'did much to raise the College to the highest place among such institutions by her skill as a teacher and by the moral influence over her pupils'.[2] 'Chessics', as Jeannette called her, not only imparted a professional tone to what she taught, but added to it a great

[2] The Home and Colonial was founded in 1836 for the training of primary schoolteachers and governesses. It was nominally Church of England, but students had to do no more than believe in the fundamental truths of the Bible. The courses were of twelve to fifteen weeks' duration and cost 8s. a week (about £12 in present-day value). Training in school method was an integral part of the programme. Anne Jemima Clough was one of several educational pioneers who trained at the Home and Colonial; she attended it in 1849, before Miss Chessar's days. A striking feature of the Home and Colonial was that at a time when primary school teachers were almost invariably single women, its hostel boasted married quarters. See R. W. Rich, *The Training of Teachers in England and Wales in the Nineteenth Century* (Cambridge, 1933; reprinted 1972).

deal of spontaneity and warmth. Jeannette wrote of her with unwonted affection: 'I like her muchly.' Mrs Marshall, too, found the stout little Scotswoman, plain of face and costume, to her liking. 'Chessics' even succeeded in wringing unprecedented concessions out of the mother, such as permission for Jeannette to attend meetings of the Royal Geographical Society, of which the tutor was a keen member.

The second was Esther Greatbatch, a near-contemporary of Jeannette's, a clever nineteen-year-old who earned a good living—Jeannette was horrified at her fee of 10s. per two-hour period—by teaching algebra and the rudiments of Euclid. She developed no liking for Miss Greatbatch, who had a 'very rude, brusque' way of saying things and the temerity to address her pupil by her first name; 'I really think it is like her impudence. I only wish I could be sufficiently cool to call her Esther' was Jeannette's response. However, what she learnt from Miss Greatbatch provided a sufficient challenge to make her continue with algebra on her own for several years as 'a cure for boredom'.

But it was without doubt the Swiss woman, calling herself at different times Mme Noël or Mme Appia, who fired Jeannette's imagination and helped develop her intellect. In her late thirties, separated and eventually divorced from a difficult husband, she came for whole days on Mondays, Wednesdays and Fridays from when Jeannette was fourteen and a half, teaching French and German language and literature. Madame's company at meal times and on their daily walk provided Jeannette and Ada with opportunities to practise spoken French and German. An integral part of her method was to stretch the students' thinking powers by setting them sophisticated compositions in French. She was a demanding teacher and a robust critic.

The impact of Madame's personality may have been greater than the Marshall parents had bargained for. Their sedately enlightened opinions did not usually manifest themselves round the dining-room table; by contrast, Madame voiced radical views and talked nothing but politics at most meals. Not since Marshall's Tudor Lodge days in the 1840s had he heard public events discussed with such regularity and with so much passion. She sympathized with the Reds during the weeks of the Paris Commune; she expressed a wish to belong to the International[3]—all this, incongruously, in the anodyne setting of the

[3] The First International Workingmen's Association had been formed in London in 1864, with the assistance of Marx. After Marx's split with Bakunin in 1872, its headquarters removed to New York in 1874, to be dissolved in 1876.

school-room and dining-room at No. 10; could her intention have been to *épater* these very bourgeois English? In a household in which eccentricity was under greater suspicion than conventionally immoral behaviour, she was the unconventional foreigner whose matrimonial status was by no means clear, at least not to her pupils (Mrs Marshall was probably aware of its intricacy). Moreover, she remained in no way cowed by her equivocal position. She even had the temerity to ask for an increase in wages, a request which, let it be recorded, was not granted; her pay, £60 a year plus lunches and sometimes tea, for three terms of about fifteen weeks each, was considered as adequate; the more so, volunteered Jeannette shrewdly, as Madame did not offer music.

If Mme Noël failed to impart to her pupil a generous response to other people's needs, she made her articulate and self-assured in discussion. The essay subjects Madame set Jeannette, part literary, part philosophical, forced the girl to reflect and, on occasion, to pass moral judgment. Their list extended from the perennial account of the unities in French drama, through trite ones on the disadvantages of life in the country, to such ambitious themes of moral philosophy as 'On tue les hommes, mais on ne tue pas les idées légitimes' or 'Peut-on rendre justice à une puissance qui nous est opposée?', or again—the last subject Madame set Jeannette—'Les vices et les vertus naissent de la société'. At intervals Jeannette rebelled against all these Gallic abstractions. 'Absolutely nothing to say' she wrote in her diary when told to comment on the assertion that to form links of affection was to give hostage to fortune; 'it's patent to anyone but a fool without further explanation!' Once she dug in her heels and refused to write on the set subject, only to discover that Madame's substitute essay theme was no improvement. After such fiascos, the end of term was met with jubilation: 'Vive les vacances, il n'y a plus de pénitence, les livres sont à vendre, les maîtres sont à pendre!'

After two-and-a-half years of Madame's regime, Jeannette's secondary education was declared complete. Madame was given a leaving present of 'a very handsome gold brooch with a star of blue enamel & tiny diamonds in the middle, in the centre of wh. ag. is a pearl. She was very pleased. P. also gave her £10 instead of the £7-10s. wh. was owing. So she ought to be satisfied, I think.'

Madame's influence continued long after lessons with her had been given up. She called at intervals to exchange news, gossip about her new patrons, shock by her *outré* views and feed Jeannette stimulating reading matter, such as Mrs Fawcett's little book on political economy.[4] That Jeannette did not acquire a sustained interest in public affairs at home or abroad, and indeed never became an intellectual, was not Madame's fault; her pupil certainly developed a few unconventional opinions of her own, such as an admiration for Napoleon Bonaparte, and learnt to defend them.

But more important than all this stimulation of intelligence and taste was that Madame, just as Miss Chessar, ultimately succeeded in making herself accepted and loved for what she was. 'I'm not very fond of her' Jeannette had written after the lessons had stopped, but at the same time admitted that she 'really felt sorry' at the parting. Two years later when Madame was about to disappear for a spell in Switzerland, Jeannette was able to confess to a 'little "serrement de cœur" ' at her departure. To set the record straight, she at once added: 'She is certainly wonderfully fond of me, & . . . "J'aime qui m'aime".'

Madame's marriage in 1876 to M. Canut, a half-Spanish, half-French lace-merchant, turned out to be another of her mistakes. Already in her middle forties, she gave birth to a girl and, fifteen months later, to a boy, and was for ever needing advice and burdening the Marshalls with the management of her savings, which she kept in England, out of Canut's reach. Mrs Marshall and Jeannette were alarmed to read that Madame was 'in favor of cold water and low dresses! she will dispose of that poor little infant in double quick time that way'; so they posted a pamphlet on babies' clothes to her and wrote screeds about the management of infants. In addition, Jeannette sent Madame a couple of pairs of baby socks, knitted on her behalf by Aunt Eliza Williams. The replies from Pau (in the Pyrenees), where the Canuts had settled, brought news of a series of catastrophes. Léon, the younger child, died before his third birthday; May, the little girl, suffered from epileptic fits. Madame herself was regularly beaten up by her man, who kept a mistress on the side. Despite their tragic essence, Madame's letters were not without an element of farce, as when she wrote that she had 'disguised herself "en paysanne" in order to track her husband to this woman's! How foreign!' A year later she reported that she had set a fortune-teller, a 'diseuse de bonnes aventures', to frighten Canut's mistress; 'as good as a novel' commented Jeannette, to whom the correspondence with Madame, and

4 Millicent Fawcett, *Political Economy for Beginners* (London and Cambridge, 1870).

also her occasional visits to London, seemed as stimulating as the lessons had been in the two-and-a-half years of her rule in the schoolroom.

John's and Ellen's views on the upbringing of their daughters had begun to diverge, just at the point at which Jeannette, at least, was ready to start thinking about how she wanted her future to shape. Ellen Marshall saw girlhood as a delightful sequence of golden days to which controlled and mild flirtation added spice. Still under forty when her eldest child reached the mid-teens, she had herself never entirely grown up. She was still enough of an adolescent to wish to participate, at one remove, in Jeannette's frivolities; courtship seemed to her, and to her sisters and sisters-in-law, to hold even greater bliss than marriage and motherhood.

Jeannette's father was more sober and much more enlightened. He intended his girls to go on studying and so gain access to all sorts of new fields of activity. His horizon had been widened by work with women who had fought to assert their intellectual equality with men, and who were beginning to make political demands. From its inception in the late 1850s he had sponsored the Ladies' Sanitary Association, a seemingly conventional beneficent cause, but one which had among its members a number of forceful women radicals to give it muscle. The activists on the Association's committees and in its rank and file were a curiously mixed bunch; some of the forces that impelled them would eventually merge with the militant movement for women's franchise. Out-and-out feminists, Emily Faithfull, Bessie Rayner Parkes, Mentia Taylor, rubbed shoulders with Parthenope Verney and Hilary Bonham Carter, both of the Florence Nightingale clan. Wives of progressive politicians (of most persuasions) such as Georgiana Cowper, Charlotte Ebury or Emilia Gurney, worked side by side with the wives of sanitary and medical reformers, Rosetta Hart, Phebe Lankester and Mrs Garth Wilkinson, whose husband, the Swedenborgian James John Garth Wilkinson, opposed vaccination and vivisection. The patronesses, from the Queen's eldest daughter, the crown princess of Prussia, to Angela Burdett-Coutts, could hardly have been more respectable.

Alongside several of his less starchy professional acquaintances Marshall took part, as honorary member, in this new venture, the prime object of which was to teach the poor the rudiments of hygiene and diet in order to help them keep well and raise healthy children.

The evangelizing was done through lectures, and *ex tempore* counselling, which the Ladies dispensed on home visits and at the Association's offices, and also by means of short, simply written tràcts. These ranged from matter-of-fact, modern-sounding advice on such topics as child-care, to texts which wrapped up their common sense on, say, the evils of drink, in verse or novelette form. Marshall's regular function at the LSA was, for a busy professional man, quite time-consuming: for at least nine years he sat on the Association's editorial committee, vetting the drafts of its publications.[5] But without doubt his chief contribution was to lay a solid scientific foundation to the Ladies' endeavours by teaching them the rudiments of physiology in a specially designed course for women at University College. The choice of Marshall was an obvious one, quite apart from his LSA connection. He had for the past seven years taught anatomy at the Schools of Art and Design, first at Marlborough House and later at South Kens= ington, where he had pioneered mixed classes of men and women; moreover he had in 1859–60 already given a course on animal physi- ology for schoolteachers (only that time the audience had been all male, composed mainly of members of the Schoolmasters' Social Science Association). The innovatory 1861 women's course of thirteen lectures given on Saturday afternoons attracted over one hundred subscribers. About half of them came from the LSA; another organized contingent were ten student teachers from the Home and Colonial, led by Jane Agnes Chessar.

[5] Over fifty LSA tracts survive in the British Library. They are not dated but were acquired between 1859 and 1872, although the Association was active until 1900. Several came out in six or seven editions; one, *How to Manage a Baby*, reached a circulation of 30,000 copies. A few of the tracts were translated into Greek, Japanese, Chinese and 'Indian vernacular'. Although most of the Association's tracts were anony-mous, several male names figured among the signed ones. Charles Kingsley, one of the founders of the National Association for the Promotion of Social Science, of which the LSA was an offshoot, contributed *The Massacre of the Innocents*, the transcript of the address he had given at the LSA's inaugural meeting; its message was that the 'laws of Nature must be understood and obeyed in order to avoid pestilence and disasters' (quoted from Brenda Colloms, *Victorian Visionaries*, London, 1982, p. 183). Dr John Challice, Medical Officer of Health for Bermondsey, wrote on *How People Hasten Death*, and the pen-name 'Old Chatty Cheerful' almost certainly disguised Edwin Lankester, whose subject was *The Black Ditch—A few words on sanitary matters*.

The peak of the LSA's activity and influence came in the mid-1860s when it spread to the provinces, opening offices in Birmingham, Brighton, Dublin and elsewhere. Its long-term importance was that it initiated a cadre of informed women who were qualified to spread the knowledge of hygiene, the pioneers of what later became the health visitors' and district nurses' profession. See William C. Dowling in *The Ladies' Sanitary Associ-ation and the Origins of the Health Visiting Service*, MA thesis (unpublished), London University, 1963.

It was among such women, the ones whom he met at the LSA and those who came to his lectures, that Marshall could have looked for models for his daughters, not to be copied slavishly but to impart a worthwhile purpose to their pursuits. The most exciting scheme was that chosen by his acquaintance Elizabeth Garrett, who was about to combine marriage (and perhaps eventually motherhood) with a career. His own Jeannette gave out signals that she had the drive and personality to do just that, and he may have interpreted as high spirits the frivolity which was becoming her everyday demeanour.

He should have noticed, and taken warning from this frivolity, not only on the part of his elder daughter, but also of his wife, from observing their behaviour towards Jeannette's first admirer. Certainly Ellen, as early as 1870, had not been blind to the fact that her first-born, not yet fifteen, was being courted, and that the suitor, the nephew of a patient of Marshall's, was adult enough to have his intentions taken seriously. The audacity with which John Wood ('Jungle', 'Forest' or even 'Lignum' in the diaries, the adolescent Jeannette being partial to puns) pursued his object had been noticed by Mme Noël: 'il ose trop' she commented to her charge. All the same, she cannot have taken the matter seriously—or was she, too, irresponsibly encouraging Jeannette to play with fire? At any rate, she did not take it upon herself to alter the route of their daily walk so as to avoid meeting John Wood.

Jeannette herself was too inexperienced to fear the escalation of the affair. Fair, good-looking, eleven or twelve years her senior, John Wood had been around for nearly seven years. She had been acquainted with him ever since she had danced with him at the party which marked the Marshalls' return to Savile Row from the exile of Kentish Town—a hot-cheeked, eager-eyed little girl of eight, hair curled back and turned over from the forehead, in pink tarlatane over pink silk. To her, his attentions had been and were still rather a flattering joke. 'What a child I was then!' she would sigh in years to come, recalling the blushes and the excitement at each new manifestation of John Wood's interest in her. That he was said to have been twice engaged only added spice to his gallantries.

His uncle, head of the family business (Cramer's, pianoforte merchants and still-extant music publishers), his actress aunt and his elder brother were in and out of Marshall's consulting room, and sometimes called upstairs to greet Mrs Marshall. His own place of work was Cramer's shop in Regent Street, on the corner of Conduit Street, which the Marshall women passed on their daily walks and where they often bought music for Jeannette's piano lessons and Ellen's singing. In addition to their main lines of business, Cramer's were theatrical agents and held the ticket concession for Drury Lane. Gifts of theatre or opera tickets from grateful patients were within the bounds of permissible professional perks. During the 1870 and 1872 opera seasons (in 1871 the Drury Lane opera season was much curtailed) the Woods sent tickets every seven or ten days. These tickets were not invariably accepted, but all the same Jeannette heard at least a dozen performances, including *Fidelio*, *Il Trovatore*, *The Barber of Seville* and *Martha*, by courtesy of the Woods. That John Wood himself was usually present on the occasion and that he made use of the opportunities afforded by the proximity of seats, the confusion of intervals, the mood of the music itself, to pursue his flirtation, Jeannette (and also perhaps her parents) accepted as part of his social graces.

The courtship consisted largely of teasing and banter which were much to Jeannette's liking. Coming from a man so many years her senior, she chose to regard them at first as almost avuncular. The prolonged handshakes, the nudging of her foot with his own appeared less innocent. When he addressed her in a letter as his 'dear Miss Jeannette' she demurred in the diary but did not voice her disapproval. Nor did she object to the fact that the note in which he addressed her so familiarly came with two copies of a piece of music bound in mauve and gold, published by Cramer's, and named avowedly after her the 'Jeannette Mazurka'. On the cover was a fanciful portrayal of herself. Its composer, allegedly one Marriott, she assumed to be John Wood himself.

It may have been the Mazurka which at last alerted Mrs Marshall to the risks which had been building up. Much to Jeannette's dismay, the next batch of tickets for opera and play were sent back to Cramer's, Marshall's absence from London serving as a courteous excuse. And on the next day, after the usual banter about John Wood's courtship, her mother 'said quite gravely that she thought it would not have been right to have gone the other night, because if J. W. had any intentions, & I was 2 yrs older, "should I be prepared to give him any encouragement"! It sounded so solemn that I said "No, I thought not!" ' Nevertheless, Jeannette professed herself alarmed that John Wood might take the refusal amiss and send no more tickets. 'That would be awful!'

Matters now ran swiftly to a climax. A performance of *Faust*, and more foot-nudging on the return journey, another batch of invitations refused ('what an awful shame & a fib too' protested Jeannette at her mother claiming a previous engagement). And then the decisive moves: an exploratory visit by John's uncle and Marshall's outraged response on behalf of his daughter.

Till then Marshall had behaved in the matter of John Wood's courtship no less irresponsibly than his wife. As early as mid-July 1870 he started teasing Jeannette about her 'intended'. The banter became part of a family ritual of which the father carried his share, paying no heed to the signs that she was becoming, to say the least, intrigued by the possibilities which John Wood's intentions offered. When in May 1872 Mrs Marshall reported that Papa was horrified, she was, it seems, constructing an excuse for the lack of discretion of both herself and her husband.

In rejecting the offer the father sought refuge in the fact that Jeannette was not yet seventeen. Teenage marriage was not customary on either side of the family and he most probably genuinely felt that this was far too soon for her to enter upon an engagement. Was there anything in his daughter's assertion that his self-esteem (his pride, she called it) had taken a knock? More than likely, for by the early 1870s Marshall had reason to be complacent. He had caught up with the leaders in the competition for hospital and College appointments, having been promoted to full surgeon in 1859 and to the chair of clinical surgery in 1866. Joseph Lister, a scientist of undoubted brilliance, had been Marshall's rival for the professorship, so that capturing it was a singular triumph.[6] In his private practice he now counted gentry as well as the rich bourgeois and the not-so-rich bohemians. Other prizes were fast in coming, especially in 1873 which brought him the chair of anatomy at the Royal Academy, as well as the

[6] In spite of his relative youth—born in 1827, he was nine years Marshall's junior—Lister had behind him six years' experience in the chair of surgery at Glasgow University. Moreover, news of his revolutionary experiments in antiseptic surgery was beginning to percolate to the metropolis. Critics of Marshall's appointment later asserted that what had tipped the scales had been the consciousness at University College Hospital that Marshall had had a rough time waiting until he was forty-eight for the chance of a chair which John Erichsen (his exact contemporary and immediate predecessor) had held from the age of thirty-two. Rumour had it that Sharpey had opted for the older one of his two favourite pupils and swung the appointing committee in Marshall's favour. Writing in 1923, more than half a century after Marshall's appointment to the UC professorship, Edward Sharpey Schafer claimed that the choice of Marshall over Lister had been 'easily the worst mistake' that the council of the College had ever made. (See Schafer, op. cit.)

membership of the Council of the Royal College of Surgeons. Another accolade dating from that year was the membership of the Athenaeum.

In practical terms, this new phase of success found expression in an innovation he was in future able to show off on his daily rounds. Two horses instead of one to the brougham he hired from the livery stables: the change in style was almost as significant as the move from Mornington Crescent to Mayfair had been twenty years earlier. And, within reach of the highest peaks in his profession, he might well have seen an alliance with a family in 'trade' and on the margin of theatrical bohemia as entirely undesirable.

After it was all over, Jeannette claimed that the pace and excitement of the exhilarating affair had caused her some loss of appetite and sleep. At the time, she kept insisting on her detachment and pretended not to hear when John Wood asked her (cheekily, she thought) when she was due to be 'finished' and if she was engaged. Yet when his intentions proved to be serious, she wrote: 'I took the matter calmly for, to say the truth, I was not very astonished.' She would have been happier if the whole business had not culminated in a tentative offer of marriage and she resented the 'meddlesome' uncle's surprise approach to her father. She had hoped for a prolonged flood of invitations to opera and play and a succession of delightful encounters at which to exchange flirtatious banter. Instead she was left without even a formal proposal, a scalp for future adornment. Because the question had not been put directly to her, she never admitted the extent to which her fantasy had been stimulated by the affair. After John Wood had been sent off—by proxy—with a flea in his ear, she had moped for a time, avowedly at the absence of further tickets. No hypocrisy, no pretence of pity for the rejected suitor, who indeed was not heartbroken. When six months later he became engaged to the daughter of a retired silversmith ('a kind of Trade's Union' quipped Jeannette) and married her in August of the following year, Jeannette's comments were rather defensive. 'I should not have liked him as a "companion for life" ' she wrote, and 'cela m'est égal now . . .' It is that underlined 'now' which bore witness to what she described as 'rather a penchant for him'. She also decided to keep all the 'various little things connected with that little "affair" because anyway he was "mon premier" '. The whole episode was for her a *rite de passage*, from being a child to being a young woman.

CHAPTER 2

DEATH IN SAVILE ROW

'I THINK P. has woken up to the idea that I am getting on, since that little affair about Jungle. I am glad it happened if only on that account' Jeannette reflected in mid-1872, as she steeled herself to face her father's ambitious plans for the further education of his girls. Within less than twelve months the process of leaving childhood would end in the trauma of a death. The year 1872 is the last time to take in the six Savile Row Marshalls as an intact family unit. The collective portrait emerging from the early diaries resembles one of those strange Victorian compositions in which each likeness, initially drawn or photographed within its own perspective, was then repainted regardless of scale to form a single surrealist group. Marshall and his wife appear with reasonable clarity, yet at disparate angles, as if their fields of vision never met. The surgeon, in his early fifties, gentle, unkempt, bewhiskered—urchins call 'Mr Whiskers' after him—hovers in the background. New medico-political demands on his time coincide with the intensification of work in his practice, and erode his leisure to the detriment of health. All the same, there are few days when his daughters do not have some contact with him, if only by accompanying him in the carriage on a round of professional visits, and at meals they hear about his patients' medical problems and a good deal of University College and Royal Academy gossip. Ellen Marshall, just over forty, a matron and yet still ready to engage in practical jokes and frivolous talk within the close family circle, continues to look forbidding to the outsider, with her short-sighted gaze which does not encompass the middle distance. Ellen's immaturity does not decrease, and not much warmth emanates from her.

She gives more of her time and attention to the girls than to her sons. The boys, Johnny and Redgepedge as their sister often refers to them, are in her accounts virtually indistinguishable; neither is very robust, both wear glasses and carry off numerous school prizes. Jeannette has little to say about John's remarkable gift for drawing; luckily he has left behind his own testimonial, a day-by-day account of the family's 1868 holiday in the Rhineland, written between the ages of ten and twelve. *Our Trip to Bonn and Back*, 195 pages of neat copperplate, is illustrated by a dozen or so pen-and-ink drawings of landscapes and antiquities, as fine and intricate as etchings, and seemingly way beyond the skill of a child. The text at times belies the precocious, staid manner of the illustrations and the little pedant becomes a recogniz-able ten-year old. He and the inseparable Reggie cast off their jackets and waistcoats; in shirtsleeves, to the despair of the genteel Fräulein in charge of the children, they chase butterflies down a woody slope or ward off attacks by gangs of German scamps. It is in fact Reggie who does most of the fighting. John is at this stage totally unassertive and also less competent physically than his brother. However, in the early pages of Jeannette's diary, Reggie is seen as rather young for his age, still playing with lead soldiers and throwing the occasional tantrum.

Jeannette herself stands out in vivid colours against the black and white of the family picture, a sturdy, self-opinionated seventeen-year-old with both feet firmly on the ground. Ada is a wan shadow of her elder sister. She has a delicate constitution—she is afraid of the least noise and apparently faints at the slightest provocation. Her artistic rather than musical gifts distinguish her from Jeannette, as do her looks—pretty, with small features, shorter stature, and a gentleness which comes from her father's and Grandfather Marshall's side of the family. Jeannette refers to her sister almost invariably as 'poor Ada'. Poor Ada, indeed.

In January 1873 Reggie fell ill of a gastric sickness which proved difficult to identify. At the onset, Sir William Jenner was called in as consultant; the day-to-day care was in the hands of Marshall himself; he was backed up by his assistant, Mr Castañeda, who often saw the young patient several times a day.

It is not clear whether Reggie's earlier bout of gastric trouble, diagnosed as diarrhoea in July 1872, was remembered when the doctors collected round his bed; if so, it may have confused the issue; at any rate it is recorded in his sister's diary as adding to the puzzle of the slow diagnostic process. The delay in diagnosis may have contri-buted to the tentative medication and nursing procedures. The thir-teen-year-old had never been of strong constitution; the stresses of puberty now added to his vulnerability. With hope rising and waning as days passed, he lingered on for five weeks. Then, on 23 February, he passed a great deal of blood, and Jenner confirmed Marshall's diagnosis of typhoid.[1] At this late stage the foremost specialist on typhoid, Dr Wilson Fox, was called in and changed the treatment radically, but the new regime did not get a chance to prove its efficiency. Within the next day or two peritonitis developed. Marshall gave his son laudanum and then morphia to alleviate the pain. Death followed in the early evening of 27 February.

During the milder phases of her brother's illness, Jeannette had shared some of the nursing with Mrs Marshall and with the professional nurse. She had helped to dress her brother and get him ready for bed; she had read to him and, as his tolerance for noise diminished, had for his sake refrained from practising the piano. When his illness got worse, she took a turn at sitting through the night by his bed in Mrs Marshall's bedroom. Dressed for comfort in a flannel petticoat and shawl, she felt the responsibility of her function, and was glad that her brother always wanted to have her at his side. She wrote about Reggie's last hours with some of the objectivity of a professional nurse:

John . . . came down to say . . . he was asking for me! I went up & going quite close to the bed & putting my face well in the light as P. told me I managed to say 'here I am, darling, don't you know me?' & P. said 'here is Jeannette'. Reggie opened his eyes very wide, raising the eyebrows, as if he was <u>trying</u> to see me, but there was <u>no</u> expression in them. I kissed him, his face & lips were cold & clammy, & then went to lie down on the sofa in the room next door . . . we were all crying, Mr C. [Castañeda] & nurse too . . . at 7.30 [in the evening] M. came down, & lifting up her hands, screamed out quite hysterically 'He's gone!' I comforted her as well as I cd. & made her take some wine.

[1] The year 1873 saw a typhoid epidemic in London. In August Marshall himself succumbed to an illness which Jenner and Dr Murchison at several points thought to be typhoid fever. Milk supplied by the Dairy Reform Company came under suspicion when Jenner told the Marshalls that over sixty cases of typhoid which had come to his notice were in families who bought milk from this source. 'No doubt the quantity of milk poor dear Reggie took when recovering fr. his first attack brought on the relapse' commented Jeannette. They now belatedly changed their supplier. Notes on Reggie's and Marshall's symptoms were handed to Dr George Buchanan who was investigating the matter of the polluted milk. Some weeks later they received a 'sort of conscience-money' gift from Mr Hope, an acquaintance or a patient, 'at the top of the Dairy Reform Company'. In December 1880, the Marshalls who had switched back to the Dairy Reform Company for their supplies of milk, had occasion to complain about 'a very questionable-looking sediment' they had noticed in it.

Milk was first incriminated as a transmitter of typhoid in 1858. In 1870 and 1873 two outbreaks in London, in Islington and Marylebone respectively, were attributed to particular dairies. See George Rosen, 'Disease, Debility, and Death' in H. J. Dyos and Michael Woolf, eds., *The Victorian City—Images and Reality* (London, 1973) ii, p. 640.

Nurse and Cook attended to the poor angel (that no doubt is what he is now!) . . . Poor P. feels it <u>so</u> dreadfully! We were all <u>3</u> now sent to bed . . .

In the days after Reggie's death, Jeannette went in to see her brother's body a number of times. After the initial shock, she found it a comfort to go in and out of the room 'where he is, poor dear. It is not much longer I shall be able.' She took her last farewell before the body was sealed into its inner coffin, 'not black (wh. looks so dreadful!), but lavender'. On the fourth day, Marshall, having previously cut off some of Reggie's hair for each of them and also, at her special request, for Mme Noël, went through the ceremony of preparing a sort of memento for posterity to put into Reggie's coffin:

In a piece of platinum plate [foil] he rolled up a piece of his own, M's, A's, & John's and my hair, & pricked on it 'The hair of his Father, Mother, Sisters & Brother'. Outside that came another piece of platinum with the advertisement fr. the Times, and below '<u>The Little Soldier</u>' pricked on it. That went into a round glass bottle with a stopper fixed in c.black wax, & over that a cover (as for chloroform & ether bottles) entirely covered with wax. I cut it, & thinned it neatly all round the neck . . . P. put the bottle in his left hand, & M's ring [a mourning ring with 'Father' on it, in memory of Grandfather Williams] is on his right . . .

She was fascinated by the detail of the undertakers' procedures: 'The lid is closed with wax! I always thought there were nails or screws, or something of that sort.'

On the afternoon of 4 March the lavender coffin was placed in the outer oak coffin: 'M, A & I were in the study, P. read Harris's (fen poet) poem on the Wind Mills, but neither M. nor I cd. attend, we felt so nervous; I heard the men bringing him down fr. M's room to the dining room (it is more convenient than the drawing room). We had supper upstairs.'[2]

Later that evening the parents visited the dining-room and were taken aback by the solemnity of the scene, the coffin 'standing under the gas light, dimly lit, with the black velvet pall bordered with broad white cambric over it.'

[2] The 'fen poet' was William Harrison (1794–1872), a small farmer who 'milked his own cows and washed his own potatoes' and became superintendent of the drainage works in the Burnt Fen district. His verse occasionally appeared in local newspapers, but was never published in book form. On 1 February, 1872, four weeks before his nephew Reggie's death, William Marshall had delivered at Ely a public lecture on Harrison and his work. 'M's room' was the parental bedroom on the second floor in which Reggie had been nursed and where he died; the parents had meanwhile used the girls' room and Jeannette and Ada presumably slept in the spare room at the top of the house.

And so, six days from the death, to the day of the funeral:

We had breakfast in the drawing-room of course. We heard the men had
come, so we sent down word for them to go into the study, & we went down
into the dining-room to say goodbye to the poor darling. There stood, in the
middle of the room, his polished oak coffin with a brass plate inscribed with his
name & age, over the head was a large star. We put all our hands together on
the lid & P. said 'May he forgive us anything unkind we have ever done or said
to him'; then we said 'Goodbye' & went upstairs agn. P. & J. (after the crape
hatbands had been arranged) left (at 9.15) in the mourning-coach, & we
watched poor little R. being put into the hearse. Uncle Startin called in, & Mrs
Cocket happily sent A.'s dress before 10, so Uncle very kindly took her to the
Station to join P. there. The mutes etc. only had small white rosettes & white
gloves to show it was a child. A.S. [Aunt Startin] came early, & talked to us, &
tried to enliven us. We had lunch & dinner. A dull day, & of course we had the
blinds down. Francis did not return till about 1, as he had followed to the
station with Watson & the carriage.—We looked at the [plaster] casts after
dinner; the one taken on Friday is not pleasant, but that of Sunday is lovely.
The photos came from Mr Watkins too; he has sent a sheet of all he ever took
of poor Reggie, & those also taken of him in his coffin; some are beautiful.
Emma brought A.E. [Aunt Eliza Williams] at about 3; she came in for a few
minutes. We talked all the afternoon till tea-time, of course principally on the
one topic, & after tea Watson came, we dressed, (I put on my black hat & veil),
& we took A.S. home, & then went to Holloway. We went in & saw Gr.ma for
some 20 mins.; she was a good deal overcome, poor thing. From there we went
to St. Pancras, & picked up P., A. & J, and drove home to supper. I felt really
so ill & 'rheumaticky' that it made P. quite nervous; I took some pills he sent
for, & some potash, & went to bed. A. told me all about the funeral; Uncle &
Aunt were very kind, poor P. got through pretty well, & A. cried her eyes
out.—Just as the coffin was lowered into the grave someone had put a lovely
little bouquet of white flowers on it; they cd. not make out who had done it.—I
believe it was Mrs Swift who had ordered it. Aunt gave A. some flowers to
throw in; Mr Bulstrode read the service.[3]

The decision to bury Reggie at Ely was arrived at after family
consultations to which Uncle William Marshall had been summoned;
more than likely, the bereaved father was settling the matter of his own
ultimate resting-place when he discussed the pros and cons of Ely
versus London. 'We have been talking about it all day, & have agreed
on Ely. There is such a nice cemetery there. Those London cemeteries are so crowded!'

Jeannette, who for some days before the funeral had suffered from

<hr />

[3] Flowers at funerals were in the early 1870s still a relative novelty.

constant headaches, was by now showing symptoms of the serious illness which would knock her flat a fortnight later, and she may therefore have been thought not fit enough to follow the coffin to Ely; for once Ada, the less robust of the two sisters, had proved more equal to the strains. Or was it that the elder daughter was deemed the fittest person to give support to the grief-stricken mother who stayed behind? For that matter, it is not clear why Ellen did not accompany her son's coffin to Ely. Victorian etiquette about women attending funerals is perplexing. Widows, one is told, were not expected to attend their husbands' burials, nor were women in general in the habit of attending funeral ceremonies. In this instance Ada went, so it was clearly not the case that their sex prevented Ellen and Jeannette from going. But Ada's mourning outfit had not arrived from the dressmaker's until ten o'clock on the morning of the funeral, after the hearse had already left for St Pancras. More than likely it was the absence of suitable mourning apparel that had prevented Mrs Marshall (and possibly also Jeannette) from joining the cortège.

For the first two days after the death condolences had been confined to those of the nearest family and a few close friends. But after *The Times* announcement appeared on 1 March, letters, cards and visitors poured in. Nearly two hundred written condolences, recorded Jeannette, when the time came to 'return thanks'; this they did, without any inhibition about personal response being *de rigueur*, on printed cards with only the appropriate name inserted in handwriting.

Among the letters Ellen received from her own people was a miserably insensitive one from her sister-in-law, William Williams's wife; the resentment it caused at Savile Row added fuel to a family row which would last till after the offender's own death, eleven years later.

The death of a child, even in professional circles and as late as three-quarters of the way through the nineteenth century, was not the unusual event it has since become in developed countries. Two out of ten children born to upper-class and professional parents could be expected to die before their fifteenth birthday.[4] Did the Marshalls bear their bereavement more easily because, at a time when to lose one of

---

[4] See the evidence in Charles Ansell's actuarial study, *On the rate of mortality at early periods of life . . . in the upper and professional classes* (London, 1874). The author, on an admittedly very inadequate sample, adduces figures to show that the death rate in medical households was particularly high, possibly because doctors came in contact with many communicable diseases and brought home the organisms which generated them.

one's children before adulthood was a common occurrence, they did
not regard themselves as singled out by fate to receive that awesome
blow? Almost certainly not: when a family loses one of its members, the
trauma which precedes the adaptation to the new reduced size can be
so severe that the organism never completely recovers. It limps along,
less vital, less efficient and more vulnerable than before the ampu-
tation. In the case of the Marshalls, they did reasonably well as a
family, and not so well—in different degrees, and with Ada, perhaps,
as sole exception—as individuals. However, quite apart from what took
place on the day of Reggie's burial at the grave itself, the homespun
ceremonials pursued by them at Savile Row, with the father usually
cast as main actor, appear to have had some therapeutic function.

Routines reappeared with surprising speed; they might have been
peasants whose livelihood demanded that the corn be threshed and the
cow milked. On 6 March, the day after the funeral, John went back to
school, Mr Horton, the Vice-Master of his school, having 'advised his
returning as soon as possible'; Marshall saw patients and in the
afternoon performed an operation. The girls and their mother had to
attend to their everyday mourning (as usual in this thrifty household,
the dressmaker had been summoned only to make the 'best' show
apparel), besides dealing with 'return thanks' and regular correspondence. On 7 March Jeannette recorded: 'I don't feel at all inclined to
cry. I only feel dazed & miserable.' There was talk of resuming piano
lessons within another week, although the usual interval prescribed by
etiquette was not shorter than three months from the date of the
funeral. Jeannette wrote to her music teacher, Miss Ward, asking her
to bring for the first lesson, which was to take place on 14 March, 'a
sacred piece, to begin with'.

In the event, the first weeks of bereavement became complicated by
Jeannette's illness. The early symptoms struck her down on 1 March:
'I have had a presentiment that I was going to be ill ever since poor
little Reggie's death.' The painful joints and the headache were
probably ascribed to grief and were not treated until after the funeral.
And it was not until 10 March that the disease was diagnosed as
rheumatic fever, a second bout of it after an attack at the age of
fourteen, this time aggravated by a bronchial cough.

Of the following six weeks of illness and slow recovery what was
hardest to bear was the incarceration in her second-floor bedroom,
from which she did not emerge till 21 April. It was a landmark to be
allowed down into the drawing-room, to try her old standby, 'The

Harmonious Blacksmith', on the piano. Many more weeks elapsed before she was regarded as well enough to resume a relatively normal life. Jenner, who had attended her throughout the acute phase of the illness, had prescribed a stiff regime for the convalescent:

to take steel, Citrate of Potash, 2 glasses of claret per day, & plenty of beef & mutton; not to take bacon, cheese, pastry, pork & veal! To go to bed early, take care not to catch cold, & take walks (& Academy) $\frac{1}{2}$ hr. at a time. Not to go to evening or dinner parties etc, Cathedral services (Ely) or out of door after 7; no dancing, running, or going much up & down stairs, must not tire or worry myself, etc, etc, etc.

Like most daughters of medical men, she thought she knew better: 'Of course I don't intend to obey all these orders; to begin with I had veal for supper . . .' But all the same, as late as the last week of June she still thought it advisable to refer to her father before she accepted an invitation to go on a boat excursion at Ely, and to her chagrin was told to forgo the pleasure.

For some weeks, Jeannette's illness re-routed her parents' emotions. During the acute enfeebling phase, they may well have thought and talked more about this new predicament than about their dead son. But as soon as she was on her way to recovery, the permanent effects of the loss they had all suffered reasserted themselves. Ellen for a time became even more prickly. It took her a year and a half to bring herself to sing again in the family circle (according to family hearsay, she had a good, trained voice which reached F in alt), and three full years went by before she added a coloured ribbon to her black dress.

   The father confronted a direct test of his having come to terms with the loss when, within three months of Reggie's death, he had to attend in his private ward at University College Hospital a young man who, after a fall on to spiked railings, had developed peritonitis, 'just what poor darling Reggie died of'. Before dying, the young man lingered for four or five days. Marshall's concern was evident from the way he reported on his patient's condition at every meal he shared with his family, and they too showed more solicitude than they usually demonstrated at his more casual talk about the cases in his ward and surgery. It was a trial run for the even more stressful weeks a year later, in the autumn of 1874, when Marshall was summoned to attend Oliver (Nolly) Brown, the nineteen-year-old son of his old friend Ford Madox Brown, in a prolonged terminal illness which involved septicemia. This time he failed to realize (or found it difficult to accept) the gravity of Nolly's condition, and thought the young man was ' "putting on the big pot" to frighten his relations'. He may have disclosed this view to Nolly's parents because, after the patient died a fortnight later, there followed a distinct cooling of relations between the painter and the sceptical surgeon.

As for Jeannette herself, it was as if the main impact of Reggie's death had been removed with the symptoms of the rheumatic fever. All that was left was a faint residual sadness, a few controlled sighs, no more than a hint of the sorrow of the past months. Music, she claimed, was more indispensable to her than ever; it helped to release the emotions that were impossible to put into words. 'Jerusalem, the Golden' heard at St James's, Piccadilly, on the occasion of a sermon by the Archbishop of Canterbury, Tait, brought tears to the eyes of Jeannette, Ada and their father alike. It was one of the rare times when Marshall went to church; neither Mrs Marshall nor John were present on this occasion.

The diaries hold no evidence of the sorrow they shared having made relations between Ada, John and Jeannette more intimate, the bond that tied them more precious; nor do they contain direct evidence of what the other two felt. Certainly, Jeannette's regard for them did not increase. Ada, she had registered at the time of Reggie's illness, slept like a top and could therefore not be trusted to give him his medicine during the night; nerves of steel and a coarse-grained lack of concern was the implication. Besides tears at the funeral and in church, there was no sign of upheaval. But it is by no means impossible that the diarist, never particularly concerned with emotions, her own or other people's, just took no notice of Ada's feelings nor of the indirect symptoms that reflected them. A degree of intimacy between the two girls was inevitable: they still shared a room and often even a bed; they also wore identical clothes (always chosen by Jeanette)[5] and were seldom parted for longer than a day or two. However, Jeannette's references to her sister do not add up to a clear picture of the younger

[5] Jeannette and Ada continued to dress identically until their mid-thirties. This was by no means unusual. Adult sisters wearing identical dresses proliferate in George du Maurier's *Punch* cartoons and in such genre paintings as Augustus Egg's 'The Travelling Companions' (1862). Princess Alexandra and her sister Dagmar often dressed alike; see Diana De Marly's *Worth—Father of Haute Couture* (London, 1980), pp. 156–7 and their 1873 photograph in dark dresses with polka-dotted tabliers and draperies, in Alison Gernsheim's *Fashion and Reality* (London, 1963), plate 111. In November 1874 Jeannette wrote of a photograph displayed 'in all the shop windows' in which the two princesses, in fur caps and boas, looked 'as like as 2 peas'.

girl; what comes over is a sense of forbearance on Jeannette's part for someone rather inadequate and boring.

John, too, Jeannette held to be of little account, apparently too young at fifteen to play an active role in the evolution of the family's tragedy. He had taken no part in the nursing of Reggie, he was not called on to read to his sick sister, he did not relieve any of the social duties connected with the receipt of condolences. No sentiments of sorrow were ascribed to him, nor did it apparently occur to Jeannette that he, more than the rest of the household, would miss Reggie.

From someone else's childhood, her father's perhaps or that of one of his brothers or sisters, Jeannette had inherited the Ely version of the familiar jingle:

> Marshall is my name,
> England is my nation,
> Ely is my dwelling place,
> Christ is my salvation.

At Ely, at least three of the eighteenth-century Marshalls had been lay clerks, and two of them also cathedral singing-men; Worth Marshall, whose talents extended to the composition of chants and hymns, sang in the choir for just under half a century, from 1763 to 1812. More recently, Marshall's younger brother Charles chose the Church as a career, and two of their three sisters married clergymen. Ely continued to regulate its clocks by the cathedral bell and at Ely the Marshalls still went to services assiduously.

But the last line of the jingle had lost its meaning. Religion, prayers, matters of the spirit hardly figured in what Jeannette remembered of her childhood. The context of Christmas and Easter was lay, a matter of family celebration rather than spiritual observance: no Child in the Bethlehem stable, no Christ on the Cross. There was also no Christmas tree; instead, the servants decorated the rooms with greenery. Presents were exchanged on Christmas Eve. Jeannette received from her parents simple useful things such as gloves or handkerchiefs, with, in addition, a pound or a guinea from each of them to extend her pocket money. In return she gave them small ornamental objects, or something practical, such as a fancy glue-bottle or a string-box or a paper-knife. Similar gifts were exchanged with her sister and her brothers. On Christmas Day there would be hot rolls for breakfast, a luxury reserved at Savile Row for very special occasions, and a dinner of roast beef and Christmas pudding, with perhaps some mince pies. In the evening came what to the children was the best part of the festivity: a great dish of snap-dragon, raisins in blazing brandy, which had to be snatched out of the flames without burning one's fingers.[6] Easter, which the girls spent usually at Talbot House, was memorable chiefly for the great number of hot-cross buns they ate from Good Friday onwards; Jeannette's record was six-and-a-half, at one sitting.[7]

Marshall himself, one guesses, was no longer a believer. If he did not reject the concept of prime cause, he had no truck with its conventional symbols. The category into which he fitted most comfortably was that of Gertrude Himmelfarb's 'placid indifferentists'.[8] His church attendance was perfunctory. He did not eschew church altogether, but it took a special reason, such as the sermon by an acclaimed preacher, to bring him in. And in his taste for a good sermon he was thoroughly ecumenical, with a tolerance that extended to non-conformist, dissenting performers. He went, and took his children, to sermons by Archdeacon Farrar at Westminster and to those of Spurgeon at the Metropolitan Tabernacle. Jeannette was always game to join in these explorations and, when she grew up, showed her own brand of undiscriminating broad-mindedness.

Most Sundays until Reggie's death the four children accompanied their mother to the eleven o'clock service at St James's, Piccadilly. When Ellen chose not to go, Jeannette as the eldest would take charge of the small party. Much later it would be said of Ellen that she forswore the God who had taken away her youngest child. In fact, her link with religion had been tenuous even before 1873. All that happened after Reggie's death was that she became an even more erratic churchgoer, and was seen at St James's almost as rarely as her husband. Though for a while she continued to insist that her children should conform to the Church's precepts, they were never confirmed and Jeannette saw her bereaved mother as of 'somewhat a freethinking turn of mind'.

Now it was no longer 'we four' or 'I & the 3 infants' who went to Sunday service; for a time it was 'we three, as usual', the trio being John, Ada and herself. Then, a year or so after his brother's death,

---

[6] This dangerous pastime appears also in Trollope's *Orley Farm* (London, 1862), xxii.

[7] The custom of competitive hot-cross bun eating was widespread, reaching even 'adopted' Englishwomen such as Karl Marx's daughters. See *The Daughters of Karl Marx—Family Correspondence 1866–1898* (Harmondsworth, 1982), p. 7.

[8] Gertrude Himmelfarb, *On Liberty and Liberalism* (New York, 1974), p. 155.

John discovered that, like his parents, he no longer felt any need for regular contact with the established church. His first assertion in the matter was not successful: he 'settled on his own responsibility not to accompany us, but appeared later, looking very red, having been despatched after us by M. He did not look very charmed, poor boy.' Mrs Marshall's attempt to push him back into the family pew succeeded for only a few weeks. Aged sixteen, he was becoming more difficult to control.

The girls, too, now became nearly as slack as their parents about attending church on Sundays. In the past only an incipient cold or really vile weather had kept them away; after Reggie's death and John's defection the threat of rain became a sufficient excuse. Dressed in their Sunday best, they would not risk the short walk across from Savile Row to Piccadilly (the Burlington Arcade was then, as now, closed on Sundays; this would have added a few hundred yards to their route). On occasion, they would even miss the service because they overslept. Reading the order of service (aloud or to oneself) in the comfort of No. 10 became an adequate mark of allegiance to the Church.

To Jeannette, as to Ellen, church attendance had never been more than a social rite, which had little to do with faith or consolation or guidance. When once or twice in her early twenties she came to speculate about the immortality of the soul, an unusual preoccupation for one who had never been devout or curious about the mysteries of dogma, she did not consider this a matter on which the Church could usefully pronounce. And one of her few explicit sentiments about transcendental matters was the rejection of the concept of hell and limbo, or what she called, in 1876, the aggravating twaddle about unbaptized infants not being saved.

At Ely, where the music was outstandingly good, going to the services at the cathedral could be a stimulating experience. At St James's there was entertainment to be got by gossiping about the congregation; this the sisters did in so uninhibited a manner as to be eventually ticked off by a zealous member of the congregation for their scandalous giggles: 'on our doorstep we had a fright by a common woman speaking to us, & saying she shd. write to Mr Kempe [the Rector at St James's] to report on our behaviour in church! I never knew such impudence in my life, & so I told her. I suppose smiling at Chickabiddy's [the curate's] fooleries was the enormity complained of, & if so, half the congregation was equally to blame. I think the woman

must be mad. M. was astounded & indignant at the creature's pre-
sumption when we told her.' They were grown-up by that time,
Jeannette nearly twenty-five and Ada also well into her twenties. To be
admonished as if they were naughty schoolchildren clearly rankled.

CHAPTER 3

PROVINCIAL AND
METROPOLITAN HAZARDS

On an afternoon of January 1873, five or six weeks before Reggie's death, Jeannette's card, the narrow piece of board with 'Miss Marshall' engraved in copperplate (inherited from the previous Miss Marshall, Aunt Lizzie, who had become Mrs Yate in 1865) was left with those of her parents at a neighbour's home. From that day she was 'out' in society, in so far as the concept applied to a young woman who was not going to be presented at Court. That the card had 'Miss A. Marshall' added in ink, so as to extend it to Ada (too young for her own bit of pasteboard), did not detract from Jeannette's conviction that she had now entered upon a new phase.

Then came the tragedy of Reggie's illness and death, and almost immediately, her own rheumatic fever, followed by six months of deep mourning. It was not until the autumn that they thought it proper to attend formal musical parties, and dancing was not resumed till early in 1874. It is from January of that year that Jeannette started to conform to the annual timetable of the upper-class Londoner, dominated by the Queen's absences and presences, and by the sittings of Lords and Commons.

Then, as now, the swell of society's tide came three times a year: in the weeks between the Christmas merrymaking and the beginning of Lent (the continentals' 'carnival'); during the Season proper in the spring and early summer; and in the late autumn with its succession of lesser revelries. The weather made its own contribution to the calendar. Fashionable weddings took place in May and June when the sun was expected to shine; so did garden parties, picnics and river excursions. Balls were planned for the winter and early spring before it got too hot.

Each of these periods made new demands in terms of dresses, mantles and accessories. The number of outfits Jeannette and Ada required eventually rose to forty or so each a year; autumn and Lent were spent in feverish activity, preparing these immense wardrobes. The Season, divided in two by the Whitsun recess when the fashionable went out of town, prescribed three sets of clothes: for the cool Easter weeks, for Ely in late spring, and for the sweltering London days that could be expected in June and July. Then there were costumes for travelling abroad in August and September and serviceable clothes in which to brave the east winds at Ely during the brief New Year holiday. As far as the Marshall girls were concerned, impressing the inhabitants of Ely was nearly as important as looking one's best at the Private View of the Royal Academy or at some fashionable London ball. They were determined to stand out, to shine in their metropolitan plumage.

Whitsun was one of their favourite times for Ely; the girls missed it only when relations between Savile Row and the Ely Marshalls were at a low ebb. And, almost as regularly, they also visited their Ely uncle and aunt for a few days at the New Year. 'We seem to make it quite a 2nd home' wrote Jeannette. Access from London was slow: most railway journeys required a change at Cambridge. Trains were often late: at a time when railroads took pride in punctuality, a half-hour lost on a journey of less than one hundred miles seemed excessive. However, the sisters travelled comfortably, usually by the afternoon express, provided with buns bought at St Pancras and the *Globe* or *Punch* to while away the tedium; in cold weather tins of boiling hot water could be hired in London or at Cambridge—Ely provided no such luxury—to keep the travellers' feet from freezing. And at Ely station there would be a pony-trap and Uncle or Aunt, with sometimes a boy in buttons to carry the trunks, waiting to take them to Hill House.

Aunt Julia and Uncle William lived not in the original Marshall home on Fore Hill, from which grandfather Marshall had conducted his business of solicitor-cum-auctioneer, but on Back Hill, in a more elegant 'nice white, plastered C18 house with Tuscan porch, bow-window on the first floor and a Venetian window on the N. side'.[1] Though rather grand by Ely standards, Hill House was not a comfortable place, with few fires to cheer the fierce Cambridgeshire winter weather, water turning to ice in the bedroom ewers, or rain dripping through the ceiling of the guest room. Aunt Julia was a bad housekeeper; she was incapable of controlling her staff of cook, housemaid

[1] Nikolaus Pevsner, *The Buildings of England—Cambridgeshire* (Harmondsworth, 1954), p.307.

and sometimes also a boy in buttons, and incapable of ordering a decent meal. Uncle William's first wife had perhaps accustomed him to better things; at any rate, he found Julia's haphazard ways hard to bear. Moreover, she was no great asset to him in Ely society, because of a distressing habit of giving offence to her female friends. For a solicitor and a coroner Uncle himself was also not quite heavyweight enough. His frequent visits to London on unexplained 'business' attracted comment; malicious acquaintances took note that in the autumn of 1872 his wife, distracted by William's wayward behaviour, herself disappeared from Hill House for a week or so. She sought refuge at Savile Row, without an 'atom of luggage, not <u>even</u> a nightgown, brush or comb', and shut herself in with Ellen and 'talked & wept for about $1\frac{1}{2}$ hrs, during wh. time sandwiches & beer were demanded & consumed!' That evening Ada overheard whispered consultations between the parents, with 'he was very wrong', 'she led him on', 'he'll have to prove himself her husband' providing clues to the nature of Julia's trouble. Eventually Mrs Marshall confirmed that Uncle William had 'behaved very badly to Aunt, & even struck her!' It took considerable tact and manœuvring on the part of relatives in London and elsewhere to mend the rift between the erring husband and the offended wife.

While she felt some sympathy and loyalty for the Ely aunt, Jeannette had never completely succeeded in putting out of her mind childhood memories of Julia's favouritism and harshness. A change of heart had taken place when Jeannette was sixteen or so, and aunt and elder niece were now on the best of terms, but nevertheless the wrongs of long ago occasionally reared their head.

There was also the matter of Uncle William's moods, related (one guesses) to this secret parallel life he was leading. When out of humour, he would despotically forbid his wife to entertain or to accept invitations, vetoing the occasions which were to his nieces the honey that attracted them to Ely. Hill House would then be becalmed for weeks on end, with tame card games—'Commerce', 'Pounce', 'Snip Snap Snorum'—as sole amusement. Ada derived some compensations from the study sessions with Uncle William whose interest in botanizing she shared, but for Jeannette this hobby held no charm. There was nothing like small-town boredom to depress the spirit, and to pass the time they were often reduced to going to church twice on Sundays. Jeannette appreciated the music, but even so complained: 'Sundays <u>are</u>

quiet here, and no mistake', and repeatedly sighed 'I am really ennuyée to death.'

Soirées at the Bishop's, sober musicals at the Deanery, sedate croquet at the Cropleys on the lawn of Egremont House—most of the Ely entertainments seemed left over from a less sophisticated era. Even the means of getting about was archaic: in winter and also on wet summer evenings ladies would be carried one at a time by sedan chair from hallway to hallway, at the cost of 1s. per journey. They travelled 'up & down, jogtrot' in the 'antedeluvian conveyance', but Jeannette admitted that she got home in pouring rain 'without a speck of wet'.[2]

In the eighteenth century a sort of 'upper middle class' of brewers, gunsmiths and rich independent farmers, with the occasional apothecary–surgeon or attorney to add intellectual tone, had inserted itself into Ely society; they fitted above the yeomen and skilled craftsmen and just below the exalted ranks of cathedral clergy. The descendants of the families in this intermediate category, the Archers, Luddingtons, Bidwells, Pates, made up Uncle William's and Aunt Julia's circle. Jeannette turned up her nose at most of them. 'Comfy people' she wrote of Ely's inhabitants, 'so small (not in stature only) and mean, & narrow!' Yet despite all the drawbacks Jeannette enjoyed the visits to Ely, no doubt in large part because here she and Ada were the centre of attention. Tongues wagged, if only because the Marshall sisters, with their London airs, were seen as dangerous competition by the local young ladies, and by their mothers or guardians. Jeannette wrote defiantly 'I am not loved "en province" ' and certainly enjoyed the role of conquering minx in which the gossip of the 'feminine female shes' cast her. She responded with gusto to the flirtatious approaches of several young men whom she had known long before they became Ely's eligible bachelors. She was glad to be wooed, but glad also that the brevity of her visits prevented any of the flirtations from developing into serious courtship. Harold Archer was entertaining and a good dancer; Martin Pate looked well on a horse. But she could not bring herself to regard in earnest any prospect that entailed settling in Ely for good, married to an up-and-coming small-town solicitor or to a prosperous young farmer.

Admittedly, she had something of a penchant for her cousin John Swift, but then he was in the process of making the transition from Ely

---

[2] The sedan chair was still used in Ely in the 1880s. It had been given up in London fifty years earlier.

to the metropolis where he was studying surgery at University College Hospital under Marshall's protective wing. His devious advances consisted of discrediting his rivals; he 'gave it as his opinion that Ely is going down, as there is not one of the rising generation to take the place of their fathers, that Harold Archer would never be half the man his father was, and as for Martin Pate, he wd. not compare for a moment with his father either!' Jeannette enjoyed her cousin's company because, having known her since childhood, he was not overawed by her fashionable manner, and teased her and baited her as if she were a sister. But he was her exact contemporary, and, as a medical student, however capable, was many years away from the time when his income would allow him to take on the responsibilities of marriage. So, although Marshall regarded him as promising and was, in theory at least, not averse to the idea of a cousinly match, Jeannette never seriously contemplated John Swift.

If local suitors did not pass muster, there were others at Ely whom Jeannette, at eighteen and nineteen and twenty, found exciting. The very fact that Ely society was minuscule made the townspeople eager to accept into their midst the officers of the Cambridgeshire militia who were frequently stationed in the city. In London, Jeannette's ways never crossed those of the army, and officers would in all probability not have found favour with her parents. Even though many of them came from county families, they were by the nature of things impecunious; a career in the army had to be subsidized and seldom led to riches. Also, officers were thought to be footloose, and their intentions dubious. From the lowest commissioned ranks to the highest, they were best avoided.

In Ely, away from her parents' direct jurisdiction, Jeannette danced and flirted with one and all, from dashing lieutenant to middle-aged colonel. As it happened, none engaged her emotions at all seriously, although she played with fire and in one instance came close to getting singed. It was splendid fun. Aunt Julia lectured her on coquetting, but was a permissive chaperone; 'a delightful chaperone' Harold Archer had called her, 'she sits by the fire & shuts her eyes'; this was when he was not complaining that she did not take proper care of her niece, leaving Jeannette unchaperoned 'in the supper-room among the redcoats'. That Julia was irresponsible enough to close her eyes even to near-embraces and walks in the moonlight compensated, as far as

Jeannette was concerned, for her absurd housekeeping and accident-prone relations with other Elyites.

Did John and Ellen Marshall find out what went on at the dances in the Lamb Hotel? At the only one the parents attended, when Jeannette was twenty-one, she had danced most decorously with Lord Colin Campbell, who commanded the Cambridgeshire regiment. To have been singled out by this notorious aristocratic beau—he had partnered her three times over—flattered her ego and had not displeased her parents. It must have made many a mother of a potential Ely suitor cross Jeannette off her list of possible alliances. Jeannette's parents teased about her distinguished dancing partner, as they also teased about major and captain and lieutenant. None of it was taken seriously, because none of it happened within what was now their home territory, London.

'I do believe (though I wd. not confess it to everyone, but you I may trust, my dear old Diary) that my long stay at Ely has rather countrified my tastes. I dislike the blacks [soot], noise & smoke & miss the flowers & little things with wh. I can ornament my room in the country, but wh. I am afraid to have out in London, for fear of their becoming as black as soot.' This is what Jeannette had written in early August 1873 when, after a long seven weeks at Hill House, she returned to Savile Row with all its memories of the painful winter and spring of Reggie's death and her own illness. That day's entry went on: 'But now is the dull time of London, & of course not going to theatres, concerts etc makes a great difference.' 'Really we are the last in town this year! I never remember seeing London so solitary' was her cry three weeks later.

Under more favourable circumstances she invariably crowed with joy at returning to the excitements of London—or of that part of the metropolis which she recognized as her home ground. In the years of her girl- and young-womanhood it was that fan-shaped segment of the city which radiates from Piccadilly Circus, its northernmost point in Holloway, extending westwards through Hampstead, Maida Vale and Notting Hill to Kensington and Chelsea in the south-west, and then returning eastwards via the King's Road, Belgravia and Piccadilly. Savile Row is all but on the eastern confine of this shape; in the nineteenth century, eastwards beyond Regent Street and southward towards the Mall, lay lands of ill-repute, stretches of clubland and the shady world of music halls and brothels.

Just as they travelled in trams and omnibuses, a mode of transport which strict etiquette condemned as unladylike, so the Marshalls, mother and daughters, interpreted the rules about where it was permissible for respectable women to walk with level-headed flexibility. If a visit to a tradesman took you to Soho, well and good; but the maze behind Regent Street, and also the lanes and courts that separated it from Savile Row, were out of bounds for the daily constitutional. And though at eighteen or twenty Jeannette may have been vague about the particular dangers of each forbidden zone, she knew exactly which routes were to be avoided. As for the 'heavenly' Burlington Arcade, right on the Marshalls' doorstep, where gloves, lace, trinkets and hats tempted in every shop-window, it was a favourite short-cut to Piccadilly in the morning but forbidden from lunch on. Without having it spelled out, Jeannette believed that it then became a warren of vice, where women of loose habits accosted men, and no lady could walk unmolested. When in March 1875 she accompanied Aunt Julia on an expedition, the ultimate target of which was a bootman in St Martin's Lane, she remarked that their walk had taken them 'into the unhallowed region of the Clubs'. And when she and Ada excursed south of the Circus, they walked briskly, descending on the east pavement of Regent Street as far as the new Co-operative Stores in Waterloo Place[3] and returning on the west side, with only a brief stop to inspect the exciting windows of Howell and James and their display of aesthetic pottery and metalware.

The weekday walk combined exercise with shopping and focused on Regent Street and its intersections. Hardly a week passed without a visit to Lewis's,[4] their chief supplier of trimmings and materials, or one or other of the sundry co-operative stores that started up (and mostly failed within a year or two) in the 1870s and '80s. From the mid-1870s they added Liberty's to the regular shopping round. A day without purchases was an exception; 'for a wonder, did not buy anything at Lewis's or elsewhere!' Jeannette noted in April 1878, at the height of a spring dressmaking spree. Their return route took them through Oxford Street and Hanover Square, or else they short-cut into Maddox Street; then back home, along the familiar side streets north of the Row, with often a last call at Kelly's, the stationer cum sub-post office,

---

[3] The Junior Army and Navy Stores, established in York House in 1879.

[4] John Lewis set up in 1864 in a small shop on the present site of the department store in Oxford Street.

The Savile Row setting:

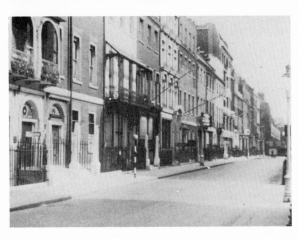

No. 10, built in the mid-'30s, was, with its neighbour No. 9, demolished *c.*1936. In their place stands a brick and stone-clad structure, three floors of offices above two shops with large plate-glass windows. Taller than its surroundings, it can be seen, two-thirds along the terrace, in this 1939 view of the east side of the Row. The general aspect on this photograph still very much as it was in the later part of the nineteenth century.

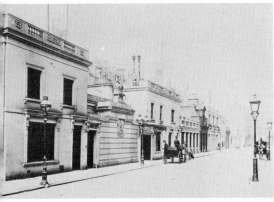

(*b*) The west side of the Row, with the premises of Poole's, the tailors. Other tailoring establishments moved into premises vacated by medical men when the original Burlington estate leases expired towards the end of the nineteenth century.

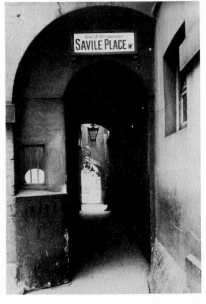

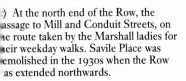

(*c*) At the north end of the Row, the passage to Mill and Conduit Streets, on the route taken by the Marshall ladies for their weekday walks. Savile Place was demolished in the 1930s when the Row was extended northwards.

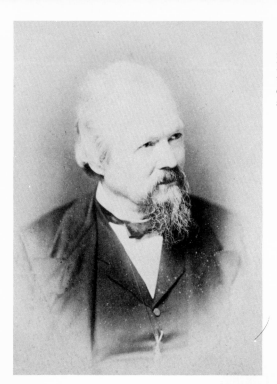

2. John Marshall in middle age. Distinguished anatomist, unassuming surgeon, capable committee-man. Indulgent father and friend.

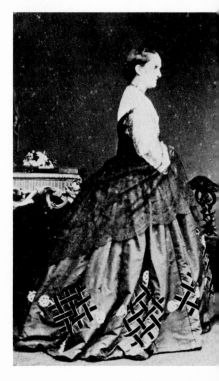

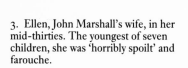

3. Ellen, John Marshall's wife, in her mid-thirties. The youngest of seven children, she was 'horribly spoilt' and farouche.

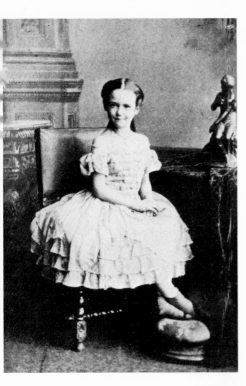

4. Jeannette Marshall, aged seven or eight. 'A boy of about fourteen . . . kept trying to kiss me under the mistletoe, a proceeding I evaded with great dexterity. This is the first flirtation I can remember.'

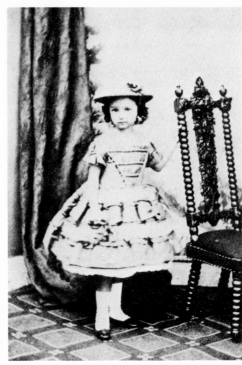

5. Ada Marshall at five. '. . . I have heard I was very jealous of her at first . . .'

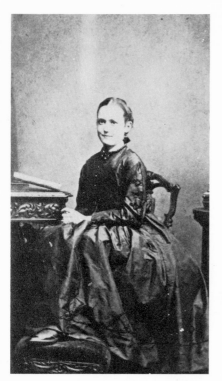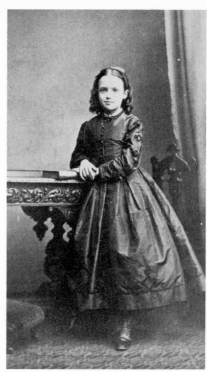

6. The young Marshalls: Jeannette and Ada in the mid-1860s.

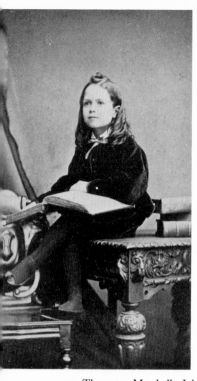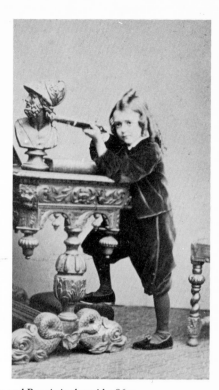

7. The young Marshalls: John and Reggie in the mid-1860s.

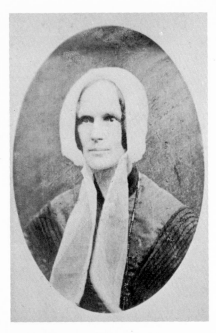

8. Anne Marshall. 'She struck me as being enormously tall as she stood on the door-step to welcome us. I liked her very much . . .'

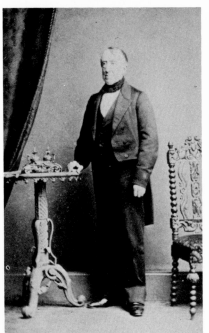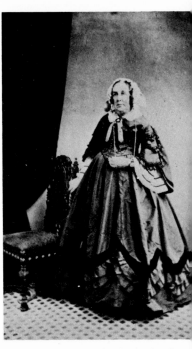

9. Charles Williams (*left*): '. . . of medium height, thin & active, always kind & lively, pleasant in manners, & a perfect gentleman.' Elizabeth Williams (*right*): '. . . much stouter, sharp & clever, but not blessed with the sweetest of dispositions . . .'

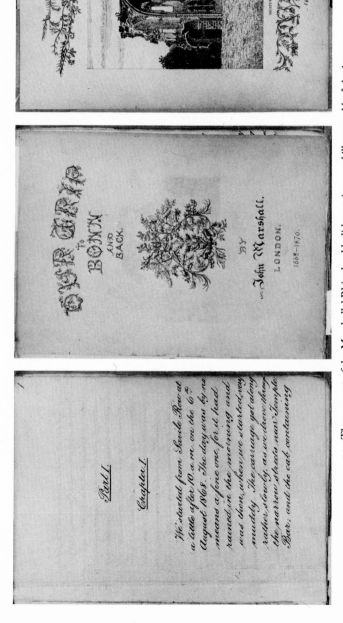

10. The account of the Marshalls' Rhineland holiday, written and illustrated by John between the ages of ten and twelve.

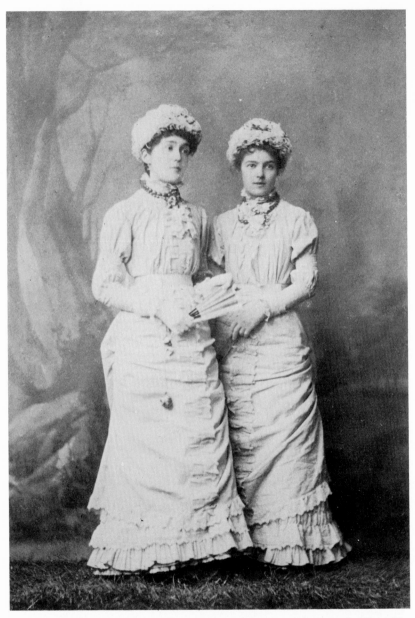

11. 'Fair Aesthetes': the dresses, of lemon cotton crêpe, were relatively simple. 'Short skirt with balayeuse, kilt, & 5 times gathered lace-edged flounce. Long polonaise with gauged neck & pli Watteau, sleeves with shoulder & elbow puffs, & gathers in between, lace collar, cuffs & down front & all round, band . . .' Both Jeannette and Ada wore their amber beads, and matching Charlotte Corday hats, trimmed with white feathers, maiden-hair fern and white and yellow jonquils, completed the aesthetic outfits.

which Jeannette had patronized since childhood and where she annually bought her Pettitt's Diary.

The houses that lined these side streets were still uniformly Georgian; as at 10 Savile Row, their façades were usually three windows wide and three or four storeys high above the level of the pavement; the basement windows of the domestic offices, the kitchen with its satellite sculleries and larders, became visible as one came close to the front area railings. Not half a mile away from Savile Row, in Welbeck Street, Mrs Haweis had in 1868 led a successful rebellion against dingy cream-coloured stucco. The fashion had spread and many staid dark-grey brick house-fronts were now enlivened by the bright colours of woodwork, railings and plaster. The Marshalls' colour scheme to which they adhered with only minor variations from the mid-1870s on had been chosen for them by Ford Madox Brown. It was of grey-green stucco, set off by white window reveals and brown (or, later, black) window-frames and ironwork. The door was a fashionable grained walnut, thin lines of gilt embellished the railings of the first-floor balconies, and, to add to the artistic effect, the larger knobs on the area railings were also gilt. On the balconies, window boxes of aesthetic blue and white tiles, filled with a lavish assortment of Victorian favourites—geraniums, fuchsias, lobelias, calceolarias and trailing ivy—completed the festive aspect.

The main arteries of Regent Street and Oxford Street were also being embellished. Successful drapers began in the early 1870s to put up grandiose stores which rapidly modernized the aspect of the West End. The areas to the east of Piccadilly and its intersection with Regent Street were also in a state of flux. Improvements in the Circus started in 1874 with the building of the Criterion. A year later, in January 1875, Jeannette reported that, after one of their rare sorties to Soho, they had been to take a closer look at the newly laid-out Leicester Square: 'I have only seen it fr. the carriage before. The figure of Shakespere is having something done to it; at any rate there is a scaffolding up. The rhododendrons and shrubs generally looked melancholy, and the gravel consisted principally of mud. I suppose the time of the year has something to do with it, but the effect was doleful.' Ten years later the zone was still in turmoil: 'Walked round by Piccadilly Circus. The pulling down of the small poky houses opposite the "Cri." is a great improvement. It is really a fine open space now, and leaves plenty of room for circulation. It will be rather a trap for the unwary in crossing.' This particular improvement made way for the Circus end of Shaftesbury Avenue. The other memorial to Shaftesbury, the statue of Eros, was put up in 1893, when Jeannette no longer lived in Savile Row.

In 1871 Jeannette wrote of her father's patients: 'they have taken to living in the four corners of the globe: St John's Wood, Hornsey & I don't know where.' On occasion he in fact ventured into suburbia, to Barnet or Norwood or Richmond, Blackheath or Peckham, or much further afield, on provincial expeditions which took him as far as Bath or Rugby or the South coast. These were exceptions, viewed with some trepidation, even by Marshall apparently, since for a visit to a patient in Wood Green he armed himself with a revolver. In the years from 1870 to 1881, Jeannette recorded only about a dozen professional visits to the outer suburbs and less than ten further afield. The remainder of the time he moved between University College Hospital in Gower Street and Savile Row, with some excursions to Brompton, where he was consultant to the Consumption Hospital, and a few domiciliary visits within a distance of two or three miles north and west of his home.

This relatively narrow circuit meant that he could arrange his days so as to be able to spare coachman and horses once or twice a week for his wife's and daughters' social calls. By the energetic standards of Victorian women, many of these were in fact within easy walking distance of Savile Row, but to call on foot was not done. This was in part because in the afternoon men—gentlemen, that is, not tradesmen or errand-boys who could be ignored—crowded the streets of the West End, released from their desks by the short working hours of Victorian officialdom. However, the chief reason for preferring to drive rather than walk in the afternoon was to protect the elaborate outfits suited for the business of paying calls.

The carriage was in any event needed to visit people who lived further out. Even so Jeannette regarded such places as Primrose Hill, or the Melbury Road side of Holland Park, or Notting Hill—in the 1870s, the 'young married couples' quarter'—as 'the other end of nowhere'; this was also what in 1883 she called St George's Square (in Pimlico) where she herself would live twenty years later. In pursuit of references for a prospective servant they would occasionally venture to the suburbs, to Highgate or Stockwell. One such expedition took them as far as Clapham, 'quite into the country'.

Jeannette regarded the round of obligatory visits more as a duty than a pleasure. So of course did Mrs Marshall, who was adept at cutting out calls that were not absolutely required by the laws of etiquette and only rarely initiated the visiting process. The rules of calling on one's hosts after a party or dinner were observed; the Marshalls also made calls of condolence and to enquire after the sick. But if they espied a friend on whom they had intended to call leaving on her own round of visits, they waited till the danger of being recognized had passed and then handed their cards to the absentee's domestic; this gave them the satisfaction of having cunningly accomplished the requisite formality with a minimum effort on their own part.

Some of the reluctance derived from the fact that even by carriage a round of visits was quite tiring on account of the time it took to travel through the traffic-congested streets of central London. In the West End weekday traffic intensified during the main shopping hours, eleven to twelve-thirty before lunch, and, in winter, two to four in the afternoon; on spring and summer afternoons people shopped later, and vehicles carrying shoppers crowded the streets up to five or five-thirty vying for space with the carriages of afternoon callers. Each carriage, each four-wheeler or hansom, took up much more space than the average modern vehicle. With no policemen on point-duty, no traffic lights, no one-way systems, rush-hour chaos was indescribable. There were memorable traffic jams round Bond Street, when it took the Marshalls three-quarters of an hour to drive from Savile Row to the Piccadilly entrance of the Royal Academy or an hour to return home from the Grosvenor Gallery in Bond Street.

Street accidents abounded: there is more art in managing a pair of horses than in driving a car. Only one of a score of accidents in which the Marshalls' carriage was involved proved at all serious. On the way back from a concert at the Albert Hall, proceeding at walking pace, the offside front wheel of their brougham knocked down and ran over an elderly woman who was taken to St George's Hospital with bruising and suspected concussion. Jeannette described the event with total recall in two pages of her diary—her own feeling of shock, Ada's hysterical crying, their male domestic's alarmist report of the victim's death. Their coachman was exonerated, bystanders confirming the footman's account of the lady having stepped down right in front of the carriage, which had pulled up immediately. There were no hard feelings. On the contrary, when their victim recovered she called on the Marshalls to thank the surgeon for his solicitude and his visits to St George's.

Only once had a coachman in the Marshalls' employ fallen foul of the police—when he drove straight into a post in Bond Street while drunk and incapable. The more usual pattern was that of a collision, sometimes strong enough to reduce one or both vehicles to 'match-sticks'—Jeannette's favourite term for total disintegration—followed by a great deal of recrimination on the part of the coachmen, while the glass of the conveyance, or their own delicacy, guarded the passengers against the foul language outside. They took such incidents in their stride, as the price they paid for living in a crowded city.

Fog added to the hazards of moving around London. In bad seasons, such as the one which spanned October 1873 to February 1874, or the winters of 1878–81, there were months of fog, with only an occasional clear afternoon to break the gloom. But winters with heavy snowfalls were an even greater trial. In frosty weather the coachman arranged to have the horses 'roughed' by putting long-headed nails in their shoes—'it wd. be tempting Providence to take them out without'—and selected routes, sometimes very roundabout ones, which avoided inclines. Snow brought havoc and disruption. After a heavy fall in January 1881, Jeannette noted that 'the milk did not come up from the country, & Swiss [tinned] milk was the horrid substitute.' The hansoms were drawn by two horses harnessed tandem, four-wheelers needed two horses abreast. Side streets remained 'perfectly unapproachable'; only the main arteries—Regent Street, Oxford Street, Bond Street—were swept clear of snow. Carts were used to carry away some of its worst accumulations. In 1889 she described a snow-plough drawn by six horses: 'What enterprise! I shd. think we have to thank the county council.'[5] According to her, the plough proved no more effective than an experiment to melt snow by steam had been three years earlier.

Walking in such weather was even more hazardous than it is today, as narrower pavements increased the risk of being hit by the lumps of snow which fell off the roofs. Women's clothes afforded little protection and every stitch down to the petticoat would be soaked

[5] The London County Council was established by the Local Government Act of 1888 and took over from the Metropolitan Board of Works in 1889.

through. So in really bad weather the girls stayed inside, and danced and pirouetted to keep warm in the icy rooms, with the indoor thermometer down to as little as 40°.

Night-time and Sundays, with only the occasional carriage or cab to break the peace, must have seemed blissfully quiet. On weekdays the double beat of horses' hooves on the granite setts which paved the roadways provided the percussive accompaniment to all activities. Then there was the rap of postman and telegraph-boy who substituted for telephone messages and were therefore constantly calling on the medical households of Savile Row. Add to this the newsboys crying the latest sensation at main crossings, the less insistent but still strident voices of itinerant vendors in the smaller residential roads; the roll of the cat-meat purveyor's drum, the whistle of the chairmender; enliven it with the occasional barrel-organ and the bell of the fire-brigade. The pre-motorized city was noisy—a great deal noisier than it is today.

It was also smellier. The subject was taboo in polite conversation, but in her diary Jeannette constantly complained of 'green water' smells in the houses of relatives and friends. Victorian noses had to tolerate different but not lesser urban pollution. The smell of any Victorian theatre or hall, with its audience in clothes which were never cleaned over bodies which knew no deodorants or anti-perspirants must have been stifling, and on occasion ladies were indeed overcome by it. Mrs Marshall carried eau de Cologne against such a contingency, and a decorative phial of smelling salts was often hung from the châtelaine worn with formal dresses. Out of doors one or two daring cranks, such as Jeannette's music teacher Miss Ward, wore respirators, gauze masks which protected from sooty fog and sulphuric emissions. The ubiquitous horse dung, effluents from drains during excavations and from open hallways and areas, the reek of cabbage and mutton from kitchens ventilating into front areas, all added up to a curious offensive urban stench, from which there was no escape even at home, for it floated through open windows and through every crack in the woodwork.

At times the pollution was so offensive that the victims rebelled. At the back of the Marshalls' home, behind the extension which in the 1850s and '60s had housed the nursery, an enterprising company installed, early in the 1880s, an electricity generating plant. The machines thudded, the chimney belched smoke and choking fumes;

the whole venture, the British Electric Light Company, amounted to an intolerable infliction on the entire neighbourhood. After suffering the nuisance for some months, a group of residents, including Marshall and several other surgeons, went to law and were eventually awarded redress;[6] the company first curtailed its activities to shorter hours and then moved out of the district. It was an early victory for organized ecologists (the case had coincided with the formation of the Smoke Abatement Society under the aegis of another medical man, Ernest Hart), and also an early manifestation of an effective middle-class tenants' movement.

Despite all these snags there was hardly a day, except in the worst of weathers, when they did not take a constitutional. On Saturdays and Sundays it took them westwards, along the edge of Green Park, carefully avoiding the masculine territory of clubs and bachelors' chambers on the north side of the street. For years, this walk was an obligatory item in their weekend routine during the Season. Their destination was *the* Park—Hyde Park, the favourite meeting-place of fashionable Londoners and of people who wanted to see and emulate them.

The concept of 'fashionable' needs to be qualified. The cream of society did not perambulate; they rode in carriages and on horseback, on weekdays only. On Sundays they stayed indoors or were out of town. But the rest, all those who, without being right at the top, were near it, might be seen sitting on garden chairs or walking up and down a relatively small area of the lawns in the southern and south-eastern part of the Park. The exact spot was determined by fashion, too: 'We

---

[6] *The Times*, 6 April 1882, reporting on the request for an injunction against the British Electric Light Company, wrote: 'The nuisance was alleged to be twofold, first by causing the exhalation of gases which were believed to be injurious, and secondly, by the noise made by the engine of the company, which it was said worked both day and night.

Mr. INGLE JOYCE, for the defendants, having asked that the motion might stand over in order to give him time to answer certain affidavits, Counsel for the plaintiff submitted that it was only reasonable that the company should undertake not to work the engine later than midnight. Mr. JOYCE, however, stated that the company had entered into contracts to supply the light to various premises, including two clubs in the neighbourhood, and that it would paralyze their business to stop so early, but he offered to undertake to stop at 2 a.m. The VICE-CHANCELLOR thought that at this time of year, when many persons did not go to bed before that hour this offer was reasonable, and the motion accordingly was directed to stand over until after the Easter Vacation, on such undertaking being given, the company, of course, not thereby admitting that any nuisance existed.'

went to the grass just beyond the Achilles statue, wh. is now the thing'
Jeannette wrote in 1880.

An important aspect of this ceremonious parading, which so resembles the evening *passeggiata* that still takes place along the *corso* of every
Italian city, was that it gave young men and women the chance to meet
with less formality than in drawing-rooms and ballrooms. The young
women were of course escorted by parents or other chaperones; an
adult brother would just about pass muster. But being out of doors
gave a young man the privilege to take the initiative. As soon as he had
been 'recognized' by the girl or by her escort (a process involving no
more than a slight nod, or even an encouraging glance) the young man
could come up and start a general conversation—and, if he wished,
veer adroitly into direct exchanges with the object of his attention.
Conversely, cutting ('not recognizing') a man who had offended her or
whom she no longer found interesting, was a powerful weapon in a
woman's armoury. Jeannette found the Park a convenient place in
which to cut people; for as attention here centred on recognizing and
being recognized, no man who had been subjected to this painful
public rejection could fail to ignore the snub.

Quite early in adolescence, a girl had to learn how to free herself of
unwanted gallants. It was important to move gracefully and in a
dignified way, yet at a pace sufficiently purposeful to remove any
misapprehension on the part of prowlers in pursuit of willing prey.
Men 'stared'; her parents noticed it too, she reported, and were usually
amused. The offenders were clearly seen as admirers, rather than
threatening lechers. The intensity of the stares was a welcome measure
of the success of one's outfit and general appearance, but it was at the
same time not to be countenanced, since to take notice was to provoke
the starer to worse excesses. Jeannette was well capable of dealing with
the nuisance: 'more than the usual no. of "creatures" stared me out of
countenance through the windows of hansoms at crossings & corners,
wh. is somewhat embarassing, though I am pretty used to it' she wrote
at eighteen. She was flattered by the attention she attracted and also
resigned to it: 'it amused him & it didn't hurt me'. A well-bred girl or
woman had to appear oblivious of her immediate surroundings; Jeannette carried this to a fine art. It was an entertaining challenge when
she happened to be out alone (if, for instance, her mother was busy and
Ada laid low with a cold): 'I had to go home toute-seule & was spoken
to by a disgusting man. I never looked at him & took no notice, tho' no

doubt I looked as if I considered him beneath contempt.' Being talked to was in fact inadmissible: 'some horrid man had the impudence to speak to me, & offer to see me across'; 'was much admired by three gentlemen, who stopped short to let me pass and murmured "splendid" greatly to my annoyance!' As she confided all this to her diary, no doubt her lack of sincerity did not make her blush.

CHAPTER 4

THE FLIRT MEETS THE CARD

IN August 1874 while holidaying in the Swiss Alps Jeannette met someone whom for several months she believed to be her 'fate'. On the evening of the Marshalls' arrival at Maderanerthal (south-east of Amsteg in Canton Uri) she wrote 'One creature took to staring at once.' She must have done her own share of ogling, for there and then she described the stranger as a 'tall man in knickabockers with a reddish beard & rather bald, light eyes of a very sharp kind, & a pleasant expression.'

Being stared at, so unprofitable when it took place in a London street, became in the setting of a hotel abroad an acceptable prelude to an introduction; it was as if sharing a foreign shelter conferred respectability and substance on every unknown Anglo-Saxon. The next morning 'yesterday's creature' was in the dining-room, breakfasting with a friend, and at once struck up an acquaintance: 'he got up to open a window first asking if we minded. I was the only one who heard, so I answered in the negative. P. spoke to him then, & soon we became quite friendly, he showed us the reading-room, library & small drawing room, piano etc., told us no end of anecdotes, & kept us all in a roar.'

Herbert Thomas ('I suppose he is of Welsh "distraction" ') was a lady-killer almost exactly twice Jeannette's age. After the sombre year of mourning and several inconsequential romantic episodes in Ely and London, she was in a mood to be wooed, but above all eager to be amused. And she found all aspects of Mr Thomas exceedingly amusing. 'I shall never forget how extraordinary he looked in his savage costume' she later reminisced; beside the knickerbockers his outfit included 'scarlet stockings, round-topped hat & puggaree[1] & the finishing touch for expeditions viz: ice-axe and blue spectacles! Such a Judy!' But it was his jokes and puns that really won her over, and his

---

[1] Pleated scarf or tie round the crown of a sun-helmet or similar headgear.

ready appreciation of her own repartee. He displayed for her delectation an avalanche of anecdotes and wit, of which every word went
down in the diary, including her own responses at which he invariably
'roared'. Early in the acquaintance, another hotel guest, Mr Crickton,
had expounded at length on the art of preparing a tomato salad: ' "You
take vinegar and—and . . ." '; as he hesitated, Jeannette took over.
' "Brown paper?" ' she suggested, 'in such an à propos manner that
everyone was in convulsions, & Mr Thomas cd. not look at me for
several minutes after without a fresh explosion.—We were friendly
ever after.'

As well as a partner in the game, she made an ideal audience. She
guffawed when he called a spider or an earwig a 'grewsome beast', or a
five-franc coin 'a fine piece of family plate'; a small lizard her brother
had caught became the 'alligator'. When she appeared at a window one
evening, Mr Thomas 'immediately struck an attitude, played an
imaginary guitar & began to sing the serenade fr. Don Giovanni!' That
he had a 'capital voice and very good style of singing', and moreover
adored the Moonlight Sonata, then Jeannette's show-off piece, was
also in his favour.

All this he served up with a judicious admixture of silent stares,
prolonged handshakes and small gestures of gallantry. No one, with
the possible exception of John Wood, had ever treated her with such
chivalry. He picked flowers for her hair on precipitous slopes, helped
her to cross glaciers, and carried her, with one arm only round her
waist—encircling her with both she would have regarded as a liberty—over a cascade. Strong, masculine, using the age difference both to
flatter and to assert his power over her, he was, it appears, quite an
accomplished gallant. Was the chivalry a preliminary to sustained
courtship? Her parents were, she thought, 'determined to counter-
manœuvre' Mr Thomas's advances: 'they think our flirtation is becoming a trifle strong.' Accordingly, neither the father nor the mother gave
Thomas leave to call on them in London. It was Jeannette, eager to
continue the game, who had failed to discourage Mr Morshead,
Thomas's travelling companion, when he casually declared their
intention to visit the Marshalls in Savile Row. The candour with which
Thomas had told her father all ' "about his birth, parentage & education" ' made her expect an offer of marriage. When he had not spoken
before his departure to London on the ninth day of the Maderanerthal
dalliance, she assumed the proposal would come when she and the

other Marshalls returned to Savile Row a month or so later. In the intervening period she filled the pages of the diary with a blow-by-blow recall of the merry doings at Maderanerthal and speculations about Mr Thomas's next move. She concluded, sedately: 'I daresay he will call.'

Within days of their return, Jeannette complained: 'I never can indulge in the slightest flirtation without being teased to death'; later she added: 'When P., M., A. & J. are all in full working order, it is no joke.' As at the time of the John Wood episode, Mrs Marshall was once again behaving irresponsibly, speculating openly about Mr Thomas's intentions. 'C'est un peu trop fort' commented the diarist one day when her mother had spoken over the breakfast table about a presentiment that Mr Thomas was to be Jeannette's husband. 'Moderation in all things. Bringing presentiments into play is a little too much!' Next, Ellen Marshall took to reporting dreams in which Mr Thomas and Jeannette were very closely linked. Again, Jeannette demurred: 'M. appears to be always thinking & dreaming about him & me, though I don't see why she shd. honor me (or him?) with such an association. I never knew her to "go on" so about anyone before. I wonder if there is a reason, & if so what?' Months later she reported another dream of her mother's about Mr Thomas: 'he came to Hol. [Holloway], & M. saw him in the dining room, & he was very pleasant to her till I came in, when he got up, & came to sit by me at once.' A fragment of a dream, and perhaps one emasculated by both the mother's and the daughter's inner censors; Jeannette thought it 'very odd' that she had been told of it by Ellen on the morning before a call from Mr Thomas; in the course of his visit he behaved just as in the dream, so that she had been 'pretty near laughing'.

On the occasion of his first call at Savile Row, while Mrs Marshall silently speculated ' "Well, you've come once, but I don't see how you'll come again!" ', Mr Thomas succeeded in what the parents later referred to as ' "the coup" of asking P. to dinner, of course to be asked in return . . . & poor Papsy was so "took-aback" that he was incapable of refusing . . . P. & M. were in full confab. on the subject as they were getting up, & I heard M. say . . . that she did not see what Mr. T. came for unless he thought of me! & P. seemed in a mortal fright lest he shd. declare his intentions on Friday', the day appointed for the Union Club dinner. His daughter appeared calm enough: ' "the why & the wherefore" of the banquet remains to be seen' she reflected, and then concluded, with the superciliousness of youth: 'Men can do <u>nothing</u> without a dinner.'

After the dinner, which had proved uneventful—' "Wittles" (of course) good, anecdotes numerous, puns many & <u>weakly</u> (Mr T's I presume!)'—Thomas must have felt that the advantage was entirely in his court. At any rate he did not hurry the next move, which was slow in coming. For two weeks Marshall and his wife knocked the matter of a return invitation backwards and forwards, in a dilemma as to how to cope with an acquaintance, who was also a potential suitor of one's daughter, and whose exact status was difficult to determine. Mr Thomas hinted at some official occupation which involved travelling as near and far afield as Durham and the Azores, and which had, he claimed, at some point in the past brought him within reach of the governorship of the Gold Coast. His entrée into clubs was impeccable; he belonged to the Alpine as well as the Union, both highly respectable. But he also wrote freelance for the *Observer* and the *Morning Post*, and a journalist's social standing was not easy to define, a freelancer's even less so. When some months later, in February 1875, Marshall told Ada that Mr Thomas held a post in the offices of the Privy Council, Jeannette assumed that this had been known to her father ever since, in Maderanerthal, Mr Thomas had been so confiding about his affairs. 'Why didn't P. say so before?' she asked, 'when he knew we were all dying with curiosity!' 'P. says the Privy Council has to do with Sanitary arrangements' she expanded, with no apparent recognition of her father's pun, and forgetting that once before she herself had, in a facetious mood, on her mother suggesting that the footloose Mr Thomas might be a government inspector, added in her diary the query 'of nuisances?'

After a fortnight's hesitation, Marshall invited both Mr Thomas and Mr Morshead to dine at short notice at the Savile Club (Thomas had given Marshall only four days' notice of the Union Club dinner). The intention was to discharge a debt—'we don't want to be indebted to strangers'—'without making too much of him or "encouraging" him.' In the event the dinner was declared to have been a 'very jolly' evening, with an uncharacteristically grave Mr Thomas being kept in his place by Victor de Rivaz, a lively scientist friend of Marshall's. Had Thomas been on the brink of proposing for Jeannette's hand, he would doubtless have been overawed by the company. In addition to Morshead, de Rivaz and himself, Marshall had asked another acquaintance, the mathematician Professor Henrici, plus two of Jeannette's maternal

uncles and the family's solicitor, Mr Bartlett—to all intents a commission assembled to determine if Thomas would pass muster as a swain.
He might of course have taken it as a gesture of deliberate
encouragement.

In fact it marked the first chord of the finale to Thomas's intercourse with the Marshalls. Before a business trip to the Azores he
called at Savile Row, on the regulation bread-and-butter visit, and left
two articles about the Swiss holiday which he had written for the
Morning Post. One of the pieces was about Maderanerthal. And there
they all were, unnamed but easily identifiable in print, Marshall as the
'distinguished man of science, but pleasant companion', Uncle William Marshall the 'enthusiastic botanist, who had never been to S.
[Switzerland] before, but knew all the Alpine flowers', Mrs Marshall
the 'charming lady who carols Neapolitan songs'. Johnny was
described as a 'capital specimen of the British schoolboy', and the
sisters were 'sweetly pretty, pleasant, lively, plucky' and accomplished.
The example of pluck was Jeannette's crossing of a perilous bridge,
her playing of the Moonlight Sonata testified to the accomplishment,
and a witticism of hers was quoted verbatim. 'Like his impudence'
fumed Jeannette. Her father was amused but thought the whole thing a
great liberty. The Marshalls' predilection for spoof now came to the
fore. Jeannette wrote an anonymous letter critical of Mr Thomas's
articles; with Marshall's connivance it was posted to Mr Thomas at the
Union Club, date-marked at Charing Cross, as if forwarded by the
Morning Post. The deception was elaborate to the point of mock dirty
thumbmarks (ostensibly the commissionaire's) on the inside envelope.
She professed to feelings of guilt but was clearly delighted, 'joyful
beyond measure' at her ingenuity; her father encouraged her: he
'roared at intervals' at what they all thought a particularly good joke.

Its victim reported back sooner than expected, the voyage to the
Azores allegedly cut short by bad weather. He spoke of the 'slashing
criticism' which his *Morning Post* articles had provoked and 'then he
roared & so did we!!' It was evident that neither postmark nor dirty
finger-prints had taken him in, and the Marshalls, too, had no intention to carry the mystification any further. The chief culprit admitted
to her guilt obliquely but unequivocally, and was relieved that Thomas
did not appear offended. This was a mark in his favour. Once again,
speculations about the ultimate intention of his visits were rife.

Some weeks later, in February 1875, Jeannette wrote down a dream
of her own: 'I very wickedly dreamt I was dancing with Mr Thomas;

highly improper, but one can't help one's dreams.' It seems for all the world as if she had looked up dancing in a dictionary of dreams—or as if she expressed, unusually for her, an insight about her own involvement. On several occasions in Switzerland, she had been made aware of Mr Thomas's attempts to get close to her with an intimacy which she found dangerous and exciting. Once or twice, as if under accusation of an impropriety, she protested in the diary that these contacts had been unavoidable. Now when she dreamt of the dancing partner's legitimate embrace she called herself, rather than him, wicked.

She complained that her father was dilatory at providing Mr Thomas with openings for continued contact; this, she surmised, was not through absent-mindedness but for one of two reasons: 'either he thinks Mr T. is "épris de moi", & that I don't return the compt., & consequently it would be "cruel" to invite him & encourage him; or, Pa wd. not approve of the "partie", thinking him too old or goodness knows what, & fears my losing my heart to no purpose.'

According to Ada, their father 'did not think Mr Thomas . . . sufficiently well off to marry anyone who had not plenty of money.' In the diary, Jeannette let her irritation boil over: 'I don't see why a person shd. be utterly tabooed because he has not a large income', and she consoled herself with the thought that he would not travel abroad for pleasure if he did not have 'something comfortable'.

She let it be known that she wanted Mr Thomas to be invited again. The request fell on deaf ears, its bantering tone having perhaps misled her parents. It is also possible that, much as in the John Wood affair three years earlier, it suited Marshall to be hard of hearing.

Her mother, she knew, objected to Mr Thomas's manner, finding the clowning totally inadmissible. Ada considered that Mrs Marshall was 'the enemy to the cause'. 'I don't know!' exclaimed Jeannette who was more incensed by her father's attitude: 'I think P. has shown pretty plainly he does not want him . . . I don't see why he [Mr Thomas] shd. do all the calling or make all the overtures. I think P. has behaved rather absurdly, "shaking him off" like that.' Her father was in her view 'the oddest individual out'.

Marshall may have been afraid of his elder daughter. He preferred the indirect approach: 'P. asked A. if she thought Mr. T. wd. "propose". A. cd. not answer for certain, but thought I preferred my liberty at present.' Jeannette recorded this exchange without comment; it corresponded to the impression she herself wanted to project.

What she failed to recognize—and what may have been manifest to her father—was that Mr Thomas was no longer in the game. If evidence were needed, it came with his refusal, in July, of a tardy invitation to join a rustic dinner-party at Richmond. Mrs Marshall held that he had never recovered from the shock of Jeannette's spoof letter. More likely, he had seen in her joke a deliberate signal to keep away.

When he called one afternoon a few days later—etiquette demanded that an invitation, whether accepted or refused, should be acknowledged by a visit—Jeannette, at least, behaved as if nothing had changed: 'I do declare he is worse than ever.' Not for the last time, she deluded herself about the tenacity of an initial attraction, while at the same time striving not to lose face even to her diary. 'I don't think P. wd. ever hear of him, & I have seen so little of him for so long that I don't like him as much as I did this time last yr., & that was not so very much.'

By the autumn, when they heard rumours of Mr Thomas's impending marriage and when her own expectations had faded, her parents twice brought up the subject, as if to convince themselves of Jeannette's indifference. 'P. actually asked M. the other day if she thought I was grieving about Mr Thomas (as I have not felt very well, looked rather pale lately).—She said she thought I had no more love in my head than I cd. kick off with my heels.' 'Perfectly true' Jeannette commented testily and was not to be pinned down. The instinct which made her guarded about proclaiming her feelings for over a year had not played her false. Within weeks they saw the announcement of Mr Thomas's marriage, on 2 December, to a Miss Mort.[2] Noting the fact, Jeannette concluded 'so much for him! certainly my experience of men has been an odd one', ending curtly: 'I have not room to discuss this point at present.' Later that winter in a general stocktaking of what, in self-mockery, she called her experience of the male sex, she returned to the subject in a review of three years' flirtations:

First, John Wood, fair, good-looking, & amusing, about 30; sent opera-tickets, & mazurka, called me 'J^{ette}.' & 'dear', squeezed my hand etc. Uncle George [Wood] put a 'spoke in his wheel', he departs, & is married in 16 months. 2nd: Harold Archer, fair, short, over 30, clever & amusing; faithful (for a wonder fr. Jan 1870, when he danced with me 6 times, to Jan. 1875, when we flirted quite 'en règle').—Being small & country-bred I kept him on the other side of an

---

[2] *The Times* 4 December 1875. The announcement supplied incidental proof of Mr Thomas's respectability: his clergyman brother performed the ceremony and their father was also a clergyman.

offer. Third: John Swift, dark, good-looking, 22, clever & getting on well; devoted since Easter 1871 till July 1875 (I only answer for as long as I know!). 2nd cousin & too young ∴ do not go beyond flirtation. Fourth Archibald Leslie Innes, [a lieutenant of the Cambridgeshire regiment] fair, nice-looking, about 24, great flirt, but entertaining; appeared to like me very much.—No money & gone to Ceylon.—Fifth: Herbert Thomas, tall red-bearded, not good-looking, but very clever, about 40; inseparable in Aug. 1874, afflicted with intense staring, makes embarrassing speeches, very nervous & awkward, in short all bad symptoms.—P. not approve or encourage—16 months after, married. There you are!

She went on to list a few less exciting and even more transient flirtations, closing the account with the usual cliché 'this will suffice to show what odd creatures men are!'

CHAPTER 5

ACADEMIC HURDLES

LESSONS with Mme Noël had stopped some months before Reggie's death; those with Miss Greatbatch went on until Ada, in turn, reached the age of seventeen. All formal education could well have finished at this point. 'Till eighteen you will do lessons, from eighteen on you will do nothing' was what Violet Asquith's governess told her charge when asked what the future held. Jeannette Marshall, just as Miss Asquith, would have taken such a 'nothing' to correspond to a hectic round of social activities with the single object of landing a suitable husband; and she was by no means certain that waiting passively for an eligible partner to turn up was how she wanted to spend the years of her girlhood. She thought that being a music critic would be fun, with all those free concert tickets as an incentive. By the time she was twenty she even began to treat seriously her father's repeated suggestions that she should apply her skills to translating or writing short pieces for magazines. After the collapse of one particular project, the translation, for publication, of a short book from the French, she expressed her appetite for some sort of remunerative occupation: 'I certainly shd like to earn some money. When girls don't marry very early they ought to try & do something.'

It was largely a matter of laying her hands on more funds. When it came to pocket money and to clothing allowances, the Marshall parents were parsimonious and Jeannette enough of a puritan to applaud their careful habits. But she was also overweeningly vain: to impress, to be the best dressed—these were aims to which she could devote herself wholeheartedly. This needed money on a more generous scale than the half-crowns and half-sovereigns meted out by Mama. In 1874, the year she began keeping a detailed account of her clothes allowances in the diary, her income had been £2 12s. pocket and glove money, 12s. for the purchase of ribbons, and 1s. a week for boots and shoes (this allowance had started in the middle of that year). 'Earnings' for making her mother and Aunt Eliza a bonnet each and three dresses for herself were 14s.; that, plus an 'extra' allowance of 5s. a quarter from the autumn onwards, and a number of gifts, brought the total up to around £12. Seven years later she still got only £11 in pocket money and shoe, glove and ribbon allowances; to her it seemed 'a fortune'. This of course was not intended to pay for her main wardrobe (apart from the specified items) which continued to be provided by Mrs Marshall until Jeannette was twenty-nine and Ada twenty-eight.

Even then, she was later to brag, at the height of her career as a young lady of fashion it had never taken as much as £30 a year (a little less than £1,000 in modern terms) to keep her in clothes and to pay for her personal expenses.[1] She derided the extravagance of her Williams aunts and cousins who went around in satin and lace. But while claiming credit for her own thrift, she longed for more abundant funds to call her own, with the freedom to budget without parental super-vision, or in years to come, the interference of a husband. 'I never <u>do</u> have any money' she wrote at the age of twenty-two. 'It vanishes, flies, dissolves, or goodness knows what, in no time—I wish I cd. make a little for myself! Shall I ever? Nous verrons! I am getting to write with much less effort that I did at first. Awful exertion to begin.' The literary venture she engaged in at that point was an account (in two parts) of a tour of Auvergne, which the Marshalls had undertaken in September 1877. It took a great deal of perseverance, and some help from Jeannette's father and his literary friends, before the women's weekly *The Queen* accepted the two articles. In February 1886 she was enchanted to receive her fee, two cheques for a total of £2 18s. 4d., 'quite a godsend' in her chronically impecunious state. It was the only money she would ever earn by her pen.

Her concept of what constituted gainful employment did not extend to the effort she put into making, refurbishing and maintaining her wardrobe. Jeannette now worked an average of three to three-and-a-half hours a day, year in, year out, holiday periods included, making and remaking dresses and bonnets, trimming hats, sewing and embel-lishing underclothes, altering and contriving mantles and wraps. Much

---

[1] This was not in fact an unusually low figure. The daughter of that other eminent medical Dr (later Sir) George Buchanan, Lilian Buchanan, some eleven years Jean-nette's junior, received in late adolescence and early adulthood an allowance of £24 a year, to cover clothing and also fares, postages and similar expenditure. See Lilian Adam Smith, op. cit., p. 20.

time was also spent on any number of ancillary activities indispensable to the conduct of this domestic industry, such as letters to dyers and cleaners and shopping for fabrics, trimmings and paper patterns. Only heavier outer garments such as ulsters and waterproofs were bought ready-made. The dressmaker would be summoned exceptionally, for Mrs Marshall's more elaborate outfits or to make sure that the young ladies' evening bodices had the desired close fit; when mourning apparel was urgently needed they would call on the dressmaker to supply the best dresses, leaving the everyday costumes to be made at home. Jeannette would have been astonished to find that by her dressmaking she saved her father something of the order of £35 a year, the equivalent of half the annual cost, in wages and maintenance, of employing a first-rate lady's maid. Nor did it ever occur to her that she was intellectually over-qualified to be a lady's maid or a seamstress.

That his daughters should earn their own pocket money was certainly not high among Marshall's priorities; it probably never occurred to him at all. When he insisted, in 1872, and again in 1874, that the girls attend classes at University College,[2] he no doubt intended not only to help them widen their intellectual experience but also to overcome the isolation of their home background. In this second purpose he did not succeed; both his daughters were, by their late teens, too set in their self-concerned ways to take much notice of others of their own sex. The provision of a formula for continued and more thorough study was another matter.

At first Jeannette had resisted her father's enthusiasms, especially as he had sprung the idea of university courses on her unawares. The plan to have her attend was raised on a Monday morning in October 1872 and became a short-lived reality by the evening of the same day:

P. came & whisked me off to the lecture (Prof. Morley on the study of English). We went there in the carriage & returned in a hansom. Inconvenient time (6 to 7). The room was cold looking with seats raised like steps, & a platform & table for the lecturer who was 10 mins. late. The pupils were principally ancient frights of governesses with specs. on nose. P came & sat by me. I had to take notes (!). The lecture was only introductory; the course is to be on exam subjects. We spoke to Prof. M. after.

The concept of examinations, which was at that point foremost in her father's mind, was what really put up Jeannette's hackles. 'P. wants me

[2] The classes were part of the women's lectures which started in the late 1860s within the orbit of the general university extension movement.

to go in [for examinations], & if I do I must make up my mind this week! I <u>don't</u> want to!' she wrote, with unusual insistence on her mutinous point of view.[3]

In the event Marshall thought better of forcing through the unpopular proposal. Jeannette scored a victory which she attributed to the fact that after the affair with John Wood, her father regarded her as an adult. ' "As for examinations," ' he had said in 1872, ' "you needn't go in for them unless you like." ' This was much to her taste. 'How wise P. is getting, that's just what I have wanted him to say!' Her exultation was premature: at intervals the determined father brought up the vexed subject; Jeannette complained he was examination-mad. 'I foresee I shall have fine struggles next year if I want not to be tied down to lessons till I am 5 & 20!' Equally resolute, she parried Marshall's arguments and succeeded in postponing the evil hour. 'A year's reprieve at any rate!' she rejoiced in 1873, just a month before Reggie's death. And then for a while no more was heard about examinations nor university lectures, as if the father, after losing his youngest child, had become more tentative in his ambitions for the girls.

Not until the autumn of 1874 did he have his way in the matter of regular attendance at university classes. Both Jeannette and Ada were entered for courses by Henry Morley on English literature and Willis Bund on constitutional history. But Jeannette once again raised objections when Marshall tried to extend her commitment to other subjects. 'I did not see the fun of being set to work as hard as a "slavey" agn!' she wrote and a few days later reported another victory: 'A. is going in for French & Italian & the Slade School. I am not. 3 lectures a week is quite enough.'

Ada's art classes were dropped almost at once. On the first day at College she 'saw an Indian <u>all but</u> unclothed at the Slade School, being drawn by men & women together.' 'P. does not approve' registered Jeannette, and this was the last time the Slade course was mentioned.

After an initial show of reluctance compounded by the bad weather which accompanied their first expedition to Morley's introductory lecture ('I wish him & his literature at Jericho!' she wrote that morning), Jeannette was immediately won over by the exciting taste of

[3] Special examinations for women up to matriculation standard were set up by London University in 1867. Access to all examinations and degrees was opened to London women students in 1878.

emancipation from the sheltered existence at 10 Savile Row. She also responded to the intellectual stimulation of the subject-matter, though it went against her nature to admit it. On the contrary, she did not resist the temptation to debunk, presenting her lecturers as figures out of Edward Lear's limericks: Bund 'tall, thin & dark, with long "Picca-dilly sweepers" ', and bouncy Morley—'energetic person' she called him—who drew diagrams on the board which he then, in the heat of the argument, rubbed out with his back. She picked holes in their delivery and quarrelled, often for no reason other than half-informed prejudice, with their viewpoint. All she derived from Bund was a very primitive classification of past statesmen and kings into good ones and bad ones, with the latter in clear preponderance. After Bund's solemnity and his 'unfortunate habit of swallowing half his words', she found relief in the facetiousness of Professor Morley, whom she referred to as the 'Englishman' because of the way he stressed the first syllable of that word. Morley, who was regarded as an excellent popularizer, clearly enjoyed the process of delivery and read large chunks of his favourite authors aloud to his class. But Jeannette scoffed at his exalted renderings of verse, especially Hallam's and Tennyson's: 'his voice husky with suppressed emotion etc. He is so unromantic looking, & the girls all sat solemnly in rows staring at him till "it was so droll, so very droll, I laughed as I wd. die; Albeit in a general way A sober girl am I!" ' She continued to prefer the 'école realiste', and fiction rather than poetry.

On Mondays Jeannette would walk home alone, an excitement in itself, leaving Ada whose Italian class did not start until half past two, to munch sandwiches or buns in the ladies' room. She did not envy her sister these vigils. But by and large the University College venture was a success. 'I certainly like going; it gives me something to do' she wrote after the first few occasions. 'I worked so hard in my schooldays that I felt the want of some writing, or learning, to do.' And she added to the time taken up by the courses by doing homework: 'P. brought us home some note books, & in the evening I wrote out the gist of Prof^r Morley's lecture from my notes. It is rather amusing, I think, though I feel sorely tempted to put little asides in parenthesis of a sarcastic description. This has become almost 2nd nature with me, cutting up my friends as I do in my diary.' After Morley's next lecture, she noted: 'Most decidedly it is fun.'

It was not just that the classes supplied a structured framework and imposed a rhythm on her weekdays. It was the very fact that this structure, this rhythm, was imposed from outside, and applied not only to her and to her shadow Ada, but to a wider category of her contemporaries that was new and stimulating. The women's classes were large, with audiences of between thirty and forty at Bund's and up to seventy at Morley's lectures. The fees, in 1875–6 two guineas (42s.) and one-and-a-half guineas (31s. 6d.) for Morley's and Bund's courses respectively, were more than most working women could afford. This time there were no middle-aged frumps of governesses present, though the young women who attended were earnest, and sat 'still as mice' while the lecturer addressed them. Before and between classes they scurried along corridors and cloisters, a 'troop of disconsolate girls' in search of the appointed lecture-room. In time she came to see herself in a prefectorial role, recording in her diary the occasions when she had supplied information about missed lectures or guided the flock of fellow-students into an unfamiliar lecture-room. Yet she never got to know the surname of even one of her companions, let alone getting on intimate terms with a chosen individual.

As the daughter of Professor Marshall, a long-standing member of the College's medical faculty, Jeannette felt entitled to obsequious respect and special consideration. On days of bad weather, Casson, the beadle, fetched cabs and offered the sisters shelter in the lodge while they waited for transport; the woman in the ladies' room could be called upon to supply information about the proceedings and so could, at a higher level, Mr Mylne, the secretary in charge of the women's lectures. And Jeannette took it for granted that the fellow-students of her brother John (who had left school in July 1874 and at the age of sixteen-and-a-half become a student of University College, winning the Andrews Scholarship for maths in his first term) would recognize her and Ada and give them special notice. She enjoyed the homage of their stares, whispers and salutations, uncouth though it may have been. Her keenness may be gauged from the amount of space she devoted to accounts of her University College experiences; in the winter of 1875–6 entire pages of her diary were sometimes filled with the blow-by-blow detail of her academic adventure:

We rushed along the cloisters to N° 18, fearing we were late. I opened the door, & half-entered (A. close behind) when I perceived an old gentleman sitting, & lecturing to about 8 boys, I withdrew in double-quick time, & started off to the waiting-room to enquire the room of the woman there, when old Casson (with his poker-like back & neck) emerged fr his box (wh. was also tenanted by about 4 students) & shouting as if we were born in a wood, asked if we wanted Prof^r Bund. I said 'Yes, please', & he showed us the way to N° 23, near the Council Room. The inhabitants of the [beadle's] box rushed to windows & door to see us pass, looking quite delighted. One nearly went on his knees to see better. I did not care, but cd. not help smiling, it was so absurd.

Instalments of the boy–girl skirmishes were noted after every visit to Gower Street:

An amusing incident occurred. 2 or 3 boys took to rushing up & down the stairs at the back of the room, bursting in at each door alternatively in a distracting manner. Mr. M. looked more & more irate, & at length 'full of righteous wrath' he rushed like a lamp-lighter up the steps to the right-hand door, & called out to one of the young wretches 'There is no class going on here now for you to attend.'—'O, indeed, isn't there?' said young impudence!—'No' said the Englishman fiercely, & returned breathless to resume de Quincey.

Most of the teasing aimed directly at Ada and herself:

About 11.20 we emerged and passed a group of boys, among whom was J. [John], to go to Morley's room. The boys dispersed as if at the approach of 2 wild animals; my dear brother evidently much overcome . . . Coming out, the Beadle's box was full of students, & one young horror waved his hat frantically! J. told me afterwards it was young Cassal, who told him he had seen the Miss FRSs! The impudence of those boys surpasses everything . . .

[A week later] Coming out a struggle was going on in the Beadle's box between someone trying to wave a hat, & someone else trying to prevent it! I understand young Cassal's hat was waved for him by a friend, & no doubt the performance was being repeated. I cd. not help laughing, & had to put up my muff.

The following Monday the porter's box 'was lined with a row of standing students, who stared greatly, but no hostile demonstration took place.' And so it went on till, some weeks later, Easter 1876 put an end to the lectures, and to Jeannette's humanistic studies.

After Morley's last lecture in March his class had voted, by a show of hands, on the 'authors to be "talked about" in the summer courses'. Jeannette was not impressed by this introduction of student participation. 'I am not going so it is not interesting to me. Morley wished us goodbye, & there is the last of him for 7 months. How time does go!' And a fortnight later at the close of Bund's cycle she declared: 'I am glad the lectures are over.' In the autumn of that year a conjunction of circumstances, illness and death at Holloway and other domestic upheavals, delayed the resumption of studies. The girls appeared committed to take up attendance at lectures; on the eve of her grandmother's death (24 October), Jeannette wrote: 'The lectures at the College begin today, but we are not going until after Christmas.' Then the end of the year visit to Ely was upon them, extended that winter until the fourth week of January. By the time they came back to London, the winter session was in full swing; the lectures disappeared by default, apparently without any explicit decision to drop them.

The subject of examinations arose again once or twice during the first year of Jeannette's attendance at the UC lectures, but Marshall had withdrawn from the fray. It was now a matter between her and the academic establishment, and therefore very easy to parry. All that she and Ada had to do was to refrain from inscribing themselves on the lists of young women who wished to be examined. 'We did not feel "called" to give our names' she wrote on the second occasion the subject was mooted, and added that the examinations on Morley's course were to take place on the day of Bund's last classes: 'his lecture & the Exam. wd. clash.' In the event the test was put forward by twenty-four hours, but she did not feel disposed to change her mind. The following year her obduracy was not even tried. The professors themselves may have decided that examinations were unpopular; at any rate there is no mention of them in Jeannette's accounts of life at the College.

Her original refusal to sit for examinations may have sprung from idleness, from a determination not to become a 'slavey' to intellectual pursuit. Doubtless she was sustained in her insubordination by her fear of the unknown: never in the nursery, never in the schoolroom had her dominance and perfection been questioned—what if she now failed? A great deal was no doubt the blurred, confused protest of the *jeune fille rangée* who has to assert that her life is her own to run. Eventually it became a more direct mutiny against the imposition of her father's will, against being cast as the Marshalls' clever girl, one of the earnest dowdies whom she ridiculed and abhorred.

CHAPTER 6

TOYING WITH STRONG-MINDEDNESS

IN the contest between Marshall's serious-minded aspirations for their daughter and Ellen's much more worldly ambitions, the latter prevailed. One can almost see the tug-of-war with Mama, Aunt Julia Marshall, and a few light-hearted Williams relations on the winning side, and Marshall with the strong-minded ladies who inspired him, and perhaps also Mme Noël surprisingly cast as losers. The fashionable and lively bluestocking of the pre-Victorian and early Victorian eras, who had exercised her intellect and wit in her father's or her husband's drawing-room, was giving way to the strong-minded woman, bent on a career and independence. Elizabeth Garrett Anderson, from way back a professional friend of the surgeon's and on visiting terms with his wife and daughters, personified Marshall's conviction that it was possible to be strong-minded and yet attractive.[1] But Jeannette and her mother remained unconvinced. In their eyes, as in popular caricature, the new strong-minded being wore drab unfeminine tweeds, sported spectacles, smoked and lived—like a young man—in chambers. Worse still, she spent her days slumming, while Jeannette had no time for typical do-gooding avocations: 'Mr. Kempe preached on visiting the sick, & assured us it was our bounden duty to enroll ourselves district visitors on the spot. Now, I shd. like to know who is to find time for that! I say (district) visiting, like charity, begins at home.'

On the occasion of a later sermon she again demurred: 'These [Scripture] readers intrude themselves on a righteous family once a month, on an unrighteous much oftener! What horrid nuisances they must be!' Of an acquaintance who lived in lodgings not far from University College Hospital and engaged in good works Jeannette wrote: 'However Miss H. can have left a comfortable home for that

---

[1] Arthur Munby thought there was some incongruity between Dr Garrett Anderson's feminist stance and her ultra-feminine appearance (see Derek Hudson, *Munby—Man of Two Worlds, The Life and Diaries of Arthur J. Munby*, 1828–1910, London, 1972, p. 293).

poky place I can't think! She has taken it into her head to visit the poor in the very lowest & vilest parts of London, wh. no doubt is well-meant, but rather cracked.' That Miss Hope, with her 'earthy complexion, plainly-worn brown hair, half-shut, rather prominent eyes, & a style of dress meant to be artistic', fell short of Jeannette's standard of presentable appearance helped no more than did the other characteristics of the strong-minded stereotype, the loud voice and 'much self-assertion wh. impresses the unsophisticated beholder'; the comment concluded sniffily: 'whether she is really clever, I am not so sure.'

The unfeminine costume which some of the liberated women favoured also provoked a good deal of sneering. Typical of the breed was Eliza Vaughan, a literary lady who 'ranted' on Poetry and the Poets at a soirée of the London Literary Society, a 'stout woman of short stature, dressed in plain tight black satin, with an Eton boy's collar & linen cuffs, red bow at the chest, blk. hair short like a boy's, & the largest amount of modest assurance ever possessed by a single human.' And the scoffing carried on even when the wearer herself passed muster or was positively popular with Jeannette. Helen, the painter daughter of Thomas and Mary Thornycroft the sculptors, old friends of the family whom even the ultra-critical Jeannette could not help liking, was regularly mocked for her eccentric attire. At one of Professor Marshall's Royal Academy lectures in 1874 Helen appeared 'more disreputable than ever' with a 'shirt front & man's hat complete'. Nor did her eccentricity cease with the passing of time. Met at the National Gallery some six years later, she wore a 'footman's coat'. In her own home she was a 'regular stable-boy' in a dust-coloured skirt, waistcoat, coat and 'absolutely no petticoats'. Many years later she was still remembered by Jeannette for 'her short hair, bowler hats & waistcoats & ties of a manly appearance. She had some neuritis in her right arm, and finding hair-dressing troublesome, cut hers off, and . . . would never grow it again. As her hair was her only beauty this was a pity.'

Jeannette herself was not entirely innocent of the unconventional where dress was concerned. This applied in particular to corsetry. In his writing on anatomy her father referred in only very general terms to the damage caused by constricting garments and lacing.[2] But a pamphlet of which he was the editor, and possibly the author, *Wasps Have Stings or Beware of Tight Lacing* was published in 1872 by the Ladies' Sanitary Association. Some of the anatomical illustrations Marshall

[2] See his *Anatomy for Artists*, op. cit., pp. 108, 356.

had drawn for it were also used in a small book, *Madre Natura versus the Moloch of Fashion* (London, 1870). This tract, dedicated to Marshall by a friend who hid his identity under the pen-name 'Luke Limner Esq.', denounced tight lacing as well as other artificial aids to beauty.[3]

In line with Marshall's disapproval of tight lacing, Ellen and Jeannette (and possibly Ada, too) avoided standard corsetry, though boneless stays were not easy to find in the shops. In 1875 Jeannette made do with a pair of conventional corsets, size 22 in., 'after removing all the bones, only 52!, I put them on & found them very comfortable.' She also protested when bustles were being reintroduced in 1882 and chose to wear light padding instead of formidable whalebone-cum-wire structures or steel hoops.

But though her father became a convert to the Woollen Movement soon after Dr Jaeger had exhibited his unbleached wool-knitted clothing at the Healtheries (the name by which the Marshalls, like most of London's population, knew the 1884 International Health Exhibition) she would have nothing to do with the new-fangled Jaeger 'underthings'. 'They are well enough for men, but the workhouse colour is a great objection in my eyes.' And when in 1883 the three Marshall ladies and Marshall himself went to view the Rational Clothes Exhibition at the Princes Hall, she found two or three of the costumes, those of normal cut, quite charming but was scathing about most of the other exhibits, 'a selection of "divided skirts" (clumsy, with kilts & polonaise) and every atrocity up to regular trowsers & blouse, wh. are sacred to America, I believe. Some of the creatures looked neither male nor female.' Faced with these androgynous outfits the Marshalls 'laughed much, & agreed to stick to the "undivided". Either the dress is downright indecent, or else ludicrous & hobbledehoyish, or else a

---

[3] Its author's real name was John Leighton. He was a friend of the entire Marshall family. Jeannette liked him for his wit and banter, but was not unduly astonished or upset when, years later, she read that 'Luke Limner', aged 65, had been arrested in Regent Street for wearing women's clothes. According to the newspaper report, the prisoner 'presented a grotesque appearance as he stood in the dock . . . He wore a blue serge skirt fringed with red, a black bodice which by its appearance suggested the presence of a corset and padding underneath, a fashionable light coloured cape with a Medici collar, . . . and a pair of large high-heeled shoes.' His head was bald and he carried a dark green matador's hat 'trimmed with yellow ribband and decorated with three large black and yellow balls, and a streamer half a yard long. This head gear contrasted singularly with the prisoner's bristly grey moustache and gold-rimmed spectacles . . . In his defence the accused said he was an artist, and as he was about to write a book on ladies' attire he could not treat the subject properly without personal experience' (*The Times*, 27 June 1891). He was bound over on his own recognizances of £5 to be of good behaviour for three months.

half-hearted thing not half as presentable & no more convenient or comfortable than one's present costume.' Nor did they amend their view when some nine months later, three acquaintances, Mrs Buckton and her two daughters, on calling at No. 10 on a Monday afternoon 'at home' showed off their own version of 'divided undergarments': 'the spectacle of Miss B standing with her skirts round her waist, in little dark blue full trousers, with a small rudimentary petticoat behind, was enough to make a cat laugh. I don't think I could dress myself such a "Judy".'

What in the end added muscle to the frivolous coterie was the adventitious force exercised by the Roaring Girl, the tousled-haired, unkempt romp who used the preposterous slang of her adolescent brothers and shared their 'strong passions and even their coarse desires'.[4] This assertive young woman had been flitting in and out of Victorian essays and fiction for over a quarter of a century. Charlotte Brontë's pistol-wielding 'Captain' Shirley Keeldar was her elder (and more attractive) sister; in the mid-1850s she was the 'fast' girl; Captain Gronow complained in the early 1860s of her immodest bearing, bad language, her make-up and the ambition to be taken for a *demi-mondaine*; she was also an outrageous flirt. A few years later Mrs Lynn Linton reiterated all the opprobrium cast on the indecorous young thing by Gronow and added a few blemishes such as smoking, together with the label 'the Girl of the Period', in an article published by the *Saturday Review* on 14 March 1868. Unlike the American mid-century New Woman who regarded the wearing of masculine dress as a symbol of emancipation, both Gronow's and Linton's Girls gave almost excessive attention to their appearance; the 'disorderly dress' and 'occasionally dirty hands' of Justin MacCarthy's damsel must have developed in the 1870s.

Overtly Jeannette rejected fastness as much as earnestness when, on the verge of young womanhood, she looked around for models. She held no brief for ladies who powdered and rouged, was shocked when her maternal cousin Jessie Startin, eight months Jeannette's senior and eighteen at the time, smoked a cigar offered by her brother-in-law, and professed herself scandalized at the behaviour of the young and flighty Mrs Warren De la Rue, a Williams connection, who went rinking

---

[4] Justin MacCarthy, *A History of Our Own Times* (London, 1880), p. 553.

(roller-skating), in itself an unladylike form of exercise, without her husband.[5]

But for all her outraged utterances, she admitted to being a flirt. She also relished that other prerogative of the fast girls, slang. Idioms from across the Atlantic held a special attraction, as she was always gratified to be taken for an American. It was not just that American girls, those that could afford visits to Europe, patronized Paris couturiers, above all Worth,[6] and were noted for their dress-sense. It was also that their entire comportment was more go-ahead, more liberated, and made them more 'visible' than politely nurtured English girls. To occupy the centre of the stage, and yet not to be classed as brazen or giddy, required quite deft manœuvring.[7]

Jeannette's slang was probably reserved for the pages of the diary. It was innocuous enough to pass unnoticed except that she herself drew attention to off-beat expressions by apologizing whenever she made use of them. There were the Americanisms, ways of expressing greater

[5] Seven years later, in 1882, when the Warren De la Rues were about to divorce, Jeannette reported that Mrs De la Rue was living in disreputable Jermyn Street: 'who with?' she speculated. Five years after the divorce, the Marshall women met Warren with a 'lady of doubtful appearance'. 'He got very red, appeared not to see us, and turned down a side street very suddenly. I suppose it is not etiquette to recognize ladies—under those circumstances' ventured Jeannette.

The womens' periodical *Myra*, in July 1877, replying to a correspondent, declared that rinking, if no gentleman was in attendance, was 'highly improper and objectionable', and that in London no lady attended a public rink 'under any circumstances'.

[6] Zuzanna Shonfield, 'The Great Mr Worth', *Costume* (Journal of the Costume Society, London), xvi, 1982.

[7] A degree of unwomanly callousness was thought to result from modern methods of upbringing. 'We have made girls sensible and clear-headed till they have grown hard' were the words Charlotte Yonge put in the mouth of one of her characters. 'They have been taught to despise little fears and illusions, and it is certainly not becoming' (*The Trial*, London, 1864, xxiii). In France, the Goncourt brothers, writing two years after Yonge, described Renée Mauperin, a *jeune fille moderne*, as the product of 'the artistic and boyish education of the last thirty years' (Theodore Zeldin, *France 1848–1945: Ambition and Love*, Oxford, 1979, p. 352). In the United States, the transatlantic sister of the Girl of the Period, the American Girl, was said by an article in *The Nation* (8 April 1880, p. 215) to be the product of 'two of the things we prize most, personal independence, namely, and education . . . since our girls have begun to receive the same education as boys there has grown up in them an imperious desire for independence and the personal dignity it carries with it . . .' The author of the piece was altogether more favourable to this new manifestation than English writers on the subject; nevertheless he could not give the American Girl uncritical approval: 'Her claims altogether transcend her concessions . . . If she were in the least introspective—which, with all her self-consciousness, she is very far from being—she would perceive that she measures other people by a standard considerably higher than her own.'

vigour and enthusiasm than was usual in educated Victorian English: going full blast, having a lovely time and loving it, choking someone off and busting up. She used language she considered simply vulgar: slap-up swells stuffed their meals and jawed (instead of politely talking) and yawned their heads off, then went to pot and became hard up. Less apologetically she used the language of the 'fast' (or 'rapid'—her own euphemism) Girl of the Period; chocolate was lummy, pretty bonnets were angelic, angeliferous or even splendiferous, new acquaintances turned out to be quite 'the go' or rather 'bébé', or, if they told 'French' jokes, simply 'killing'; any crisis was dismissed as an 'awful muddle'. At times the different modes of speech overlapped, as when she summed up, in a curiously mixed sentence, a plan for a joint Swiss holiday with her uncle William Marshall: 'He seems to "cotton" to the idea, but I dare say at the last moment he will slip out of it unless P. "nails" him.'

All this was interspersed with a generous sprinkling of rather pictur-esque expressions for which she did not apologize, perhaps deriving from the provinces and strangely out of place in the diaries of a young lady living in Savile Row. When it rained it poured 'heavens hard' or 'like Wilkes' and gave her 'the dismals'. She then felt 'as yellow as a pagle' or as 'queer as Dick's hatband' or again 'as green as a quarter of soap after a week's washing', but before she got used to it, 'like eels to skinning', matters improved 'by degrees like lawyers go to heaven' and she was once again 'tol-lol', 'as brisk as a bottled gooseberry'. An offended aunt, 'in the tantrums' instead of 'on the broad grin', looked as if 'she could eat us up with a grain of salt'; it made her 'as loving as Ball's pigs who sucked each other's eyes out'. Rare occurrences were to be noted 'with a piece of blue chalk'; shops decked out for Christ-mas, for instance, looking 'as gay as a gardener's dog with a rose in each ear'. Impatient people 'whipped the cat about'; unexpected guests, who turned up 'like a regular three days ague', were wished 'in Pepperland'.

Despite frequent whimsy—'drumsticks' for domestics is a startling example—the general effect is one of robustness. What she reported of the exchanges with men had, on her side, a rumbustious aggression which to the meek and self-conscious must have been quite daunting. Older, more experienced men were amused (and often clearly attracted) by her playful onslaughts, and for her part she found them better sparring partners than the boys of her own age. And she made quite sure that none of them, young or old, got an inkling of the short distance that separated her from strong-mindedness.

Underneath the levity there was a more sober core inherited from the Ely side of the family and nurtured, let it be said again, by the two or three serious women who taught her. In spirit, if not through much practical action (save an occasional donation), she inclined towards the women's rights movement; so did they all, at Savile Row. They cheered when in 1870 Elizabeth Garrett and Emily Davies were elected on to the London School Board and again when in 1873 their own Miss Chessar became School Board member for St Marylebone.[8] Inevitably, some of her father's professional contacts occasionally brought her to the periphery of the suffrage movement. In 1876 they became friendly with one of its acolytes, the middle-aged Miss Williams, 'a women's rights lady, but not an exaggerated variety of the species'. It was through Miss Williams's mediation that Ada and Jeannette, many years later in 1884 and '85, attended two suffrage balls at the Kensington Town Hall, pleasant if tame and, in Jeannette's reports, entirely non-propagandist occasions.

A franchise procession in July 1884 provoked the debunking which was her second nature; together with Uncle William Marshall she watched it from the vantage point of a first floor in Piccadilly, as it made its way up St James's Street:

A more untidy & straggling procession I never saw. The crowd of the spectators was the best part of it. Some of the men carried poles with blue ribbons, & a few banners & brushes whatever _that_ meant, while the bands played & the people sang 'For he's a jolly good fellow'. Even Uncle said he never saw such a lot of riff-raff. Sir John Bennett looking quite drunk, & Newman Hall were the only two _celebrities_ we saw. That was enough to stamp the whole thing.

For all her lack of enthusiasm about the political manifestations of the suffrage movement, she was a feminist by instinct and would on occasion stand up to be counted in support of the women's cause. In 1874, faced with an unenlightened relative, Aunt Yate, on a visit to the capital from Long Buckley where her husband was rector, she resorted to proselytizing: 'told Aunt many things à propos of the advance

---

[8] The School Boards were administrative bodies created by Forster's Elementary Education Act of 1870. As a result of Jacob Bright's 1869 legislation, members of the Boards were chosen by popular election by ratepayers, who included some women.

women have made the last few yrs. in education etc. If my beloved relative had been living in the depths of Central Africa, she cd. not have known less of what is going on.'

On occasion an obscurantist man would provide her with an exciting target. One such was a surgeon, a descendant of Sir Humphry Davy, whom she met at a medical dance in 1877:

clever in his way, but perfectly demented on the idea of women entering the profession. He said he was pleased to find anyone to defend the cause so well, as I stuck to my guns, & several times rather non-plussed him. His arguments were decidedly weak. Notwithstanding our difference of opinion he seemed glad enough to dance with me, begged me to stay longer, and saw me to the carriage. I cd. not pretend to agree with him, though he was quite 15 years my senior. I thought it my duty to open his mind a little.

When the Women's Disability Bill was defeated in April 1875 she wrote, forgetting for once that she regarded herself as a conservative: 'the Bill was agn. thrown out but only by a majority of 35, wh. shows it is coming slowly but surely, notwithstanding all those narrow-minded men can do! "Public Opinion" gives a most disgusting article fr. the "Morning Post", written by one of those horrid old Tories I'd lay any money. They'll have to change their tune . . .' She applauded when Morley, in his lectures on contemporary fiction, revealed his intense admiration for Charlotte Brontë, Mrs Gaskell, and above all George Eliot, 'whom he spoke of as Mrs Lewis, so I suppose she is married now' commented Jeannette hopefully. And she enlarged on her own approval of Morley's views: 'I will say this for him: he is one of the men who recognize the fact that women are not all fools; such men are few & far between, so I feel grateful to poor little Morley.'

Given the degree of her self-esteem, it was inevitable that her most consistently pursued goals had to do with improving her status as a young woman of parts. This she did by concentrating on activities at which she knew she would not fail. Though intellectual education (in the guise of the University College lectures) had come to an end, she diligently continued with her musical studies under Edward Dann-reuther which had started in 1874. At its onset, the project to substitute a musician of European renown for the familiar Miss Ward who had taught her the piano for nearly as long as Jeannette could remember, made her very apprehensive. To be tested by such a critic was as petrifying as the thought of university examinations. But though Dannreuther found fault with the flat way she struck the keys and the fingering Miss Ward had taught her, he was flattering and encouraging about her talent. His charges, high by the standard of the day even for an outstanding teacher, were a guinea for a lesson in one's own home and 15s. for a generous hour's tuition in the music room of his house at 12 Orme Square, Bayswater. The Marshalls, always careful about getting good value for their money, preferred the cheaper formula. So on Friday afternoons, at first weekly and later fortnightly (in series of six lessons), Jeannette played her pieces on the very same Broadwood on which Wagner, a friend of Dannreuther's, would practise during his London visit. It was good to hear that the maestro considered her as both industrious and gifted. 'She is a very interesting pupil' he told Ellen who almost invariably chaperoned her daughter at Orme Square, when the second series of lessons were about to end in the spring of 1877. 'I like her!' Jeannette reciprocated the partiality and found his quaint English and his sense of humour to her taste. 'Mr. D. quite improves on acquaintance' she noted midway through the 1876 course of lessons. Eventually, in 1878, the lessons stopped, much as the university courses had been discontinued in 1876, without any explicit decision being recorded. Perhaps she became discouraged: for a while there had been less enthusiasm about the tuition, and she cancelled the last lesson of the series on the plea that her summer holiday had left her 'awfully out of practice'. Nevertheless, she was glad to have had the advantage of first-rate tuition and boasted after playing to the Misses Gray, cousins by marriage on the Williams side: 'I went up 100 per cent in their estimation when they heard Mr. Dannreuther was my master. A good card to play!'·

Another way in which the sober side of Jeannette manifested itself was through the catholicity of her reading matter, an eclectic mix borrowed from Mudie's, in most years at the rate of a volume a week. Little of what she read was particularly mind-stretching, though Carlyle, Darwin and Taine made an occasional appearance. English titles predominated, but French and German books, nicely balanced as to quantity, accounted for up to one half of her reading. The novelists she chose were by and large the obvious, fashionable ones, from Dickens, Thackeray and Wilkie Collins to the Kingsleys, Hardy, Miss Braddon, Ouida and Mrs Humphry Ward. Even before Morley had applauded them, the Brontës and George Eliot were among her favourites, but she did not read much Jane Austen, and Trollope was represented only by *The American Senator*. In twenty-five years she never touched a single novel of the eighteenth century. Of the American novelists, she read Mark Twain and Howells; among the French, Mme de Staël, Dumas and Hugo were at the top of the list, although she also read a good many less obvious ones such as Erckmann-Chatrian, Edmond About and Pierre Loti. The Germans she favoured were the now largely forgotten E. Marlitt, Georg Ebers, Gustav Freytag and Berthold Auerbach.

Her parents made little attempt at censoring what she chose to read. She was nineteen when Marshall lent her Pushkin's *The Captain's Daughter*, bound up, she noted, with Hawthorne's *Scarlet Letter*, 'wh. I am supposed not to read'. Disregarding the veto she read it and listed it baldly in her 1874 reading list. The lack of intervention allowed her to lay her hands on works of one or two authors usually considered as unsuitable for unmarried young ladies, such as Ouida and Paul de Kock. Her own prudishness intervened after she had read de Kock's *Sœur Anne* so that she listed him in the diary by his initials alone. No impropriety could have been associated with Sacher-Masoch, for his name appeared in full when, admittedly at over thirty, she came to read *Der Judenrafael*. A few of her choices showed her to be experimenting with the new and not then widely known: she read Henry James's *Washington Square* in 1881 and his *Portrait of a Lady* in 1882, both within a few months of publication. She came to Kipling's *The Light that Failed* in 1891, E. F. Benson's *Dodo* and Gissing's *The Odd Women* in 1893, and *The Time Machine* by H. G. Wells in 1895—all four in the year of their publication. The 'aesthetic' trend was represented by several of William Morris's utopias, a number of titles by Vernon Lee, the newly published *Prudence, A Story of Aesthetic London*, by Lucy C. Lillie, and Ethel Coxon's *A Basil Plant*, both in 1882, and the *Yellow Book* in 1894.

Superimposed on the literary sampling were a few attempts to impose a rather more rigorous pattern on her reading. Like the true obsessional that she was, she would for many months on end without any warning concentrate on one author or one genre. In adolescence, she worked through all the dramatic works of Corneille and Racine, and also through Molière's comedies, and hardly a year passed without some Shakespeare being included. The year 1887 and the early part of 1888 were devoted to Russian fiction, when, in addition to *War and Peace*, which she knew as 'Peace and War', and *Anna Karenina*, she tackled a great deal of Dostoevsky and Turgenev (often in German). In 1889 nine novels of Walter Scott's appeared on the list. This was also the time when she developed a taste for Scandinavian authors and read them avidly for two or three years. It was as if at last she had discovered the key to structured self-education which had eluded her in her twenties, and was once again hovering on the brink of strong-mindedness.

CHAPTER 7

PAPERING OVER THE CRACKS

IN some respects Ellen Marshall had never entirely outgrown the North London of her early years. Familiar shops in the Holloway Road neighbourhood retained her allegiance, possibly because better bargains were to be had there than in the West End. Each Thursday, back on the Williams home ground, its limits set by the landmarks of the Red Cap and the Brecknock, the Nag's Head, the Cock and the Britannia (which also marked the omnibus terminals), the girls with or without their mother or Aunt Eliza made the round of local tradesmen. They bought braid or filoselle from Allice's, the mercers, and footwear from an unnamed shoe shop in the Holloway Road. In season, they ordered pelargonium and pots of mignonette from Parmenter's, the nursery opposite the Brecknock. They called at Mr Watkins, their accredited photographer, in his home at Torriano Avenue. At their regular sweet shop they spent their pocket money on jumbles, coconut-ice and ginger-beer, or refreshed themselves at Beale's, the bakers; no other buns tasted as good as the Holloway ones. Jones Brothers, the large drapers, as yet independent of the retail chain which eventually engulfed it, was another objective. And at intervals they excursed eastwards on the 'tremendous long walk' to Church Row, Islington, where Mrs Ford ran a Servants' Registry Office, to state their requirements for cook or housemaid, and to complain about those supplied on earlier occasions.

Jeannette and Ada had spent one or two days a week at Talbot House ever since they remembered, and also Christmas and Easter holidays. To children, the scale of the Holloway existence must have been reassuring. The house was spacious and, though semi-detached, bore some resemblance to a country villa, with a drive and a circular flower-bed on the street side. There were fruit-trees and currant-bushes in the long back garden, and an arbour large enough to shelter the tribe of Williams grandchildren. Beyond the walls of Talbot House were quiet, safe streets. The traffic was still so thin in Holloway that Jeannette from the age of four or five had been encouraged to act as guide to her blind Aunt Eliza, 'leading her across the roads with the greatest sang-froid'.

As the girls grew older, they found the familiarity and informality burdensome, the food appalling and their grandmother's callers—mainly elderly neighbours and impoverished dependants, with the doctor as sole male—home-spun and exceedingly boring. There were also other snags about visiting Talbot House, connected with the old lady's character. Elizabeth Williams, who had never been an easy person, in her old age remained true to type: unmellowed by marriage and motherhood, she continued to act the spoilt heiress, with no consideration for others and a brand of verbal aggression which at times made her seem positively evil. She suffered from that particular form of deterioration which emphasizes the invalid's negative qualities: 'G'ma goes at it "hammer and tongs" ', 'G'ma highly waxy', 'not open to reason', 'sharper and sharper, bless her!'—Jeannette was unremittingly realistic about Grandmother Williams, though in recognition of the inevitability of decline, her comments were good-humoured and indulgent.

There was doubtless an element of *Schadenfreude* in the granddaughter's indulgence. She happened to be a favourite at Talbot House, and Ellen, who at Savile Row sometimes displayed the unpleasant temperament inherited from her mother, here often felt the sharp edge of the old lady's tongue. But the real victim was Aunt Eliza, ageing, single, guileless, and, because of her blindness, entirely at her mother's mercy. Jeannette was fonder of this aunt than any other relative outside the immediate family circle. And the widespread sympathy for Eliza was one of the reasons why, when in the autumn of 1876 Grandmother Williams succumbed to the progressive ravages of heart disease and sclerosis (and possibly also of cancer), no one was particularly sorry to see her die.

In her mid-seventies, a series of falls and 'attacks'—perhaps minor brain haemorrhages—had reduced her to a state of permanent invalidism. A few months before her death another problem arose. 'The fact is that she has got into the way of taking too much brandy with her champagne & that makes her so cross that there is no bearing her. She really is not responsible at all.' Eventually the drinking was controlled, but her condition continued to give rise to constant anxiety. Throughout the first half of October bulletins were recorded daily. A fortnight before Grandmother's death, Ellen and her daughters confronted the problem of their winter wardrobes: 'The fact is that we are afraid to buy anything colored, as we fear we shall have to go into mourning before long. It seems dreadful to think of these things beforehand, but at the same time it is no use buying a lot of dresses wh. one can't wear.'

Jeannette took to writing of her grandmother as if she were already in her grave: 'though peculiar, she was always very kind & fond of me' was the entry for 19 October. A day later, on the 20th, came a telegram. Ellen Marshall who opened it 'came back into the drawingroom as pale as a sheet'; she handed the telegram to Jeannette with the words 'she's gone!' 'On the paper I saw "Moritura est Mrs Williams".' After she had told her father who was attending to a patient, Jeannette sat down at her desk and 'wrote to Lewis & Mrs. Hardie for mourning as one must order those things directly.'

In the carriage in which he accompanied his wife and Jeannette to Holloway, Marshall suddenly realized that the telegram had been misinterpreted. 'Why,' he exclaimed, ' "moritura" means dying or about to die, not dead!' At Talbot House they found the blinds up, and by the next day the patient was conscious, comfortable, free from pain and had taken a great deal of wine and beef tea. 'Really it seems like a resurrection!'

Meanwhile the fabrics for the mourning dresses had been delivered. 'We chose a dress of Barathea for M., 2 of french twill for A & me, as they were there. It seems dreadful but we cd. not send them back' wrote Jeannette, down-to-earth as usual. The old lady died four days after the misleading telegram, on 24 October. As once before, after Reggie's death, Jeannette, though not present during her grandmother's last hours, recorded the sequence of events with the detachment of a trained nurse: 'her breathing got higher & higher, and with 3 faint moans (like a child dropping to sleep) she was gone.' Again, as after Reggie's death, she did not attend the funeral, but wrote about it with a mix of practical detail, shrewd comment and pious sentiment. 'Poor Grma is buried in the family vault at the Chapel of Ease, Islington. She is the 8th person laid there . . .' There followed an enumeration of the others buried in the sarcophagus of the proud soap manufacturer, great-grandfather John Williams, and she continued: 'The funeral was <u>without</u> mourning coaches, scarves or hatbands . . . every one going in their own carriage. In order that people shd. not think it was meanness that prompted them doing so, they had four horses to the hearse, and a very handsome polished oak coffin. It is so horrible, the idea of saving every penny of what one's relations have left . . .' The Marshalls' coachman, too, appears to have been concerned to keep up appearances; 'as a mark of respect' he put a mourning band around his hat, and wore black buttons and gloves.

Jeannette's 'best' mourning clothes were not delivered until ten days after the funeral. And it is within the bounds of the literal interpretation of 1870s etiquette that she and Ada stayed away from the funeral because it would not have done to wear their everyday mourning on such a solemn occasion; a dark-grey tweed bought earlier in the month before the bereavement was just not formal and black enough to pass muster. John, whose first term at Cambridge had begun a few days earlier, was another absentee. However, this time, unlike in 1873, Ellen Marshall attended the funeral, supported only by her husband. Tears were shed before and at the funeral, they talked 'a great deal about poor gr'ma', and Jeannette, for one, reflected about the relief of an easy death and the mystery of the hereafter: 'May the solution of the enigma be a happy one! Amen.'

Though not grieved over, the old lady was sufficient of a character not to be easily forgotten. When many years later Jeannette wrote in her Commonplace Book that in her old age Elizabeth Williams had been 'very tyrannical & disagreeable', and 'desperately unkind' to Eliza who had been 'absolutely martyrised' by her mother, this harsh re-evaluation was clearly tinged by the bitterness she felt, in adulthood, towards her own mother. But in the months which followed the death, Jeannette often referred to happier memories of her grandmother's partiality—'I was her favourite'—and the many gifts which resulted from it.

Moreover a degree of havoc in the Williams family was sufficient to keep the old lady's memory green. The customary ambiguities of Victorian family trusts which surfaced after her death led to a fracas between the Williams heirs and the Hall family, who were beneficiaries of an earlier will, that of Jeannette's Aunt Annie Williams, the widow of Uncle Charles. Jeannette reported the row with Dickensian relish:

before Aunt Annie died she made a will leaving all she died possessed of to her family [the Halls]. These terms seem (by an idiotic piece of legal foolery) to include any money wh. wd. have come to her later; thus handing over her expectations as well as her possessions to her family . . . evidently the lawyer (Aunt Annie's brother) made the will with full knowledge of what he was doing. Of course poor Gr'ma was very indignant that her father's money shd. go to utter strangers, but there was no help for it. Uncle Charles's share of her property amounting to £1,400 [c.£42,000 in modern terms] must go. Of course everything that cd. be secured, was. M. wrote to the Hs. very warmly & intercourse ceased fr. that time.

In the event, the Hall heirs acted with exemplary propriety, declining to profit from the loophole in Annie Williams's will. The only assertion of their moral right to Uncle Charles's share of the family trust released by Grandmother Williams' death was to stipulate that one-tenth of it should go to charity, 'that being one of the directions in Aunt Annie's will'.

Other tempests arising out of old Mrs Williams's testamentary dispositions (and out of the arrangements of Grandfather Williams for the division of the Williams wealth) rumbled on for a decade or longer. To begin with, Ellen Marshall questioned the size of the inheritance which her brothers had calculated to be her due; her own arithmetic had led her to expect an annual income of £400 (on a principal of some £8,000–£10,000, or over a quarter of a million pounds in terms of today's values), twice the amount allocated to her. Oil was poured on the fire of her suspicions when, at a family meeting held ten months after the old lady's funeral, 'Uncle W^m. handed round a paper for everyone to sign to say that they were satisfied, wh. looks "fishy"!' However, no more was heard of this particular problem after 1877. Instead a shadow of misgiving about the way the trust monies were invested descended on the diaries: 'Uncle [William Williams] told M. that her money is in Uncle Edwin's and John's business, wh. piece of news she did not receive with unalloyed pleasure. Of course both M's, AE's & A.S's money will be taken out and invested by Uncle W. (who is the Trustee) but if in the interval (wh. Heaven forbid!) the business "goes to pot" (elegantly speaking), where are their little fortunes?' Eventually Ellen's share was safely settled in bonds and investment property (in Lordship Road, Stoke Newington). But Jeannette, whose own savings remained in the Williams coffers, established a habit of watching and commenting on her uncles' financial affairs.

After the death of Reggie, Mrs Marshall had worn strict mourning for over two years. To put on bright colours when a member of the close family was still in deepest black was considered ill-bred, so out of courtesy to their mother (though no doubt also out of thrift) Jeannette and Ada had worn their mourning dresses until well after the first anniversary of their brother's death. 'Much longer than is usual I believe, but I feel as if I never cared to put on colors agn' commented

Jeannette. The pattern was repeated after the death of Elizabeth Williams, with Ellen in black for eighteen months, and the granddaughters for almost as long, although they could have cast off all sombre apparel after nine or at most twelve months.

Rebellion was in the air: the year 1875 saw the formation of the National Mourning and Funeral Reform Association, in articulate protest against the rigours and extravagance of fashionable mourning etiquette. But the Marshall women were not iconoclasts; they studied the edicts of fashion journals and then steered a deft course between complete disregard and inflexible observance of the rules. Common sense held sway. Crape was what etiquette ordained for deep mourning, but crape was impractical, unsuited for travel or exposure to rain. So only one crape-trimmed costume, their 'best', would be ordered and as soon as fashion declared crape to be no longer an essential adjunct of grief they were glad to dispense with it. For everyday Jeannette and Ada made do with retrimmed old black outfits or put on plain sober-coloured dresses of homespun, tweed or some washable fabric such as écru holland. Jeannette wrote of one such costume: 'Of course I shd. not be <u>visible</u> in it, but it will save my other.' Wearing black was in any case lowering to the spirit. On the occasion of a later bereavement, in 1883, she wrote of herself and Ada: 'we looked like animated ink blots, the effect of new black being particularly striking.' A year later, after yet another death in the family, she trimmed her travelling hat with grey gauze and a positively frivolous little tuft of crimson feathers, asserting: 'Really one can't travel quite like a crow, abroad.' If challenged she would have argued that some fashion commentators regarded crimson ornaments as suitable for complimentary mourning, and that complimentary mourning was adequate after the death of a scarcely known uncle.

One of the side-effects of being in mourning was that they had, that winter of 1876–7, time on their hands. With social activity curtailed, the time-consuming business of devising outfits and dolling up for evening occasions was sufficiently reduced to allow them to divert their attention to home improvements. The few bits and pieces, principally of china, inherited from Talbot House, had to be fitted in. In any case the mid-Victorian furniture and décor of No. 10, dating back to 1854, when Ellen and John first moved in, needed refurbishing and updating. That goods of nineteenth-century manufacture lasted a lifetime is a figment of modern nostalgia. Then, as now, chairs occasionally

needed respringing; even the best quality soft furnishings and upholstery eventually had to be replaced. So Mrs Marshall and her
daughters set out, on a modest budget, and with the usual 'Marshallic'
contriving, on a programme of modernization in line with the latest
aesthetic precepts.

Jeannette's earliest experience of aesthetic décor was confined to a
few *outré* examples and her devotion to high-art was not a matter of
love at first sight. When at sixteen she had been invited to lunch at the
Clapham villa belonging to Greek patients of her father's, the Spartalis, where the floors were covered with matting and the furniture
stained light blue and dark green, she described the effect grudgingly
as 'very <u>artistic</u> but pretty'. In 1874 she derided the 'peculiar' home of
the Ford Madox Browns: 'The drawing room (I suppose) is carpeted
with cocoa-nut matting, like our kitchen, with common gas burners, &
the most extraordinary pictures on the walls; cane-bottomed chairs & a
kind of divan in the centre, wh. I dignified by the name of the
"woolsack".'

'I don't altogether admire her drawing room' she wrote three weeks
later, after calling on an acquaintance of her mother's. 'The walls are
too cold a color, & I don't like either the stained floor, the mixed
furniture or the peacock feathers.' This was the last display of resistance. By the mid-1870s she had become a devotee of 'artistic' decor
and enthused about the 'most tastefully furnished' country home their
old friends, the Spartalis, had acquired on the Isle of Wight: 'the most
exquisite artistic papers (designed by Walter Crane) that ever I set eyes
on. All the doors are blk. & gold, the mantel pieces the most lovely
marbles, and the fire-places enlaid with Minton's tiles. Windows over
the fire-places, & the bed-room furniture Japanese in blk. & gold.'

Lavish interiors such as the 'Japanese' rooms designed by Thomas
Jeckyll for Aleco Ionides or Frederick Leyland were beyond the
Marshalls' means, but many aesthetic effects had the merit of being
inexpensive. The Marshalls' approach was similar to that which gov-
erned their interpretation of fashion in apparel. Rather than pay hard
cash for professional help, they went in for what could be achieved
with their own talent and application. In a rush of do-it-yourself zeal,
mother and daughters re-upholstered chairs and sofas, and then
protected their fresh glory with loose covers of Liberty chintz or
cretonne in cheerful floral patterns. Ada and Mrs Marshall performed
wonders with paint-brush and varnish pot. Later, at the height of the
aesthetic craze in the 1880s, Ada would be delegated to embellish the

tall drawing-room shutters and improve on the shade of the staircase dado when the greeny-blue of the professional decorators was found wanting. But for the moment such major tasks were left alone. Instead, they stripped and grained the floorboards and converted suitably frail tables, sets of shelves and corner brackets into modish gems by coats of blackest japan varnish adorned with gilt fillets.[1] Jeannette's special contribution consisted of divers art embroideries. From the fairly conventional tickwork of her mid-teens, running and darning stitches on striped canvas alternating with appliqué ribbons and braids, she graduated to complicated, very individual designs. She covered all sorts of dark or neutral, firmly woven, cloths (originally intended for prosaic domestic use as towels, dusters or stair runners) in intricate all-over geometric mosaics, worked in filoselle silk and bright wool yarns. Her needlework adorned every horizontal surface and hung from thin brass rails on either side of every fireplace; as antimacassars, it protected the backs of newly upholstered easy chairs. She called the designs 'oriental' and reported with pride the admiring comments of family and friends as each new piece went on display.

The third drawing-room (first-floor back, recently promoted from schoolroom) now boasted a paper in a 'wonderful kind of Morris pattern, with pale greens, yellows, mauves etc, & little gold lines'. 'Sweet!' was Jeannette's verdict. Even the relatively new drawing-room floor-covering had to be brought into line with new fashions. In 1872 she had thought the new fitted green carpet, its yellow trellis enclosing roses and buds, 'very pretty'. But in aesthetic interiors wall-to-wall carpets and all-over designs in garish colours were anathema, so Persian and Indian rugs (usually from Shoolbred's, for Liberty's were pricey) now lay on matting or stained boards. Eventually the new look of the floors would be emphasized by the removal of the typically mid-Victorian circular table from the centre of the room and by a much less formal, scattered arrangement of furniture.

The only completely new piece of furniture, the indispensable bentwood rocking-chair, belonged to the dining-room. Upstairs, the aesthetic effect was enhanced by numerous displays of small blue and white 'oriental' china. A 'beautiful piece of Japanese embroidery on

[1] As always, they were enthusiasts rather than pioneers. Paint-pot mania was in the air, encouraged by women's journals and popular books on interior decoration such as Lucy Orrinsmith's *The Drawing Room, Its Decoration and Furniture* (London, 1878), which recommended that young ladies take to staining and polishing, rather than 'dabble with watercolours'. See Isabelle Anscombe, *A Woman's Touch, Women in Design from 1860 to the Present Day* (London, 1984), p. 28.

fine blk. cloth' was made into a screen, in a black bamboo frame streaked with gold, and took pride of place in the main drawing-room. It came from Whiteley's, which competed with the newly opened Eastern Bazaar of Liberty's in supplying Oriental handicrafts. Even the summer garb of the drawing-room grates underwent an artistic transformation; the 'long & melancholy tresses of shavings as if an old person had been combing her head over them' were replaced by more wood shavings, but this time 'dotted with green leaves in a very eccentric manner. P. calls it Leightonesque.'

Innate caution would make the Marshalls stretch the process of refurbishing over a decade or more, but by 1877 the entire drawing-room floor was already considerably lighter, more up-to-date and altogether closer to that high-art look which was the object of their endeavours. The total effect was pleasing and they felt they wanted to show it off. To do this, they decided, required hospitality on an unprecedented scale. In June 1877 they gave a ball, an affair at which some fifty-five or sixty guests, mainly family and close friends, danced quadrilles and waltzes to the sounds of a piano, cornet and harp trio (the harp 'by P's wish'), and feasted on 'first-rate' refreshments 'including green gooseberry ice by P's special order'. Hired wax-candle chandeliers (for which special hooks were provided in Victorian reception rooms, where no permanent central fittings existed) and banks of house plants, also on hire from the nurseryman, added to the festive aspect of the drawing-room floor. Jeannette, still in half-mourning for her grandmother, pale mauve muslin with black ribbons and pearls, thought the *tout ensemble* a 'capital size' and 'extremely pretty'; she christened the new third drawing-room 'Paradiso', and was delighted when 'all the artistic people went into fits' over its Morris-style wallpaper.

The following year there were, in fact, many more genuine 'artistics' among the 125 guests who attended the Marshalls' Soirée Musicale. For this elaborate occasion, they engaged seven professional musicians, large mirrors and fifty 'nice little chairs' and a profusion of rout-seats were hired in addition to flowers and chandelier, and a 'grand' from Pleyel's. The programme, largely vocal but with some solo violin numbers and a piano duet, ranged widely from Mozart and Handel through well-loved contemporaries such as Verdi and Meyerbeer to compositions by Signor Catalani, an acquaintance. Ices were served in the interval and an 'excellent supper' at 1 a.m. (the Marshalls had providentially partaken of a 'heavy tea' in the parents' bedroom while the house was being made ready). Among the visitors there were many who had never been to the house before and would never come again, except perhaps to consult Marshall professionally: the Alma-Tademas, the Holman Hunts, and two Jones's, who may have been Edward and Georgiana Burne-Jones. With some lesser lights, the Thornycrofts, Graily Hewitts, Spartalis, William Rossettis and the Rossettis' brother-in-law, Dr Hueffer, the artistic coterie was large enough to dominate family and medical friends, and make the evening into a truly fashionable occasion. Even the exotic was not missing: 'Mrs Dadebhoy Baramgee created a great sensation by coming in a most blazing green Indian dress, trimmed round with a gold band set with diamonds! Everyone asked who she was, some thinking she was a princess.'[2]

Both ball and soirée were attempts by the Marshalls to penetrate into the fashionable aesthetic circles and to integrate artistic with medico-scientific friends. The one obvious absentee, Ford Madox Brown, was in Manchester at the time, painting frescoes at the Town Hall: had he attended the 1878 occasion he could, with some justice, have cast back Marshall's remark, made in an 1874 letter, about the Browns being 'indefatigable' hosts. At the time the quip (if quip it was—it may have been intended as a compliment) caused great offence to the thin-skinned painter. He responded with a 'shamefully rude . . . most insulting letter saying that they [the Browns] never trouble themselves about who comes, or who stays away fr. their evenings . . .' This was the first in an exchange of letters, two shots being fired by each of the contenders, which over a few days threatened to put an end to a friendship of nearly thirty years' duration. Then Brown 'came down a little fr. the high ropes' and Marshall decided to 'smoke the pipe of peace' with his old friend.[3]

The propensity of quite serious Victorians to take umbrage at relatively unimportant slights often expressed itself in such time-consuming correspondence; pen and ink perpetuated aggressive or careless comments which would soon have faded from memory if uttered face to face or over the telephone. The Marshalls were adept at

[2] The diarist's version of the name may hide that of a relative (possibly mother) of Maneckji Byramji Dadabhoy (1865–1953), the Parsee lawyer knighted in 1921 for services in India. Four days after the musical soirée Jeannette noted that the border on the Indian guest's sari was 'of filagree gold, & at intervals of about 4 inches, there was a large diamond!' It was estimated to have cost some £8,000–£10,000.

[3] For the heterogeneous company frequenting the Browns, see Oswald Doughty, *A Victorian Romantic—Dante Gabriel Rossetti* (Oxford, 1960), pp. 334–5.

such sparring by letter, usually against adversaries in the wider family circle. A potentially deadly duel between Ellen and her sister-in-law Julia Marshall was contained only because the 'seconds', John Marshall and his brother William, had much to lose from the protracted rowing of their womenfolk. Marshall himself took offence when at a Williams wedding breakfast he had been 'stuck at the very bottom of the table among mere boys & girls'; this time Ellen's 'plain, but very temperate and polite letter' of expostulation was countered by an 'unsatisfactory letter fr. Mrs. John Williams, in wh. she neither explains nor apologizes, excepting in a half-hearted fashion', and relations with this in-law never completely recovered.

This contretemps paled in comparison with the family quarrel which lasted from early in the 1870s until the end of the 1880s, and of which an early salvo was heard when Mrs William Williams chose to write, when condoling after Reggie's death, a 'most cold-blooded epistle' which thoroughly 'roused' Ellen's 'monkey'. Although a failure of the girls to pay the customary courtesy call after a small ball at their aunt's had been at the origin of the conflict, Jeannette thought it 'really very mean & paltry of them, keeping up that rubbish about calling at a time of such grief & trouble.' For three years Ellen with her daughters expended considerable effort avoiding encounters with 'the enemy' as Aunt Mary Williams became known at Savile Row. The tittle-tattle about the quarrel by fast-circulating maiden cousins and the ever-gossiping Aunt Eliza did not help matters. However in 1876 hostilities were suspended when after the death of Grandmother Williams the warring factions met unavoidably at Talbot House:

A knock came at the door as we were ready to depart, & Sarah announced 'Mrs. William!'. Auntie Eliza rushed out, but it appears the old creature intended to come in, & in she stepped! It was an agonizing moment. We had already said goodbye to Uncle William Williams, who was evidently in the greatest consternation, so had only to make our escape. Young Mary entered first, then her Ma. M. shook hands with both (out of deference to Uncle's feelings) with the iciest 'How de do'. I did likewise. Aunt Mary stood petrified, & did not seem to see anything; I saw her hand hanging flabbily, shook it and made my exit.

Soon relations returned to their previous icy mode. In 1882 when they heard that Aunt Mary was suffering from cancer, Jeannette wrote: 'I am so sorry for them, the more so as we cannot show them any kindness.' Her mother was adamant about remaining in dudgeon and Jeannette did not at this stage feel free to dissociate herself from

Ellen's intransigence. Nor could she do more than express pious regrets two years later when Aunt Mary died: 'I am extremely sorry for them all, tho' I have not seen her for 8 years, so cannot grieve personally. In addition to a wreath of white flowers, I sent a note to Mary with a line expressing A's & my sorrow for them. That is all we can do, the uncomfortable relations considered. M. wrote a note to Uncle, & sent a cross of white flowers.' Eventually she became less tolerant of her mother's obdurate stance. 'I believe short-sighted people are short-sighted in their minds as well' she wrote in 1888. Later that year she reported with approval—'wonders will never cease'—an amiable visit from Uncle William Williams. After having raged for over fifteen years, this particular storm had blown itself out.

Ellen Marshall was in fact not only stiff-necked in her quarrelling, but accident-prone and petulant in the relations which led up to conflict. She went into the fray with a volley of invective and, when the counter-attack proved dangerous, expected her husband to extend his protective umbrella over her head. Such a situation arose when, soon after old Mrs Williams's death in the autumn of 1876, she was called to account for an alleged affront by an Elyite, who had recently married and was now living in London:

a letter at breakfast-time . . . considerably electrified us all. It was fr. Mrs Eyre Thompson, whom it appears we were guilty of passing (or as she thinks "cutting") in the [Westbourne] Grove on Friday. She enquires if it was intentional, reproaches M. for not calling, as good as tells her she ought to have asked the pair of Eyres, & winds up by asking how it is that she has forfeited her claim to being M's old friend. A most intemperate effusion altogether.

Mrs Eyre-Thompson was known to be thin-skinned and relations with her had for many years been less than cordial. When the newly wedded Eyre-Thompsons had called at No. 10 on their return from their honeymoon, the Marshalls received them without enthusiasm: 'Mrs. (got up regardless of expense) gave herself such airs & graces, & putting on such a patronizing way that M. gave her a little snub.' A return call on the Eyre-Thompsons in Notting Hill confirmed that affectation and airs were on the increase.

Nevertheless, social niceties (of a lukewarm variety) were maintained and in due course, the Marshall ladies inspected Cherbury, the young couple's infant son. Jeannette wrote of Mrs Eyre-Thompson being 'distressingly affectionate' and of her pressing invitation to call on her. This was not taken up and a year later came Mrs Eyre-Thompson's resentful missive. Mrs Marshall's return shot was a 'stinger': 'she begins by showing her that <u>she</u> passed us, & not <u>we</u> her, as we neither of us saw her, repudiates the idea of old friendship (wh. is nonsense, M. only having <u>met</u> her 12 times in <u>all</u>) & gives her to understand, in a ladylike way, that she has taken a great liberty in writing in that fashion. Serves her right.' When they did not hear from Mrs Eyre-Thompson by return of post, the Marshalls thought her 'utterly squashed'. Jeannette commented: 'in <u>her</u> place I shd. have replied somehow or other. <u>Any</u> answer is better than none at all!' But when the reply, 'the result of nearly 4 days meditation', eventually reached Mrs Marshall it was 'most insulting in tone, & very inconsequential': 'She . . . tackles the "<u>old friend</u>" point, & says that in a former letter M. excuses herself on that ground for offering advice "wh. fr. a slight acquaintance wd. have been an impertinence". Then she says that if M. said this without meaning it she was "guilty of an insincerity" of wh. Mrs. T. wd. "be sorry to believe her capable".'

At this point, perhaps to mark that Mrs Marshall considered the whole thing 'low' and would not sully her hands with further exchanges, she brought out the big gun, Marshall himself. He returned Mrs Eyre-Thompson's second letter, adding a note for himself: 'he quite refutes both her charges, & tells her that she herself asked for that advice, wh. she now calls impertinent. It was capitally put, & will quite stagger Mrs. T., we flatter ourselves. She always imagined herself a great favorite of P's, but she is now undeceived.'

The enemy side also responded with heavier ammunition, in the shape of a letter addressed to Marshall from Mr Eyre-Thompson. Jeannette, for one, was unimpressed: 'It is very weak, as might be expected, considering who wrote it; he repeats all about the not calling & the "old friend", & says Mrs. T. did not know <u>I</u> was near-sighted too (wh. is as much as to say, <u>I</u> am a liar in saying I did not see her) & takes us to task all round. He encloses the whole correspondence for P. to read over carefully etc. I never knew such impudence! One thing is that he probably cd. not help himself, being, no doubt, ruled with a rod of iron by Mrs. T.'

Marshall then treated Mr Eyre-Thompson to a letter which was intended to be, and which in the event proved final: 'He goes over all the charges, those of untruthfulness, insincerity & impertinence, lets them know that <u>they</u> worried P. to go when he did not wish, says agn. that we did <u>not</u> see Mrs. T., but if she had accosted us, we shd. have

received her as usual, in short quite does for them on all points, &
finishes by saying that he "requests that all correspondence &
acquaintance cease fr. this time."—He returns his own first and M's
letter wh. Mr E. had sent back, with the remark that it was unnecessary
to have sent them, as P. had already read them. P. was writing & we
[were] talking about what he shd. say till 12 o'clock.'

After this last salvo the Eyre-Thompsons ceased to exist in Jeannette's reports of the Marshalls' life in London. Ely was a different
matter. Though Uncle William considered Mr Eyre-Thompson's
impudence excessive and tried to correct it with a 'considerable snub',
he and his wife continued to 'know' the family. Eventually the inevitable happened. At a musical evening at the Archers Jeannette found
herself in the presence of the enemy: 'I drank my tea side by side with
Mrs E. Thompson, of whose existence, except as a perfect stranger, I
seemed to be totally unaware.—I moved my train out of her way,
without moving a muscle of my countenance.'

Snubbing people was an accomplishment which was proving very
useful.

CHAPTER 8

THE BROWN MOOD

JEANNETTE was not above an occasional skirmish of her own, and inclined to stand on her dignity just as much as her parents. At the age of twenty-three, in a fit of pique about 'most disagreeable remarks' emanating from the Edwin Williams household, she and Ada took their revenge by arriving after midnight at a soirée of Aunt Bessie's. They ate an ice, danced a couple of waltzes and, refusing supper, ostentatiously departed within the half-hour. As their uncle saw them off with a grim ' "Goodbye, I shan't <u>thank</u> you!" ', Jeannette 'at once turned round & rejoined, with a small bow: ' "Well, then, <u>I</u> shall thank y<u>ou</u>, Uncle", & departed.' This bit of saucy repartee, as well as the initial snub, met with approval at No. 10, where the Craven Hill Gardens set was never very popular; it led to some recriminations on the part of Aunt Bessie and her daughters, but to no breach of relations.

For full-scale affrays she would have to wait till much later. Meanwhile, she was learning to bear with attacks on her self-esteem from an unexpected quarter. After some hesitation, because initially the matter appeared so trivial, she noted in the spring of 1877 a 'strange phenomenon' which had been going on for some days: 'opposite us is Poole's counting-house, & the clerks etc. are visible fr. the drawing room, so I suppose we are ditto ditto to them. As soon as ever I sit down to play, some man over there gets up, comes to the window, and gazes for a quarter of an hour together. Sometimes he varies the entertainment by waving about a sheet of paper. What he means I don't know. Possibly he is demented. Of course I appear totally unaware of his manœuvres.'

The last sentence was naïve or not entirely candid. The man *vis-à-vis* would almost certainly have noticed that Jeannette, in turn, stared sufficiently to note his appearance: 'He is tall, rather thin, dark, with brown hair cut short, and reddish whiskers & moustache. Neither ugly nor handsome.' She concluded that he was thirty-five to forty years old and that he appeared to be one of the senior clerks in the outfit.

Appreciative glances and signals addressed in the direction of the Marshalls' drawing-room windows continued throughout spring and summer; only Sundays brought respite. She expressed herself exasperated, but was no doubt also somewhat flattered and amused. With the hot weather, the Venetian blinds at the front of the house were let down, greatly to her relief, she wrote, 'as really that man opposite is more plague than profit. It is wretched not to be able to look out at a passing vehicle without finding a pr. of admiring optics fixed on one.' It made her self-conscious about practising the piano, which stood in full view of his worshipping gaze.

Then, on rising late one morning in late August, she found her mother, Ada and John speculating about the contents of a fat letter addressed to herself:

I found it to contain an enormous sheet of paper covered with writing on all four pages, & one of them crossed also. . . What shd. it be, by all that's horrible, but an offer fr. that <u>wretch</u> over the way! I was so astonished at the beginning that I said to M:—'this cannot be for me,' then I looked at the signature 'Edward Saltwell', & handed it to M., who read it out loud among the horrorstricken exclamations of the victim, & the roars of the whole family . . . The letter shows the most crass ignorance, with an attempt at fine writing . . . P. was shown it & enclosed it in an envelope with a note saying 'Sir, I have read, & return you the enclosed communication, & beg that you will send no other. Yrs etc. John Marshall.' . . . This being the case I have only my and M's memory to draw on; we wrote out all we cd. remember as an epistolary curiosity.

She then paraphrased what Saltwell had said, larding it with her own tart commentary:

He begins Dear Miss Marshall, & excuses himself for not having written before, & tells me I am far above him in position etc. etc. (wh. I am fully aware of) & also that there is a disparity in our ages, wh. he seems to think still more serious. He feels, natheless, that he has a right to address me, even shd. I reject him wh. 'Heaven forefend!' Then he goes on to say he has been staring at me for several months (what news!) & has endeavoured to prevent his 'confrères' knowing what he was about (I doubt if he succeeded). Also he fears he has sometimes taken M. or A. for me, whom he compares to a 'star in heaven'! He feels he is not good enough for me (<u>quite</u> right!) but offers to put on livery & be my footman, or proposes a compromise: (o! horror of horrors!) to be my lackey & my husband too! 'if so it wd. please you!' O! immensely!!! He goes on with a lot more twaddle & ends 'Yr. obedient servant', wh. is the only sensible part of the letter.

Jeannette tried to take the family's teasing in good part. 'What tickles M's, P's, etc. fancy is that such an epistle shd. be addressed to me, who am considered rather "high & mighty", & always go by the name of "the magnificent".' Only the visits to Ely and the holidays abroad brought relief. In London Mr Saltwell's adoring gazes continued to dog her, and he featured in the diary nearly every day. Her fear of meeting him in the street became obsessive:

Having just crossed Regent Street opposite [New] Burlington Street, who shd. I see within half a dozen yds. of me but the Horror. He evidently saw me as he was crimson. Without 'waiting for repairs' I crossed the road with one bound, narrowly escaping being run over by a passing hansom. It was very idiotic no doubt, but the impulse was too strong, & I found myself at Duvelleroy's[1] before I knew where I was. M. & A. thought I had gone mad.

She occasionally wished her father would take the matter more in earnest and complain to the clerk's employers, to 'have him sent off'; but common sense prevailed, and both she and her parents preferred to avoid a 'set-to'.

Exactly two years after Mr Saltwell's first offer, while the Marshalls were holidaying at Bel Alp, in the Valais, another letter from him was forwarded to Mrs Marshall with an enclosure for Jeannette: 'I have not seen my communication & do not intend [to], but M. tells me it is a repetition of the last one, & hers is to ask her to read & destroy the one for me if it contains anything that would "grieve me". I am to be told the purport. I feel quite savage about it, & do not know what P. intends doing.'

Her father's reply to the 'enemy', 'perfectly plain & dignified', threatened legal proceedings if he molested Jeannette any more. It calmed her down, so that she gave only cursory mention to Saltwell's note of apology to Marshall and his promise to leave off troubling her. In fact, the lovelorn glances from the counting-house continued and the name of Saltwell did not altogether disappear from the diary for another four years.

Withdrawal from the social round when in mourning (twice over, after Reggie's and Grandmother Williams's deaths) had carried penalties; each time the re-entry amounted to a new launching. Even the holidays brought Jeannette little in the way of affairs of the heart. In 1878 they spent four days in Venice and in the company of Mr Pearson, a

[1] A fan-maker at 167 Regent Street, on the south side of its junction with New Burlington Street.

not bad-looking unattached civil servant met at the Grand Hotel, where he and they were staying. There was much staring (ogling is what Jeannette called it on this occasion) and satisfactory exchanges of banter: 'He takes to remarks of a flattering description in a low tone. The smartness of my replies seems to somewhat astonish his weak nerves.' When two years later they ran into him again, this time travelling with wife and sister-in-law, at Mürren, Jeannette expressed no regrets; in Venice in 1878 she had thought him a little 'épris', but to her he had never been more than a passing fancy. In any case, circumstances had now changed: a man met in 1879 had made her heart beat faster.

At Bel Alp, a tiny Swiss resort high up in the Valais, in August 1879, two or three days after Mr Saltwell's second missive had caught up with the Marshalls, Jeannette was asked by a 'very good-looking young man about 6ft. 2 high' for the name of the piece she had just finished playing on the piano in the hotel's *salon*; it had been Rubinstein's Barcarolle. Into her middle age and after she would recall in detail this first meeting with the handsome stranger and would speak of the flirtation that ensued as the only significant affair of her younger years. Yet from a distance it seems as devoid of promise as all her other frustrated hopes.

The shortage of genuine suitors had made her eager for some dalliance. On arrival at the Bel Alp Hotel she at once noticed the admiring glances cast in her direction by another guest, a presentable but plain middle-aged Scotsman, Mr Sutherland. He immediately became 'so very attentive as to alarm P. & M. much . . . I hear nothing but the probable views of Mr. S., & how he "follows me up" & how careful I must be, until I was downright savage.' Marshall especially held out against Sutherland, perhaps because of the disparity of ages. Jeannette believed him between forty-five and fifty: he was in fact forty-five precisely, to her twenty-four. That he meant his attentions to be taken seriously she was certain, as he told Mrs Marshall a great deal 'about where he lives, his house, furniture, pictures, etc., wh. no doubt is meant to come round to me.' Then the younger man, the one with a taste for Rubinstein, appeared on the scene. Mr Sutherland's role was reduced to acting as foil for the newcomer, who met with much more favour in Jeannette's eyes.

For once she did not insist on the exchanges of wit and ready repartee which had made flirtation with John Wood or Herbert

Thomas so attractive. She allowed herself only the faintest of sniggers when she discovered, on the third day, his 'unromantic' surname of Brown, and again, when three months later she found out that his first name was Harry, her 'favorite aversion!!' She dwelt at length on his pleasing appearance: 'It is time I described Mr. Brown; he is, as I thought, 6 ft. 2, good figure & walks well, about 30–2, brown hair a little wavy, lighter moustache, wh. he wears long, & very nice blue-grey eyes. His nose is not exactly perfect, but the tout-ensemble is really very pleasing . . . he is the neatest man in his dress I ever saw, & habited in light grey, looks "assez grand".'

They all took note of his good manners—'he is extremely polite, & jumps up every time a lady enters a room'—and she returned again and again to Brown's 'irreproachable costume' which, she claimed, impressed her parents as much as it did her. They, and Ada too, approved of Harry Brown, Ada even contriving to afford him one or two (exceedingly short) tête-à-têtes with Jeannette. She found out a little about his profession and avocations in the seven days of hotel life at Bel Alp and later at Monte Generoso, a tiny resort high up between the lakes Lugano and Como. He claimed to be a barrister (though perhaps only aspiring to the Bar, as after their return to London Marshall could not find Harry Brown's name in the Law List). He was, she thought, very clever and exceptionally well-read; he sang and was, 'for a gentleman', exceedingly fond of music; all affinities strong enough to act as bond. Every morning he greeted her with a warm, grinding handshake; last thing in the evening he again shook hands, lingering over the process. Mrs Marshall declared him to be 'very much taken' with Jeannette. 'C'est possible' was Jeannette's coy comment.

In London he played his cards ably, with his paths continually crossing those of the Marshalls as if he intentionally chose the routes of his Saturday and Sunday walks so as to meet them. Jeannette missed the first of these meetings; it was aggravating: 'I might go out for months & never meet a soul & then stay at home once, & that's what comes of it! Dégoutant!' A fortnight later they ran into him again and this time Mrs Marshall told him how to obtain a ticket for her husband's Academy lectures and demonstrations, about which there had been some talk at Bel Alp. Much to Jeannette's disappointment, Brown was by no means regular in his attendance, despite the fact that he was invariably invited back to 10 Savile Row after the lecture. After the first of these visits Jeannette wrote 'I cd. see M. was most grinny, &

dared not look at her. Mr. B. seemed nervous, & carried on a rather
spasmodic conversation.' The next time they were all more relaxed.
Jeannette kept her countenance, working at her needlework. 'P. had
his supper, & M. & Mr. B. wine & biscuits, A. & I the latter only. I sat
demurely at the opposite end of the table, & was (M. says) quite meek.
My natural character, of course. Mr. Brown talked with far less effort,
. . . & looked the picture of content.' He extended the duration of his
visits till after the fourth evening Jeannette exclaimed in feigned
horror: 'he stayed till nearly 11-25! Where will he draw the line?
Midnight?' Earlier, she admitted, she had been 'sufficiently idiotic to
shed a few bitter tears of woe' at being made to stay away from that
evening's lecture: 'the impropriety of hearing P. describe the muscles
of the trunk in Mr. Brown's presence is considered "quite too awfully
shocking". I really am not horrified myself at the prospect, but all are
not artistic, I suppose . . . It did seem an aggravation to be kept away fr.
P.'s lectures wh. I have faithfully attended for three years because of
those most unfortunate gluteal muscles! There is a serio-comic aspect
of the case, I must say.'

The demonstrations which followed the course of lectures were in
any case out of bounds for ladies, so Harry Brown's lack of assiduity in
attending them caused her fewer pangs. His last visit to No. 10 was
after the only one to which he did go, the second of the series; he was
'refreshed with curaçoa wh. he seemed to appreciate' and left behind
Whymper's *Scrambles amongst the Alps* which he had promised to lend
her. When he did not reappear for three weeks, she returned the book
by mail with what was, by Marshallic standards, quite a polite informal
note; she referred to the pleasure her father and she had derived from
Whymper's amusing book, explained that because of Marshall's attack
of severe bronchitis, there would be no more demonstrations for the
time being, and concluded: 'With our united kind regards, Believe me
Sincerely Yours E. J. Marshall.'

Mrs Marshall, as was her wont, kept talking of Brown's intentions. 'I
don't see it has come to anything as bad as that yet' commented
Jeannette early in November, when her mother told her to make up her
mind 'one way or the other'. 'Perhaps he may come once and never no
more. Anyway what is to be, will be & it is no use worrying oneself
about it.' After his first evening visit Ellen again attempted to gauge
Jeannette's feelings: 'M. asked me today what I think of Mr. Brown's

attentions. I dare not yet commit myself to an opinion, but it seems to me that he was rather taken with me abroad, & the other night seemed very delighted to see me, and A. even says that he looked beaming as he sat by my side . . . I own to not objecting to the person in question.' And when Brown's fickle attendance at Marshall's lectures should have counselled caution, at the end of November 1879, the diary entry recorded Ellen's lack of prudence: 'M. still persists in thinking that Mr. Brown is contemplating a serious step à mon égard.'

The father, too, unwittingly added fuel to Jeannette's interest in Brown. He led the teasing ('Brown, Brown, Brown fr. morning to evening') and referred to his daughter's admirer as Ellen's 'future son-in-law'; then, as if to compensate and show the importance he attached to the matter, he spent time on premature enquiries into Brown's background. Worse was to come. When Brown, about to discontinue his visits, failed to turn up at the third demonstration, Marshall, as well as Ellen, completely misjudged the situation: 'Both P. & M. say now there is no doubt of his intentions, & both like him, so that if he asks & has sufficient of the "Needful" for a decent maintenance, he has a very good chance.'

Though by the New Year she professed to have given up all hope of the erratic Harry Brown, her parents' ambivalence kept reviving her expectations:

P. is much exercised in mind about Mr. Brown, & thinks there must be some explanation for his silence. He was so 'honest-looking', 'so polite' to M., 'so deferential' to P., was without doubt 'so much taken with me' etc, that P. cannot make it out. No more can anyone else, but so it is. I begin to quite forget all about him. The question whether I shd. like a Royal Institution ticket to be sent him, I answered promptly in the negative. He had been seen & commented on by quite enough people at the Academy without introducing him to a fresh set at the Instn. Besides, I wd. not go a single step, out of my way, after him.—P. cannot find his name in the Law List for this year either. Whatever can be the reason?

A couple of days later her mother told her that Marshall continued 'to "harp" on the Brown subject'; 'he cannot think how he cd. behave so, or take such a liberty with him & his family. I feel I can scarcely believe I ever knew him.'

There was a lack of consistency about all things connected with Harry Brown with which neither the parents nor Jeannette knew how to cope. That he did not appear in the Law List was certainly puzzling.

His rooms were in Somerset Street, parallel with the north side of Oxford Street (on the present site of Selfridge's), and his father lived in Belsize Square. A perfectly acceptable set of addresses; indeed, much later, after it was all over, when Jeannette found occasion to locate Brown's parental home, she was impressed by its grandeur: 'It is really a beautiful house, a double & detached one, with stained glass in door and windows &c, & artistic blinds & curtains!' But they could discover nothing about the income which sustained those stylish abodes. Besides, the one acquaintance Brown shared with the Marshalls had volunteered a most unfavourable judgment of his character. In conversation with Ada, young Johnson, the son of a Savile Row neighbour and medical colleague, had explained that he had for a short while worked in the same office as Brown, but knew very little of him, and 'did not like him at all'. This, added Jeannette, had been repeated twice, with emphasis. 'P. thinks Mr. J. must have some good reason for his remarks. Mr. Brown is consigned to the lower depths of infamy.' As usual Ada had proved ineffectual, too delicate to follow up the matter with young Johnson. 'I wish she had!' wrote Jeannette in irritation.

In June 1880 she exchanged a few sentences with Harry Brown in Hyde Park, their first conversation since the evening when he had come to Savile Row early in December 1879. After some generalities about how unlikely one was to chance upon acquaintances in the vastness of London, he 'suddenly remarked:—"You sent my book back in a great hurry!" in a tone wh. makes me think that was the offence!!' She thought her explanation mollified him. But speculating about the reasons for his baffling retreat was no longer material. Henceforward, contact was restricted to casual meetings in the street or the Park, and later to curt greetings and occasional exchanges of superficial pleasantries.

Eventually Jeannette decided that the time had come not to 'know' Harry Brown on meeting him in the street or elsewhere. The process of cutting him out of her life was slow, and cost her some effort, even to the point of declaring 'Hyde Park tabooed on Saturdays', and diverting the constitutional to Regent's Park. In May 1881, when the wound to her self-esteem was still fresh, she admitted that her heart, too, had been touched: 'It has made a difference in my life, I believe (without any ridiculous romance), and I am never going to get married to anyone else.' Six years later she repeated much the same sentiment:

'I can't help feeling he really cared for me. However all this is past &
gone, & I shall never marry <u>now</u>!'

Despite her genuine disappointment, Jeannette continued to keep her
eyes well open for any signs of 'intentions', even from men whom she
considered as hardly eligible. She took stock of Elyites, but they did
not answer. Harold Archer, her favourite sparring partner there, was
now married to a Miss Luddington; out of pique, thought Jeannette,
because she had not responded to his advances. The others did not
come up to him. She was in any case not sufficiently desperate to
contemplate a provincial exile. In London in the past two or three years
she had several times run into a Mr Roby, whose attentions had
thrilled her at balls when she went back into society a year or so after
Reggie's death. He had since put on weight, and she no longer cared
'2d about him'. Then there was Hamilton Cartwright. His father, 'old'
Cartwright, who lived in Old Burlington Street, just west of Savile
Row, was the Marshalls' dentist. The younger Cartwright, also a
dental surgeon, highly qualified and on the staff of King's College, in
his spare time haunted the neighbourhood.

   Once or twice during light-hearted interludes at the height of the
suspense about Harry Brown's intentions, she had referred to Hammy
Cartwright as the second string to her bow. 'P. does not object to Mr.
Cartwright, excepting his profession, as he has no doubt had an
excellent education, is clever, well-off, & very respectable-looking.'
Her father laughingly proclaimed himself ready for either, the up-and-
coming dentist or the conjectural barrister. But Cartwright's profession was the rub. When in 1880 the older Cartwright was put up for
membership of the Athenaeum he was blackballed; 'inspite of his
popularity & because of his profession' wrote Jeannette. The Marshall
parents discouraged Hammy, afraid that Jeannette might be tempted
by his alleged future income of £2,000 a year; she herself thought him
conceited and, according to Ada, did not care a rap about him. All the
same, she was piqued when in 1880 he appeared to lose interest, a fact
which at the time she ascribed to his belief she was engaged to Mr
Brown. Years later she wrote about Hamilton Cartwright: 'I certainly
might have had him, if it had not been for M.'

   This was less than fair to Ellen, as Jeannette had felt no enthusiasm
(or had not shared it even with the diary) for Cartwright, and it is by no
means clear that on his side there had been any serious interest in

Jeannette. Also, her own judgment occasionally made her pin her hopes on a dud, or reject a reasonable candidate, such as Brown's rival, Mr Sutherland. Three years after the Bel Alp episode, with the pangs about Harry Brown already dulled, Jeannette learnt a great deal more about the now newly married Scotsman. He had risen from plebeian beginnings to be chairman of the P. and O. shipping company: 'still not v. rich & draws a salary'. The source of this information, a patient of her father's, was himself immensely rich, so Jeannette concluded: 'I suppose Mr. S. is well off according to our ideas, but his lowly birth wd. have stuck in my throat.' That Thomas Sutherland was about to become Member of Parliament for Greenock and would eventually glean first a KCMG and then a GCMG might have made the humble origin (he was the son of an Aberdeen house-painter) somewhat easier to swallow.

Even leaving aside the unproductive holidays of the years 1876–8 and the callowness with which she frequently lent the respectable garments of matrimonial intentions to a flimsy dalliance, her progress towards marriage was strewn with obstacles. Two of these catch the eye. First of all, there was little communication in the Marshall family and none of the intimacy which would allow any one member of it to know for certain what another might feel or want or intend; delayed and impaired intimations, near-guesses and surmises were all inadequate preliminaries to action. Secondly, although the daughters had by this time succeeded in overcoming some of Mrs Marshall's aloofness, and were attempting to keep an open house, the means of doing this—the afternoons 'at home', the once-a-year reception—were too formal to serve as setting for the early stages of a courtship. Matters would have been easier if they had been in the habit of entertaining guests impromptu, as they did with the Startins or the Ely Marshalls. But as a rule, they did not go in for such casual entertaining.

No help could be expected from the ten aunts: Aunt Eliza's set of friends consisted of tedious left-overs from the days of Grandmother Williams; Aunt Mary was not on speaking terms with the Marshalls; Aunt Startin, Mrs Edwin and Mrs John Williams had their own worries with crowds of marriageable daughters. Four of the aunts on the Marshall side moved in excessively provincial circles. This left Aunt Julia, too tactless to be trusted with matchmaking, but at least aware of the problem: 'I hear that Aunt Julia attacked P & M both very violently on the subject of my getting married,' wrote Jeannette in 1881, 'and said I shd. not be too particular etc.' The advice was not well received: 'I do wish she wd. leave me alone & let me be an old maid in my own way. Both P & M quite agree that it is better to remain as I am, unless I meet anyone whom I like, wh. seems most unlikely as far as I can see.'

A brother, even a younger one, ought to have been an asset. But John, since Reggie's death the youngest in the family, had grown first into a farouche adolescent, then into an unpredictable undergraduate, and was beginning to cause problems. From late adolescence on, his life had run separately—though always in parallel, as if on a minor road—from that of his parents and sisters. As early as 1873, a matter of months after Reggie's death, when John was only fifteen-and-a-half, separate arrangements were being made for his summer holidays. Thence on he never spent more than a week or ten days travelling abroad with the rest of the family. His new status of youngest child secured him none of the privileges of that position. The Marshall parents were not in the habit of spoiling their girls and they certainly did not cosset their adolescent son.

Until the age of nineteen John was signally successful in his studies, winning prizes and scholarships at school and at college. His academic gifts ranged from classics to science and mathematics. What is more, he seemed set to become a competent artist. The two Rossetti brothers, Gabriel and William, had praised his talent when he was in his mid-teens,[2] and a little later Jeannette reported that Mr Pickersgill, who as Secretary of the Royal Academy had a practised eye, was astounded by the quality of John's work.

No one, least of all himself, was clear about the direction he was going to take, but options abounded and there appeared to be no pressing hurry about reaching a decision. Jeannette reported ambitious plans on his behalf: 'J. will go up to Cambridge & take as many degrees

---

[2] William Michael Rossetti's *Some Reminiscences*, op. cit., contains, in i, pp. 144–5, a thumbnail sketch of John Marshall, which concludes: 'one of his sons showed, as a mere boy, a singular turn for landscape painting, by which Dante Rossetti was greatly impressed.' In an entry in his own diary (*The Diary of W. M. Rossetti*, 1870–1873, Odette Bornand ed., Oxford, 1977, p. 229) dated 16 February 1873 W. M. Rossetti also referred to John's drawings: 'Called at John Marshall's to see about some more chloral for Gabriel [see Chapter 9]. He was not in; but I saw for the first time his son, now aged (I suppose) twelve or thirteen, who from a very early age indeed has distinguished himself by executing very clever landscapes. He told me that he used to wish to be a painter, but does not now particularly; he was engaged in some geometric work when I entered.' Young John was in fact just a few days short of his fifteenth birthday. The visitor is unlikely to have confused him with Reggie, who by mid-January was already very ill and, according to Jeannette, looked 'like a ghost'.

etc. as he can, both at the London Univ. & at Cambridge. Then in 2 or 3 years he might take a fellowship & get £3 or 400 a yr. to start with. Of course that wd. be very nice if it cd. be carried out.'

At first, it was exciting to have a brother at Trinity. He brought college friends to Savile Row and some of those, the early ones, Jeannette thought entertaining enough, though, as usual, she was apt to comment scathingly about shortcomings in their looks, manners and conversation. If the sisters had been adept at taking advantage of new opportunities, and the brother in turn ready to devote time and thought to their entertainment, there might have been more fun to be reaped than the one or two teas in his rooms in Trumpington Street and the evening service in the college chapel, to which he invited Jeannette and Ada in his first year at Trinity. Not that he could, at this stage, have laid on anything much more exciting; they were, after all, still in deep mourning for Grandmother Williams. But when in May 1878 he failed to get his sisters invited to the Trinity Ball, on the disingenuous plea that it was slow and not patronized by Trinity men, Jeannette was exceedingly put out and relieved her anger by referring to John as 'that stupid idiot of a brother of ours'. To compensate for his daughters' disappointment Marshall procured them invitations to the Masonic Ball held at Cambridge's Guildhall two or three days after the Trinity occasion. 'Fr. intense dismals, we mounted to joy of the most violent description, executing war-dances of the most startling character' wrote Jeannette on receipt of the tickets. Chaperoned by Aunt Julia and escorted by their subdued brother, Jeannette and Ada found themselves in a crowd of splendidly apparelled Masons, in knee-breeches, aprons and jewelled insignia. Jeannette had a glorious time:

Almost directly we got there a steward came up to Aunt & said 'will you allow me to introduce some partners to your young ladies?' She gave her permission & in a moment up they came very willingly. One introduced the other until they were standing round three deep waiting for their turns. By the 4th or 5th dance I was filled up to the end . . . J. was quite delighted, & insisted on my staying till 'God Save The Queen' was played (at 4.30!). With extras I danced 26 dances & was regularly worn out . . . I must say it was rather a triumph.

This success encouraged John to get them invited to the next Trinity Ball, in 1879. His nerve gave out at the last moment and he failed to accompany them, but made up for his desertion by arranging breakfast the next morning in his rooms—he had by now moved to the College—and taking them to see a polo match and rifle-shooting.

Evening service at King's, followed by tea, again in Trinity, crowned
the occasion. After this effort, no more invitations were issued though
he remained at Cambridge for another two terms.

His early results at Trinity had been in line with the plans for an
academic future. However, in April 1877 the spell of success was
broken when he failed to win a college scholarship on which he had set
high hopes. Almost simultaneously, a painting of his was rejected by
the Royal Academy, and this caused perhaps the greater disappointment. His father instantly pulled strings to get the painting accepted by
the recently opened Grosvenor Gallery, but this too proved unsuccessful. John's prospects of an artistic career faded after this double fiasco.

Did these failures precipitate a process of rebellion of which the
occasional fits of 'obstinacy' reported by Jeannette had been the earlier
signs? 'Johnny got into disgrace,' she had written on Christmas Day
1875, '& was sent to bed by P. before tea, about 7 o'clock. He refused
to read a little pro bono publico & was very obstinate till he put P. out.
We were sorry, but it really served him right.' A puzzling incident, out
of keeping with the general tenor of parental behaviour at 10 Savile
Row, and also with John's age: he was at that point a few weeks short of
his eighteenth birthday. There were other manifestations of immature
stubbornness—or perhaps assertions of independence. In August
1876 Jeannette recorded that John 'was to have gone to Ely in the
morning, but . . . was so obstinate & disagreeable about a whole library
of books he wanted to take that his departure was postponed till the
afternoon. He was very rude, & both P. & M. were very angry.'

Despite such isolated vagaries, Jeannette, for the time being, continued to accept him as an integral member of the family circle; in
frequent long letters, she kept him informed of events at Savile Row
and she looked forward to his replies about life at Trinity. Her diary
entries were at times positively affectionate: 'Poor Jack left after tea
with his box & hamper containing more china etc. He was sorry to go
& we to lose him, but we shall settle down, & so will he in a day or two';
at the beginning of another term, the crucial one of the double débâcle
described above, she noted that he did not like returning to Trinity,
although in her view 'the absence fr. home is doing him good. He is
decidedly much more agreeable than "he used to was".' All of which
was to make the rift which would shortly occur more puzzling.

'Existence is the tamest thing out just now!' she complained in the
autumn after their return from Bel Alp and Monte Generoso, before

Harry Brown's attendance at the Royal Academy added spice to the routines of her daily life. 'Nothing but music & work & reading to keep one going at all! Ahimè!' It was beginning to dawn on her that, in the shrinking household (with John at Cambridge, there were now for months on end only four of them left at No. 10), with no more university classes and no music lessons, she missed any sort of framework for her daily life. Only her wardrobe continued to make regular demands; with balls and soirées, dinners and garden parties crowding in, she spent more time than ever planning and executing her costumes.

As the '70s turned into the '80s, brown became one of the most fashionable colours for women's clothes, particularly a rich reddish shade known as 'Etna'. Jeannette made two or three brown dresses, starting with the travelling dress which had served her in Switzerland and Italy in September 1879, and enjoyed the pun which linked her outfits with her musings about Harry Brown. The second brown number she described in April 1880 as 'of deep chocolate <u>brown</u> (still my fate!)'. It cannot have been a success as it was discarded with unwonted haste six months later: 'I am gradually eliminating everything <u>brown</u> fr. my possession. I have always <u>hated</u> the color.' Next spring she changed her mind, but wrote of the newly acquired summer sateen: 'A warm brown (ugh!)'

Thoughts of Mr Brown continued to assert themselves, not only in her waking hours but also in her dreams. Her diaries of the early 1880s contain references to a number of dreams, almost without exception comforting ones, with engagement or marriage as central theme and Harry Brown as usual protagonist.

She could have done with some more tangible solace. Ever since the let-down of the Brown affair she had shown signs of depression. What she wrote was disheartened to the point of bitterness; 'I hate men!' she exclaimed. 'Dismals', a new word in her vocabulary which now kept recurring, headed the entry, in April 1880, on the day when the Royal Academy had disappointed the Marshalls by sending only two tickets for its Private View: 'it is no use repining but this does seem a horrid year, instead of being a lovely one, as I had hoped. Mr. Brown vanished utterly, A.D. only seen once, & for an instant, Mr. Cartwright invisible agn. after two evenings' flirtation, & <u>now</u> Private View. It <u>is</u> very hard!'

She was wrong about Harry Brown, who made a few further appearances before his definitive exit. A.D. was a near-mythical figure, a nameless admirer whom she occasionally saw from afar and to whom she ascribed the initials A.D., because this was how the unidentified sender of a valentine received some years earlier had signed himself.

'Why can I not like people?' she asked later in 1880, and, convalescing after measles in May 1881, reflected: 'Perhaps this illness has been for my good, to give me something to complain about . . .' As late as February 1884 she grumbled (in an irreverent reference to Queen Victoria's John Brown, in *More Leaves from A Journal of Our Lives in the Highlands*, which the Marshalls had borrowed from Mudie's nine days after its publication on 12 February): 'The Queen's book is wofully silly, I think, and one mass of Brown!' Nine months later—five full years after the star-gazing of Bel Alp and Monte Generoso—she finally exorcized Harry Brown from her dreams by acknowledging his haunting presence: 'I cannot think why it is I am continually dreaming of Mr. Brown lately. I am sure he is not worth the trouble, but so it is.'

CHAPTER 9

IN AND OUT OF AESTHETIC
CIRCLES

To get over her disappointment about Harry Brown she needed a sustained distraction—and, at the age of twenty-five, what better than another romantic affair? More than ever, she looked critically at all the men who came her way, and speculated about her chances with anyone in the right age group, thirty upwards, with sufficient means. Various 'medicals' and 'artistics' whom she met on her ever-widening social round were thus inspected. For a week or two, for a month or two, she would pin her hopes on a dinner partner with whom she had exchanged banter or a proficient waltzer who had squeezed her hand at the end of a dance. Then she discovered that he lacked money or perseverance in courtship, that he was committed elsewhere or, worse still, proved to be a bore. She was ready to experience genuine ardour, which did not come her way, or to be charmed by exoticism.

Dr de Jankowski, a Russian (or, to judge by his surname, Russianized Pole) whom she met at the International Medical Congress entertainments in 1881, filled the need for someone new and colourful. They conversed in French, 'cracked jokes, and even got to a little flirting wh. I think was very clever of me in a foreign language.' She found him attractive; his pleasant appearance was somewhat marred by a slight squint and 'double eye-glasses', but a 'very handsome <u>order</u> outweighed this little drawback.' Once again her mother and father teased, calling her 'Mme. la Comtesse'; Jeannette thought the doctor 'un peu épris', and altogether prematurely dreamt of sleigh-rides. He came to lunch at Savile Row and then disappeared, returning presumably to his Moscow practice, never to be seen again. The whole episode had lasted eight days.

A few weeks' acquaintance and more flirting of an equally mild variety led her to speculate about the intentions of Henry Finck, an American art critic met on yet another Swiss occasion. By now Jeannette was impatient of her sister's continual chaperoning—'a proper talk à deux seems an impossibility'—and beginning to look for more than just witty repartee: 'I own he is one of the few men I have met who is superior, and who knows more than I do.' 'Oh why is he a Yankee!!' she sighed. 'He wd do so well! Just my luck.' She returned some books he had lent her with what she called a 'Billy Ducks' which she hoped he would appreciate. Then he called to take his leave before departing for America, murmured 'I am so pleased to have met you' with a warm, prolonged handshake, and ten weeks later she was able to write: 'I liked him much at the time, but now (such is the soothing influence of time) . . . I shd. not mind if I never saw him agn. Anyhow America wd. be exile.'

For one who enjoyed foreign travel, Jeannette was in fact curiously ambivalent about people who came from abroad or who, though living in Britain, were just not British to the core. Some she rejected with a hostility amounting to xenophobia; those she liked or tolerated she treated on the whole as freaks, amusing specimens caged for her entertainment. One such curiosity was the sculptress Mary Zambaco, a Londoner of Greek parentage, whose mother Marshall had known as far back as the 1860s.[1] Separated from her husband, Mme Zambaco had notoriously blemished her reputation by entanglements with, first, Edward Burne-Jones, and subsequently, with at least one other extra-marital partner. In spite of her bad name Marshall continued the acquaintance and eventually introduced Mary Zambaco to his family. Even when, in the late 1880s, they suspected her of continuing the affair with Burne-Jones, which had allegedly been laid to rest some fifteen years earlier, their disapproval did not result in her banishment. 'We are rather exercised about Mme Zambaco' wrote Jeannette in November 1888, and continued:

When M. & I went to her studio in Campden Hill Road the other afternoon, & found it all shut up, a man offered to ring the bell for us, and while waiting, he volunteered some information. There are only 2 studios side by side, and one is Mme 'Zambago' 's (like lumbago!) & the next Mr. Burne Jones', 'Royal

[1] Mary Zambaco was one of the trio of closely related Greek beauties whose likenesses recur in the paintings of Rossetti and Burne-Jones; the other two were Aglaia Coronio and Marie Stillman. Mrs Coronio was the sister of Constantine, Luke and Aleco Ionides; the youngest of the family, another sister, Chariclea, had married Edward Dannreuther, the same Dannreuther who had given Jeannette her advanced piano lessons in the mid-1870s. Mrs Stillman, the daughter of Consul Spartali, and Mrs Zambaco, born Cassavetti, were also in the Ionides clan; see Dorothea Butterworth's 1936 family tree of the descendants of Constantine John Ionides, in the British Library and at the Victoria and Albert Museum.

artist' added our informant with a flourish. Now knowing that B.J. has a large studio at the Grange, & that Mme Z. did not know <u>we</u> knew of her studio there, (wh. P. found out by many enquiries at her former rooms,) & remembering the set out there was between them before, it looks <u>very</u> odd! I feel quite disgusted to think that she is going on agn. in the old style. It is a shame! If I were Mrs. B. J., I wd. soon have her wig off!! P. actually mentioned the man's remark when he & M. called at Shepherd's Bush to Mme Z., who looked uncomfortable, wh. I don't wonder at. How very inopportune!—I don't like the look of it at all.

All the same, when the sculptress, announced by the chambermaid 'as Mlle Coucou!', paid them a visit at Savile Row six months later, she was once again received as if her name had never been besmirched.

Mary Zambaco came into the category of 'artistics', to whose vagaries the Marshalls were inured. Scandal had on occasion touched them quite closely. Even respectable Elyites had skeletons in their cupboards, such as Uncle William Marshall's adulterous propensities and his calamitous neglect of professional business, as well as, a generation earlier, the glossed-over irregularity of great-aunt Charlotte's marriage to her sister's widower. On Jeannette's mother's side, too, all was not well. The fast Mrs Warren De la Rue who went rinking without her husband was admittedly only a remote connection by marriage. Much closer in the family, Jeannette's cigar-smoking first cousin, Jessie Startin, was the respondent in a divorce case, Forrester *v*. Forrester, which caused some stir not only among the relatives but also in the press. Though the evidence was deficient and Jessie eventually went back to her husband, the fact alone that the case had been reported in *The Times* gave them all a jolt. However, adultery was something the Savile Row Marshalls frowned on and tut-tutted about, but had come to accept as one of the realities of life around them.

John Marshall's dealings with Dante Gabriel Rossetti, for one, provided a massive schooling in tolerance. Rossetti's part in the uncomfortably lop-sided association of the artist and the surgeon is adequately documented in Pre-Raphaelite papers and biographies: he regarded Marshall as his 'habitual doctor'.[2]

Jeannette's diaries bring home Marshall's share of the relationship,

---

[2] Although Dr Gordon Hake usually attended Rossetti on a day-to-day basis and was constantly by his side during major illnesses, 'habitual doctor' is what Rossetti himself called Marshall, in a letter to J. A. Rose, dated 1869. See *Letters of D. G. Rossetti*, O. Doughty and J. W. Wahl, eds. (Oxford, 1965–6), p. 683.

his forbearance, and also the extent to which she herself came to terms with the irregularities of the artist's domestic arrangements. She had been less than seven when Ford Madox Brown had summoned her father to the bedside of the dying Lizzie Siddal-Rossetti, and did not comment about the events of that tragic day in February 1862 until twenty years later, after Rossetti in turn had died: 'No doubt he had a wretched life since his wife's death fr. poison she took herself! They had only been married 2 years, & she found herself superseded, & took laudanum. No doubt his grief was remorse, & for 2 years he saw her ghost every night! Serve him right too!' In March 1883 she completed the Marshall version of what had led to Lizzie's overdose. At the Academy, where she had gone especially to look at the Rossettis, in front of the 'brilliant-colored lady in green dress, with blue tiles & passion-flowers behind her head',[3] whom should she see but the model who had sat for the picture in 1865. 'It was "Fanny", who lived with Rossetti, & because of whom his poor wife committed suicide.' On this occasion she had not a word of blame for Rossetti's share in the tragedy. Of Fanny she wrote 'Nasty, common-looking creature.'

The only trace in her 1872 diary of Rossetti's own breakdown and suicide attempt were two cryptic sentences on 10 June: 'Poor P. was called up at 2 o'clock in the morning and did not get back till 8.30! He feels dreadfully tired.' Ford Madox Brown, panic-stricken because Rossetti was still in a state of collapse after a dose of laudanum ingested twenty-four hours earlier, had that night once again summoned Marshall to the rescue.[4] Nine months later Rossetti had forgiven his medical adviser for officiously bringing him back to life and wrote a letter condoling with Marshall on the death of his son. A month later he declared himself willing to support Marshall's application for the chair of anatomy at the Royal Academy and was genuinely pleased when the surgeon carried off this prize.[5] Moreover, it was Marshall who was called in whenever Rossetti's health collapsed, which it did with alarming frequency from the mid-seventies on.

[3] *The Blue Bower*, No. 132 in the catalogue of the 1984 Pre-Raphaelite Tate Gallery exhibition.

[4] There is enough in the diary about Marshall's movements during the ten days preceding the summons to Roehampton to suggest that, contrary to some biographers, he did not examine Rossetti until after the aborted suicide.

[5] Cf. *Letters of D. G. Rossetti*, op. cit., in particular No. 1313 dated 4.3.73, No. 1314 dated 7.3.73, No. 1317 dated 16.3.73, No. 1328 dated 9.4.73 and No. 1341 dated 22.5.78.

However, in contrast to Marshall's relations with the Ford Madox Browns or with the William Rossettis, there was no hint of intimacy between the medical adviser and the difficult patient at Tudor House, Cheyne Walk. When in March 1875 the Marshalls, parents and daughters, were bid to Rossetti's studio, to inspect his new paintings, Jeannette was guarded in her description of the host: 'rather short, stout, greasy, & spectacled', but praised the energy with which he shifted the easels to afford a good view of his recent work. About the paintings she enthused: 'They are totally different to any others I have ever seen, & altogether I admired them very much . . . The last, and best is "Proserpina" . . . She is dark, & (P. said) a glorified portrait of Mrs Morris . . . The face is <u>wonderfully</u> painted, but her figure is not nice; <u>so</u> long-waisted!'[6]

On a later visit, in 1878, she again complained about Rossetti's treatment of the figure. This time the subject was Fiametta, for which Marie Stillman, a patient of Marshall's and friend of the family, had been the model; 'tho' the neck is ugly & figure too large, yet it seems a shame to find fault with anything.' They were also shown *The Blessed Damozel*, a 'quaint conceit' thought Jeannette, and added: 'Mr. R. was very agreeable, & talked very cheerfully & was very nice altogether, but he looks more baggy & untidy than ever, & a great deal older. If it were not for his eyes, wh. are very observant, one wd. never take him for a genius.'

A year or so after this second encounter Jeannette had proof that Rossetti had indeed used his eyes to good effect:

P. & J. [John] went to see Mr. Rosetti, & brought back the astonishing news that he wishes to take my face for a picture! He says if P. & I will consent, he will give P. a chalk drawing of me! (wh. wd. be worth quite 100 guineas). He is very much struck with my appearance, & evidently fr. the way P. & M. grin said something very flattering, wh. I have not been told. It wd. be something to go down to posterity under D. G. Rosetti's wing, tho' I shd. not have thought my style sufficiently melancholy.

In fact, taking her likeness, or that of another member of the Marshall family, was the way the artist intended to rid himself of his feeling of indebtedness to Marshall. Years back he had already contemplated making a portrait-drawing of the surgeon, 'the best head in

---

[6] Besides *Proserpina* and a few sketches, the pictures on show were *Dante, in a dream, seeing the death of Beatrice, A Roman Widow, L'Improvisatrice, La Ghirlandata, Lady Lilith* and *A Girl putting a bowl of yellow flowers on a mantelpiece.*

the family', and presenting that in lieu of payment. Instead he hit on the more straightforward solution of offering cash: 'I at last to-day sent 50 guineas to Marshall, which I ought to have done long ago; but partly have been always short of tin, and partly Brown thought it would be better, if possible, to paint or draw some family-portrait for him—but this would never come about, now I live here' he wrote to his brother from Kelmscott, the Oxfordshire house he borrowed from William Morris. To Brown he boasted that with the cheque had gone a 'letter putting everything in as delicate and friendly way as I can'; he must have been aware that hitherto all the generosity had been on Marshall's side.[7]

Six years had passed, and, after meeting Jeannette for the second time, Rossetti reverted to the original idea of offering a drawing in recompense for Marshall's medical skill. But ill-luck haunted the project. First, Marshall dithered for some eight weeks about how to respond to the offer. When he eventually accepted on behalf of Jeannette, he and the rest of the family were about to go off on their annual holiday abroad, and the venture had to be postponed. After their return to London, six weeks later, no sooner had they shaken off the dust of travel than Rossetti fell ill again, 'from the old cause, I am sorry to say'.

It proved a false alarm, but the artist was busy drawing Mrs Stillman for a painting of Desdemona and working on a commission for Constantine Ionides from a portrait of Janey Morris which eventually became 'The Day Dream'; the plan to take Jeannette's likeness went into oblivion. When Mrs Lea Merritt, a painter acquaintance and patient of Marshall's, talked in early November of how delightful it would be to sit for Rossetti, Jeannette wondered 'I don't know if I shall now', and then made no more reference to the matter until, a year after the artist's death, Marie Stillman mentioned that Rossetti had 'often talked to her of his great wish to make a drawing of me!' 'I always regret that last chance of being immortalized!' sighed Jeannette; she and Ada had just then been sitting to a less august patient of their father's, Paul Rajon, the engraver, for drawings of their heads in sanguine. In 1885, Marshall and his daughters ran into Rossetti's friend Theodore Watts-Dunton at the Royal Academy. When the surgeon referred to Rossetti's plan to sketch Jeannette for the head of

---

[7] Cf. *Letters of D. G. Rossetti*, op. cit., in particular: No. 1250 dated 9.10.72, No. 1252 dated 11.10.72, No. 1253 dated 17.10.72, No. 1313 dated 4.3.73, No. 1317 dated 16.3.73, No. 1337 dated 6.5.73, and No. 1338 dated 6.5.73.

Joan of Arc, 'Mr. W. smiled & bowed, & said there was a Miss Marshall (he would not say which, but stared at me all the time) whom Rossetti used to rave about, he was in perfect raptures etc. Really most trying, & made me quite uncomfortable.'

This was the first intimation of the subject for which Rossetti had intended her likeness to serve. Her feelings would have been hurt had she known that in 1882, just before he died, Rossetti had completed an oil of Joan of Arc, based on a much earlier watercolour resembling Mrs Morris.[8] The face of his beloved Janey which had inspired him for a quarter of a century haunted him still in those last weeks in Birchington, on the Kent coast.

Marshall had sent Rossetti to Birchington that winter in a last-minute bid to save his life. Earlier, at the end of October, he had instructed his most reliable nurse, Mrs Workman,[9] to join the Cheyne Walk household and make sure that the routines prescribed in order to keep Rossetti off chloral were being observed. But in spite of the supervision the artist's condition continued to deteriorate. At ten o'clock on the evening of 11 December a messenger from Rossetti informed Marshall that he 'had had a paralytic stroke, one arm & leg being powerless!' Nurse Workman confirmed her patient's self-diagnosis. 'I am sure I hope not' wrote Jeannette of the stroke, 'but wish he wd. send at reasonable hours', and added on 12 December: 'I hear that Mr. Rosetti is in a queer state but had exaggerated his symptoms.' A few days later Marshall asked a newly qualified doctor, young Maudsley,[10] 'to spend a quiet month' with Rossetti. Writing on 28 December Jeannette quipped 'Mr. Maudsley must be getting quite aesthetic by now' and enlarged on the scheme: 'He is trying a new treatment under P's direction, trying to break "Dante" of his love of whiskey & chlorate by injections of morphia. At present it seems to answer.' A few weeks later the Rossetti household, with or without the custodians appointed by Marshall, transferred to Birchington.

The final act started on the evening of Maundy Thursday, 6 April, when William Rossetti who had received a telegraphic message that his

[8] This is R.3 in Virginia Surtees, *The Paintings and Drawings of Dante Gabriel Rossetti* (1828–1882), *A Catalogue Raisonné* (Oxford, 1971), not to be confused with the oil of Joan of Arc painted in 1863. The 1882 painting is a replica of a water-colour dating from 1864, R.2 in Surtees.

[9] Cf. Ch. 17 below.

[10] Nephew of the Henry Maudsley after whom the hospital is named.

brother appeared drowsy and that the nurse (no longer Mrs Workman) thought him to be sinking, came to ask Marshall to accompany him to Birchington. Because of the late hour, they decided to put off the journey till the following morning. On Good Friday Marshall realized that the trains, running on Sunday schedules, would fit awkwardly with his London duties, and again postponed the visit to the coast; instead, he did a round of his patients and, in the evening, accompanied his whole flock, including young John, to a 'Stabat Mater' at St James's Hall.

On the Saturday, alerted by another telegram, this time from William, who had gone down to Birchington on Friday and now reported Gabriel to be very ill, Marshall took the midday train to Kent. When he returned twenty-four hours later, incongruously carrying a bunch of geraniums, Jeannette reported:

Mr. Rosetti was absolutely blue when he got there, the doctor etc. had given him up, & he was really dying fr. blood poisoning arising fr. congested kidneys. P. packed him in wet sheets etc., & in 4–5 hours brought him round, virtually saving his life. Of course he is still dangerously ill, but there is a chance for him, though P. doubts if he will ever be fit for anything agn. He is more plague than profit, poor creature. The place is too cold for him, & the East winds P. thinks were the final cause of the attack.

The next day, 10 April, a telegram, received at 3 p.m., informed Marshall that all was over: 'Poor Mr. Rosetti is dead, & his friends wish it to be kept quiet until Friday! How odd!! What a wasted life his had been lately! It is very sad to think of. If he had led a good & proper life, instead of drinking whiskey & chlorate, he might have flourished for years . . .' On the 12th she reported that the news of Rossetti's death was that morning in *The Times*, 'so his friends have not kept it very secret'. She added that her father had been invited to the funeral on the Friday, '& may perhaps go'. He did not go; he had himself been on the sick list for most of the winter and early spring and found east winds trying.

Jeannette's own epitaph of Rossetti followed two or three days later, on the occasion when she referred to his sad life after the death of Lizzie: 'he was punished by having a miserable existence, so let us hope his is happy now.'

He died without having cleared his debt to Marshall. A year or so later William brought two of his brother's drawings, for Marshall to choose. A sketch of Janey asleep over a book by William Morris was rejected;[11] the one Marshall retained was a 'Scotch girl with small eyes & rather pouting lips . . . not a particularly good specimen'.

For all her niggling pinpricks, Rossetti was one of the few 'artistics' whom Jeannette treated with respect. Her usual commentary about the avant-garde met on 'artistic' occasions was quite different. Leftover acquaintances from Marshall's bachelor years in Mornington Crescent and current patients of the bohemian variety—in this amorphous crowd which embraced both rich and destitute, both society successes and suicidal failures, she saw only ridiculous and often unsavoury 'guys'. She met them in their own setting when she accompanied her father on Studio Sunday (the annual occasion when artists opened their workrooms to critics, patrons and friends to show the selection they intended to submit to the Royal Academy), or, with the rest of the family, attended the artists' 'at homes'. They were to be seen on neutral ground, at the Royal Academy soirées and Private Views, or, in even greater numbers, at their sanctum, the Grosvenor Gallery. They also came to Savile Row to consult Marshall, or to put in an appearance at one of the Marshalls' annual jamborees.

Jeannette's comments were uniformly caustic: 'The flood of "artistics" in everything hideous in the way of costume was appalling' she wrote at the age of nineteen about an 'at home' at the Ford Madox Browns, and four years later, after a reception at Brown's daughter Lucy's (Mrs William Rossetti), sniggered that her visitors had been 'most singularly attired, the ladies sad & the gentlemen mad-looking'. As she got older, her comments grew bold and personal. The wife of the minor Pre-Raphaelite painter John Brett was 'as usual in mouse-color & very sloppy'; the young Graham Robertson, later one of the chroniclers of aesthetic London, she saw as 'frightful & all but imbecile'; Holman Hunt's (second) wife 'looked a regular Judy'. One or other of the Morris women, William's wife and their two daughters, Jeannette invariably singled out for particular lashings; after a dance at Aglaia Coronio's in 1883 she wrote:

Mrs Morris and her 2nd daughter May were there, and the former looked very well, I thought, though very sloppy, in a cream crêpe, sparingly trimmed with old gold satin, & made high to the throat. Her hair was fuzzy, and she had a white Indian shawl over her shoulders. When her face is quiet, it is fine & fascinating, but when she speaks she is spoilt. The daughter, in a brown-red bedgown with no tucker, was a guy everyone voted. She is excessively ugly.

[11] Probably No. 388 in Surtees (1971), op. cit.

At another meeting at the Coronios, on the occasion of a tennis party in July 1886, she thought that the elder girl, Jenny, and Janey herself looked 'such horrid frights'.

'I do heartily object to the aesthetics, but otherwise it was not bad' was her summary of a Burne-Jones garden party, also in 1886. Under the apple-trees in the 'dissolute' (her father's *bon mot* malapropism) garden of the Grange 'a ghastly & aesthetic company was assembled'. It included 'Mrs. Stillman & Effie (who is a telegraph post!), Mrs. Morris (who looks like a maniac) & her eldest daughter (who is out & out the ugliest person I ever saw), Mme Coronio (looking awful!)' She was equally trenchant about another aesthetic garden party, that of the Holman Hunts in 1889:

Found the usual gathering of artistics more or less loathely, but leavened with some fairly clean & respectable folks . . . Poor Mr. Hunt looks pale & old, and his wife in an awful embroidered garment of dubious cleanliness, looks untidy and gaunt. Spoke to Mr Wm Rosetti, who was wandering around with his solemn little family . . . I spoke to Mrs Stillman & Effie, and was introduced to Mr Strudwick who was unexpectedly un-aesthetic in appearance & manner. Plain & pleasant, in fact. One rather dreadful incident occurred, viz: a poor youth either fainted or fitted in the hot studio, and A. & I saw four gentlemen carrying him by the legs & wings to a remote part of the garden. It was done with such a horrid air of haste & secrecy as to give one quite a turn. We told P, who went to assist, and found him pillowed in a hollybush! How original! The 3 Morris women looked more witchlike than ever. We left about 6.45 or so. Not even as amusing as the Ionides'.

The Luke Ionides garden party, four days earlier, had ranked as more entertaining chiefly because it was the second occasion within less than a week—the first being a Royal Academy soirée—at which Jeannette had met and played off against one another two of her lukewarm beaux. Even without such a challenge she did, in fact, usually derive some mild entertainment from her visits to members of the Ionides clan. But this is how she summed up her attitude after another garden party, at the Coronios in 1888: 'I like to see these queer folks now & then, but I do not like Greeks, and never shd. They are a set of "furriners" of doubtful cleanliness.'

It was becoming a phobia. Aesthetes and Greeks and also Jews—all unfamiliar people she saw as sloppy, greasy, dirty, in short repulsive. And she expressed her aversion in particularly violent terms when its objects were male, and of marriageable age and status. Of the men at the 1883 Coronio dance she had written that 'they were nearly all 5 feet nothing & as "black as the hakes" '—an expression which defeats interpretation, but which was clearly not intended to be complimentary. That the prejudice was selective and its direction not always predictable—she did not for instance object to some of her father's Jewish professional friends, nor to many of his foreign patients—only highlighted its irrational foundations. In a minor degree the xenophobia and, in particular, the anti-semitism had always been there, a grating deposit in the fabric of Jeannette's diaries, but around her twenty-seventh or -eighth birthday it became much more pronounced.

Much of it may have been due to a particular susceptibility to the increasingly conspicuous society anti-semitism of the 1880s. It was probably that which permitted two outbursts in early 1883 about her aunt-by-marriage, Mrs John Williams, the only relative whom she knew to be Jewish, and her daughters by an earlier marriage. Within a few weeks she first wrote of Aunt John as 'that nasty Jewy woman', and then, after accidentally meeting her with two of her daughters (and accompanied by Uncle John), 'Quite enough Jews for one day.'

A few months later in November, she saw her erstwhile admirer, Harry Brown, at a concert in the company of two women 'one fair and the other dark, the latter rather "Jewy".' This set her anxiously speculating about the reason for Harry Brown's defection, now three years away: 'I guess he must be engaged to that Jewy person of concert fame.' And when in 1886 she saw the death at the age of seventy-nine of Harry Brown's father, Samuel Simon Brown, announced in the paper, she concluded: 'They must be Jews! wh. is enough for me.' She had in fact known of Mr Brown senior's first and middle names ever since December 1879; 'his names are the extraordinary ones of Samuel Simon! Gott im Himmel! What were his parents about?' she had commented, but had not at that stage re-classified the Browns, father and son, as unacceptable Jews. It was now, in the mid-1880s, that fiascos and frustration had turned her into something of a bigoted misanthrope.

In one respect Jeannette was always ready to emulate and learn from the avant-garde; this was in their perception of fashion. By 1879 aesthetic fashions in dress and interior decoration were quite the thing; it was the year of 'green serge gowns and Morris papers . . . Every lady of true culture had an amber necklace . . .'[12] Jeannette, as usual, succeeded in being in the vanguard: the earliest sage green dress in her wardrobe (and also in Ada's, for Ada's outfits were, as always, the exact replica of Jeannette's) dated back to 1878. By the following year seven new dresses, out of a total of eleven acquisitions, were distinctly aesthetic in detailing, such as tight sleeves with slashings at shoulder and elbow, and colour—more sage, peacock, old gold and the reddish-browns of her 'Brown' mood.[13]

As for amber, Aunt Julia Marshall had given her a string of beads as early as in 1873. Jeannette started wearing it as soon as she came out of mourning for Reggie. She then twice added more beads to the neck-lace, paying for them out of her spending money (a reasonably priced string cost 7s. 6d.) and at the height of the aesthetic fashion, 1879–82, wore her amber almost incessantly. The third requisite of aesthetic fashion, Morris wallpaper—or an imitation of it—had graced the third drawing room at No. 10 since 1877 (see p. 87).

She did not demur when in 1881 the weekly *Pictorial World* pub-lished an impressionistic sketch of her and Ada, in the dresses they had worn at the Grand International Bazaar held in aid of the Society of Friends of Foreigners in Distress late in June, over the caption 'Fair Aesthetes'. The pale yellow crèpe dress was a signal success. One of the advantages of aesthetic dress was its relative cheapness, and this aesthetic number fitted comfortably into Jeannette's restricted budget. Home-made, at next to no expense, of cotton bought at the 1880 John Lewis sale, it was the outfit in which the sisters were depicted in the group painting of Baroness Burdett-Coutts' garden party given in honour of the 1881 International Medical Congress, and in which Jeannette and Ada were photographed in 1882.[14] Jeannette thought this likeness of herself at twenty-seven 'really good & not by any means hideous'. She described it in some detail: 'I stand in a very haughty attitude with my arms folded, & an expression of entire nonchalance & contempt of the world in general wh. is quite a surprise to <u>me</u>. A. says it is just like me, & P. says I look as though I had just

[12] Elizabeth Wordsworth, *Glimpses of the Past* (London, 1913), p. 149.

[13] For details of Jeannette's aesthetic wardrobe see Zuzanna Shonfield, 'Miss Mar-shall and the Cimabue Browns', *Costume* (Journal of the Costume Society), xiii, 1979, pp. 62–72.

[14] The artist of the painting, now in the Wellcome History of Medicine Museum, was A. P. Tilt and it was painted from photographs; Jeannette's and Ada's successful likenesses were taken for that purpose.

dismissed an old beau I did not care about!' She was so pleased about it that she condescended to note that Ada's photograph was very nice indeed.

While Jeannette was amused by the 'artistics' and looked to some of them for lessons on what to read and how to dress or how to furnish one's house, she (and her mother and sister too) got little else from the contact with the avant-garde. They did not appear to notice, and they certainly showed no desire to emulate, the loyalty and devotion of the circle round Rossetti and Brown, nor the easy, unstinting warmth characteristic of the London Greeks.[15] No. 10 Savile Row might have been a happier place if some of this liberating generosity had rubbed off, if not on Ellen then on the young Marshalls. Instead, all three, Jeannette, Ada and young John, were, for the time being, in the early 1880s, caught between the uncertainties of their parents, mainly matters of professional pride and of not being sure where you belonged, and their own assumptions of superiority and self-sufficiency. Friends, suitors, good matches would seek them out, they believed. What they failed to recognize was that they might be handicapped through the very fact that they were all (with the exception of the father) bad at giving. Their stinginess manifested itself in the strained family relationships, in the meagre circle of intimate friendships, in the lack of political or charitable involvement. Too mean to pay the club subscription, too timid to take the plunge into unfamiliar social circles, they were left in a curious limbo.

[15] See George du Maurier's appreciative comments on the Ionides connection in three letters to his mother (June 1860 and January 1861) quoted in *The Young George du Maurier*, Daphne du Maurier ed. (London, 1951), p. 5 ff.

CHAPTER 10

THE OUTSIDER

HER brother John had become sufficient of an obsession to Jeannette to figure almost daily in her diaries of the 1880s. Her accounts convey above all else an impression of someone born a century too soon into a setting where less store was set on personal fulfilment that on achievement measured in terms of accepted labels and honours. Had he been our contemporary, the vocabulary of psychoneurosis and such concepts as alienation would have been used to describe his condition.

In his late 'teens some of this condition manifested itself in periods of hyperactivity which alternated with weeks, sometimes months, of debility. The earliest bout of physical prowess against a background of being below par was recorded during a holiday in 1876, when he was eighteen. Within a fortnight of arriving at Freshwater on the Isle of Wight, 'mealy-faced' after cramming intensively for an examination, he surprised his family by a twenty-five-mile hike with a fellow-student. Such route marches were repeated and lengthened until at the end of his first year at Cambridge he astounded them all by arriving home one mid-June morning at the beginning of the summer vacation after a walk 'fr. Cambridge having left there at 2 [p.m.] yesterday & been on his legs all night!' 'Stupid boy;' commented his sister, 'it is 60 miles! He seemed quite done up, & had had several adventures. A fellow idiot had accompanied him. He had a bath & breakfast, & then lay on his bed. He has burst a vein on his ancle, so is obliged to rest his leg.' When six months later he once again started a vacation 'having carried his portmanteau fr. the station' (presumably King's Cross or St Pancras), she called the exploit his 'latest fad', with no trace of understanding of the symbolic nature of these assertions of athletic maleness in a youth who as a child had suffered from a weakness in the legs.

The patches of ill-health, which contrast so noticeably with these feats of energy, first came in the wake of exceptionally hard work before tests or exams. As the years of his early manhood progressed, the pattern changed: spells of physical malaise and reduced vitality, 'dawdling about with his feet on the fender all day', became noticeable when stressful decisions or anxiety-provoking tests loomed ahead. After four terms at Cambridge the symptoms were sufficiently pronounced to give cause for anxiety:

We are a good deal worried about John. He looks pale & thin, and has a very bad appetite for a long boy of his age & size. He also seems very 'glum', and is occasionally unpleasant, and extremely contradictory. If any one says one thing, that is the very reason why he says the exact opposite. After dinner, because he eat [ate] very little & refused pudding, dessert etc., P. spoke very gravely to him & told him he wd. injure his health if he went on so, and to our surprise he began to cry! He can't be well, I am afraid. He certainly does not look so. It is a pity that he is so obstinate.

She continued to complain at intervals about his proneness to obstinacy and contrariness, but for a year or so there was nothing much in her diaries about the general state of his health.

Then in January 1879, after her brother's twenty-first birthday, Jeannette wrote that their father was once again worried about John, 'who behaves very badly, & seems to me as if he must have a screw loose.' A week or two later she returned to the subject:

He behaved in a very rude & disrespectful way to M., & at last was so insulting that she complained to P., who took him out in the carriage & gave him a good talking to. J. wept & sobbed like an infant of four, said no one liked him, that he wished he was dead, had been miserable for years, & so-forth, going on like one demented. He quite upset both P. & M. by his extraordinary behaviour. He now says he wishes to be a surgeon, but as this means another 6 years living on P., before he can even begin to hope to earn something, neither P. nor M. see the fun of it. I hope P. will make up his mind for him, & give him the choice between an artist's & lawyer's professions.

This was the first reference to John's future since the confident speculation about academic income and honours four years previously, when he had been about to sit for the Trinity scholarship. Now that he was of age the choice of career became pressing, and even more so when, in January 1880, the results of his finals were announced: 'he is a Senior Optime,[1] & No 23 in that class, wh. is not very high, but he has done his best & that's enough' wrote Jeannette, indulgent for once. This disappointing outcome put paid to the idea of a future fellowship. By this time all talk of an artistic career had also been

[1] Second class in Mathematical Tripos.

abandoned, though not before Marshall had introduced his son to several artist friends and other people in artistic circles, presumably to get their views of the lad's talent.

Within days of John's telegram announcing his Cambridge results, it was provisionally settled that he should become a barrister. The decision was most probably forced on him, for his sister noted that 'P. says he will keep him up to it; I only hope he will!' John's own suggestion, that he should study surgery, was never again mentioned in the diary, although it may still have floated around at this time, for on the next day Jeannette, in chronicling the debate on John's future, recorded that he had been that day to University College, 'making arrangements for classes as he is to prepare for the Science Tripos in June & December, & the 2nd BA at the London Univ. in October.' She added that she was thankful he would have something to do but hoped he would soon also be entered at the Temple. 'He will not make a penny for ever so long I am afraid.' The Bar option was confirmed a fortnight later, with Uncle William Marshall signing a bond for John at the Middle Temple, and the father himself enlisting the support of three legal acquaintances to get his son accepted.

When they decided to turn John into a barrister the thought may have been at the back of the Marshalls' minds that this choice would consolidate the family's standing on the professional ladder. As a category barristers ranked higher than medical men, and the foremost barristers especially, much higher than even the most successful sur-geons. It was also, given John's age, the more practical step. As it turned out, the idea was a complete failure. All the evidence of the next six years confirms that the choice was imposed on him against his wish and that he did not try (or perhaps tried and failed) to overcome his reluctance for the law. The pattern which had established itself in the early terms at Trinity now accelerated. His sister wrote of glum inactivity and escape into frequent bouts of ill-health. This delayed the taking of exams; once, in 1882, he did not turn up for the oral part of a test, thus failing the exam altogether. By the time he was called to the Bar in January 1886, not only John but also his family had given up any thought of him ever practising law.

In the wake of this inadequate performance came trouble of a dif-ferent kind. As the parents and sisters openly voiced their disapproval and disappointment, so John's behaviour at home became increasingly uncouth, with the main force of his aggression turned against Mrs Marshall. In 1881 and early 1882 Jeannette reported three major clashes between mother and son, and hinted at many more, with John being 'horribly hateful', and insulting to his mother 'as usual'. Nor was Ellen Marshall particularly adept at handling the situation. She cried and complained to her husband and, like Marshall himself, treated her adult son as a child. But at this point the father, at least, used fairly restrained terms to describe his son's behaviour; he spoke of John's 'lack of affection, gratitude, & a sense of duty'. However, he also hinted that these might all turn out to be signs of underlying mental instability.

In early July 1882 matters reached crisis point: 'Fr. a letter M. found', wrote Jeannette, without explaining whose letter it was nor how it came into Ellen Marshall's possession, 'there is no doubt that J. is not only most rude, insulting & disagreeable, but filthy & disgusting in every way into the bargain.' Perhaps she had not been told the details of her mother's discovery; at any rate she added nothing more specific on the subject. However, soon after the incident of the letter the parents cut John's allowance and decided that he must no longer live at home. Arrangements were made for him to move in with Mr Horton, who was Vice-Master of University College School during the years when John had been a pupil there.

There followed an unhappy period during which John, after the almost immediate failure of the Horton scheme, tried sharing rooms with several of his college friends in turn. That these set-ups kept breaking down was to be expected, since recent graduates are often volatile in their living arrangements and friendships. What was less usual was that first Mr Horton and later two or three of John's own friends, after initial bouts of enthusiasm, soon professed themselves disillusioned with his wayward behaviour. Indeed, Jeannette reported that Mr Horton, who combined the function of host with that of coach (the intention being that John should prepare for exams under Horton's supervision), called his guest 'a nightmare' within some three weeks of his moving in.

As to John's own choice of friends Jeannette, for one, was scathing. In July 1882, at the time of the letter from which they had concluded that John was 'filthy & disgusting in every way', she reflected: 'He has evidently got a set of vile friends who give him very bad advice.' And each time she now met her brother's Cambridge contemporaries she found little or nothing to their credit; everything about them—looks, comportment, intellectual capacity—came in for a lashing. Some she declared immature, others too old for their years, others still altogether too grown-up both in age and in manner. Several were indeed approaching middle age; what she did not appreciate was that one or two of these more mature men in John's Cambridge set, such as Sidney Colvin and Walter Raleigh, whom he brought home alongside the newly graduated, were on their way to becoming acclaimed men of letters. And because she did not attach any importance to them, she failed to discover the nature and strength of their relationships with John.

The situation continued to worsen for two years, with John at times completely at odds with and absent from Savile Row for months at a stretch, and then, when tempers simmered down, visiting home several times a week. In mid-February 1884, after some weeks of such an attempt at reconciliation, came another crisis. A week or two previously John and Davey, a friend with whom he happened to share rooms at that particular time, moved to Hampstead. The new domestic arrangements had already earned them a black mark: 'they actually sleep in the same room! They are two disgusting, good-for-nothing, lazy wretches!' Then, on 14 February, Mrs Marshall received a packet which so hurt her feelings that all attempt at a dialogue between mother and son was effectively cut. The offending missive consisted of 'a Valentine in the shape of an old rusty screw in a box, & inside is a scrap of paper with "You are, you know you are a —" '.

The authorship of this valentine held no secret for Jeannette: 'We all are pretty sure it comes fr. J., and are in a more disgusted frame of mind with him than ever. P. sent him a note the first thing this morning to postpone his visit, as he says he cd. not sit at table with him till the matter is cleared up. The writing is wonderfully like J.'s, and we think the box in wh. the screw was sent is the very one M. gave him the gold pin in! Awfully low insult, I think! He & Davey together, probably.'

Three weeks later Mrs Marshall and her daughters ran into John during their customary walk. Ada, who like her father was inclined to be conciliatory, bowed. Mrs Marshall 'did not see'. Jeannette, it would appear from the very fact that she did not note her own reaction, cut him dead.

The affair of the valentine was never entirely clarified. Victor de Rivaz, a friend of Marshall's, who acted as something of an intermediary between John and his parents, and who was an amateur graphologist, declared the handwriting to be John's. When eventually tackled by Marshall, John first denied all knowledge of the matter, and 'was very insulting & in a white rage'. In his anger he exclaimed that he would take no more money from his father. 'So much the better' commented Jeannette. He perhaps thought better of his threat because later on the same day he called again and, after exchanging a couple of messages, was admitted to his father's presence. This time he said he thought he knew who had sent the screw. 'So do I!' wrote his sister. It is not clear if she, or indeed her parents, reflected on the hidden message of the valentine. Had John not repeatedly accused his father and mother of tight-fistedness, one's guess would be that the symbolic screw was chosen solely for its sexual connotations. As it is, there remains an ambiguity about the exact meaning of the offensive missive.

Rivaz, discouraged as most other friends who had tried to help, soon withdrew from the case, advising the parents to 'let John go', as he was never going to be a credit to anyone. 'He has found John out, thinks he is a blackguard, & told him so.' The *coup de grâce* in this instance had been the son describing his father as a liar, and a cipher in his own home.

Marshall had long since returned to the idea, which he had mooted some two or three years earlier, that John was mentally unstable. There had in particular been an episode lasting ten days or so in 1881 when John had shown great excitement about a philological theory of his which he thought would 'explain all philosophy, ethics, religion, language, besides proving everyone wrong, enabling anyone to master mathematics, law, every language . . .' At the time Jeannette had commented that his ravings were of such violence that it 'really may become very serious if his attention is not diverted in some way. P. is going to see what he can do, but is much worried.' And she continued on the next day: 'He is not quite so excited today, but has a very strange look & manner. P. says a stranger wd. really pronounce him mad!' Since then the father had once or twice thought he detected signs of suicidal tendencies in the young man. Marshall's assistant and shadow, Mr Castañeda, another friend who had volunteered help, added to these fears his own view that John was 'behaving like a hysterical girl'.

Perhaps because he saw his son as someone suffering from a sickness rather than as a sinner, Marshall never quite abandoned his naturally permissive manner towards the young man. There were of course occasions when he too became desperate. Jeannette's view was that some of the bouts of ill-health which hit Marshall in the 1880s were caused by strains brought on by John's behaviour; for instance, she surmised that a bad attack of gout in August 1884 was the result of her father learning from John's friend and new flat-mate, Bourne, that John 'is as full of vice as he can be'. At times Marshall became 'quite savage' about John's vagaries; despite all his tolerant liberalism he would despair of his son and express his disappointment and fears aloud: 'P. is quite depressed, & declares he [John] is not fit for the Bar, or any honourable profession.' But even during the worst periods of estrangement and non-communication the father would still on occasion arrange to meet the son, usually inviting him for a meal at the Metropole Hotel. And it was the father who advocated conciliatory moves and tried to find ways round John's apparent inability to become financially independent.

Of the women at No. 10, Ada was the only one who sympathized with the father's interpretation of John's vagaries, and who on occasion appeared to side with Marshall when he tried to get his tactics accepted by the rest of the family. Jeannette, and for the most part, her mother too, saw in John's aberrant behaviour nothing beside moral turpitude. In fact, Mrs Marshall for the most part diverged from her husband, advocating drastic punitive measures, especially where John's allowance and the repayment of his debts were concerned. The tension between the parents led to disagreements which at times bordered on major scenes: 'It is a wretched house, instead of a happy one, as it used to be.' On these occasions Jeannette changed sides according to which protagonist, father or mother, happened to be the more intransigent at the time.

The persistent disturbance at home threatened the even tenor of her life. The only escape route she knew or found acceptable led into marriage, but she did not put it beyond John's malice that he might try to put a spanner into the courtship works. Had he not some years ago caused her annoyance and pain by his uncalled-for comments about Mr Brown? 'J. was hateful as usual' she had written in August 1880, '& made some disgustingly rude & coarse remarks about Mr. B., & his not coming etc, wh. I was foolish enough to care about.' John was in any case not someone she wished to introduce to a prospective suitor; she did not think him incapable of cadging money from a comparative stranger. Since the failure of the Brown flirtation there had in fact been no one for whom she cared sufficiently, or who pursued her with enough fervour, to test these fears. For the moment she raged and ranted, deeply frustrated at home and not within sight of getting away:

'I do declare I feel sometimes as though I wd. accept any reasonable offer!'

The years of the John débâcle were bleak in other ways. There were three deaths in the family in less than two years—Aunt Julia, Uncle Charles Marshall and Uncle Startin. None of these deaths hit Savile Row emotionally. Nevertheless, losing Aunt Julia seemed equivalent to giving up the social amenities of Hill House. For several years to come contact with Ely faded; all that remained was an occasional snatched visit to Uncle William and to his widowed sister, Aunt Wilkes (Wilkinson), who came to keep house for him. It was not until 1886 that the Ely habit was re-established, and then only in a modified, curtailed form. 'I must say Ely is not exciting now' wrote Jeannette at the end of a visit over Easter 1887. 'Still I have a weakness for the poor old place, and like to be here for a short time.'

No more dances, and, at least for a time, no more ogling in the cathedral and at Deanery socials. After 1883 several of the Ely potential suitors all but vanished from the diaries. Harold Archer was married. John Swift by the early 1880s qualified as a surgeon and left Ely permanently; Jeannette thought he had 'gone off', and on seeing him from afar at a private view in Suffolk Street in 1888 declared that he looked 'dreadfully common & vulgar' and that she 'shd. not have cared to be seen speaking to him'. The Bidwells, the Luddingtons, also no longer figured; some were engaged, some married, and in any event she had never thought any of them interesting except as dancing partners. Only Martin Pate remained faithful, throwing glances at her over the cathedral hymn-book, or riding by, a stalwart figure on a stalwart horse, to make her speculate what being married to a rich farmer would be like. Still, the possibility of Jeannette marrying into Ely, which had earlier tantalized Aunt Julia, now tantalized Aunt Wilkes, and to an even greater extent, Ada.

As once before in the '70s, after Grandmother Williams's death, unproductive holidays contributed to the social hiatus of the recent bereavements. In 1884 they travelled in Scandinavia, visiting Sweden and Norway after the International Medical Congress had brought them to Copenhagen. The journey, in the course of which they covered much ground not usually included in such family holidays, was a touristic success but a complete failure in terms of meeting eligible bachelors or widowers. It ended with a call on Aunt Startin's daughter,

Eliza Nyström, in Göteborg, who in the best Startin manner had nine children to show to her London relatives. A year later they had stayed in the British Isles and moved speedily through the Lake District, Scotland and Yorkshire, never resting long enough in any one place to make friends; besides, British hotels lacked the relaxed atmosphere that helped to break the ice in the alpine resorts.

That winter Marshall found time for a winter vacation, taking his wife and daughters to the South of France for a holiday in the sun. A patient, Mrs Richardson, invited them to spend Christmas and New Year's Day in her house, Villa Zima, two miles outside Cannes. They travelled in style, taking a *train de luxe* down to the Riviera and returning by sleeper, and enjoyed the new experience of meals in the restaurant car. But living in luxury was a tame excitement when it offered nothing in the way of marital openings. A Mr Woodroffe met at Mrs Richardson's proved to be a married man; it was just as well that Jeannette regarded flirting with him as only a *faute de mieux* occupation and remained relatively unmoved by his admiring glances.

Once or twice some latent ambivalence about the prospect of marriage worked its way to the surface. After reporting a dream about being a married woman, she added a convoluted sentence about her misgivings on the subject: 'Not but what I shd. not want to be, if it were not for that disgusting boy, who really makes our lives a burden for us.' A little later, in yet another outburst about the wretched state of family affairs, she wrote: 'M. said the other day that she wd. like to see me married, though she wd. be sorry to lose me' and sighed stoically: 'At one time I thought I shd. be married, but now I think it most unlikely.'

The abrasions left by the frustrated involvement with Mr Brown were beginning to heal. Having decided that he must be engaged to the Jewish-looking woman in whose company she had seen him at the 1883 concert, Jeannette reaffirmed that she was now 'resignée or even content to settle down into an old maid . . .' That these were indeed sour grapes became clear when she added 'certainly Mr "Right" seems as far off as ever.' On the eve of her thirtieth birthday she wrote: 'Every dog has had its day, & I have had mine' and, after listing the names of fifteen admirers, added 'Kismet!' Then on the day itself she completed her reflections with a complacent 'I still wear well', reiterated that she was likely to remain single and, making a virtue of necessity, concluded: 'I prefer my liberty to the title of Mrs.'

There was by now something of the soured ageing spinster about

Jeannette's entire outlook. As a rule, she had never shown much concern for public affairs. Issues sporadically reported in the diaries —the women's cause, the Franco-Prussian War and the Commune, the Tichbourne trial or the Phoenix Park murders—elicited only a very few sentences. But now she no longer devoted quite so much space to the detail of everyday life, and her comment on general news became a little more regular. What she had to say was a curious amalgam of a superficial radicalism—a vestige perhaps of Mme Noël's influence— when it came to events abroad, and an out-and-out conservatism about what was happening in her own country. 'How disappointing!' she wrote on hearing that the March 1887 attempt on the life of Tsar Alexander III had failed. But when in February 1886 a clash of unemployed demonstrators with the police in Trafalgar Square ended in rioting which for three or four days convulsed the inhabitants of the West End, Jeannette's response bore witness to her ambivalence. After first reporting that the shuttered shopfronts and the crowds of sight-seers contributed to a 'most curious Bank holiday effect' in the streets of the capital, she concluded grimly: 'Really, London will be uninhabitable if this goes on.'[2]

Meanwhile there had been new developments concerning John. Though Jeannette probably did not recognize it, and certainly did not admit it, the crisis and estrangement of 1884–5 marked the beginning of a process of emancipation, with John gradually becoming independent and the parents slowly letting him go his own way. Fearing a permanent withdrawal of financial support, or perhaps genuinely offended by the threat of it, he had some months after the fracas over the valentine made a pre-emptive move and in one or two stages taken his entire savings from the keeping of Uncle John and Uncle Edwin Williams. At about the same time he began taking on small jobs, a succession of coaching, holiday tutoring, and marking exam papers at University College: 'Rather him than me. I shd. think it must be very stupid work' wrote his sister about this last task. His total earnings were still paltry. Aged twenty-eight, a fully qualified barrister with two degrees after ten or eleven years' higher education, he was as yet incapable of earning more than a fraction of his keep. Although the

[2] Compare Jeannette's 'Bank holiday effect' with the 'utter panic' of *The Times* news column report on 11 February. Constance Woolson (see C. Benedict, *Constance Woolson, 1840–94*, London, 1932, p. 239) thought London during the days of the riots resembled the 'doomed Babylon'.

allowance had been stopped once or twice, Marshall continued to pay for most of his son's expenses. In addition, on several occasions John brought home unpaid accounts which his father had to clear. The debts were never enormous, a matter of £30 or £50 at a time; the payment of them was an irritation rather than a heavy burden.

It is not clear whether it was John or someone else in the family who first conceived the idea of a job abroad. Jeannette had once or twice mentioned in desperation Australia (her own idea of the other end of the world) and New Zealand (her mother's) as sufficiently distant exiles for her reprobate brother. In 1882 there had been some talk of a dragomanship[3] at the end of his law studies, which would take him right out of the country. This idea was revived soon after he had been called to the Bar, and over a period of nearly three years Marshall and John himself tried to enlist the help of friends and acquaintances to find work overseas. There were one or two near-misses: after some talk of the post of secretary to a judge in Hyderabad and a well-paid lectureship in Canada, John was interviewed for neither.

Eventually he made do with something a great deal less ambitious. In 1888 he decided to accept a four months' engagement as private secretary in St Petersburg (the total pay to be £35 with presumably everything found), and to look for something more permanent once he became established there. There followed some tense weeks, with John on the brink of going, but delaying his departure from one day to the next. When at the end of June he finally made up his mind he wasted no time on farewells. It was from his flat-mate Bourne, met accidentally at the Botanic Fête in South Kensington, that Jeannette, who had been waiting impatiently for the confirmation of her brother's departure, learnt that there had been no last-minute hitch, and that John had safely left for Russia.

[3] Dragoman: interpreter or professional guide in the Middle East.

CHAPTER 11

AT THE PEAK

'P. was examining at the Coll. of Surgs, so I did not see him after the usual morning visit' wrote Jeannette on the fifth day of the measles which had laid her low in the spring of 1881. 'I hear he has caught a cold, wh. is a very great pity' she continued. 'He is dreadfully careless. M. tells me his income last year was between four & five thousand. Very comfortable too!'[1]

She was, at twenty-five, considered old enough to be apprised of the family's exact financial standing. Earlier, there had been hints of increasing affluence, usually after some bonanza: a cheque for £400 in recompense for Marshall's ministrations to a rich Cambridgeshire patient in 1872, a fruitful day's takings in London of £20 plus in 1874. But never a computation of a whole year's earnings, until now when Ellen could boast on her husband's behalf that he was well within reach of the high flyers in the medical profession.

The top men commanded incomes two or three times as great. They were mostly the fashionable physicians and just a few surgeons with a reputation for the skilful performance of complex and delicate procedures. The laryngologist Morell Mackenzie who attended Queen Victoria's son-in-law, Frederick William, the crown prince of Prussia, in his terminal illness, was in that category. Writing in July 1888, weeks after Frederick (who had succeeded his father as emperor in March that year) had died of throat cancer, Jeannette reported that 'Mackenzie got 50 guineas a day & £1000 for each operation. Not bad pay.'[2] But the circumstances under which he earned these fees were unique. Of some 15,000 medicals, only a very small number, say no more than

[1] Income tax in 1880, at 5*d.* in the pound on incomes of over £150, reduced Marshall's earnings by no more than £100. In terms of 1986 value, his annual *net-of-tax* income was in the £125,000–£150,000 band.

[2] The same entry, on 9 July 1888, reported gossip which accused the German crown princess (Queen Victoria's eldest daughter) and Morell Mackenzie of fraudulently suppressing the terminal character of Frederick William's complaint in order not to prejudice his succession to the imperial throne.

twenty, were in that class, with incomes ranging from £5,000 to £12,000 a year.[3] To be, as Marshall was, a runner-up, was beyond doubt amply sufficient. His income corresponded to his status at the top of the medical establishment and put him squarely into the upper regions of the upper middle class.[4]

Marshall respected money. If a well-off patient was tardy in paying the surgeon's fee, a lawyer's letter would be dispatched to extract what was due. But nowhere in the diaries was there evidence of that 'near-obsession with income and fees'[5] which has been ascribed to late-Victorian doctors. His current income would have seemed adequate to him; he and his kind, who postponed fulfilling their social aspirations till late in their careers, found it difficult to expand their relatively frugal demands in line with their rocketing earnings.

Somewhere between £1,000 and £2,000 a year lay the line between middle-class comfort and gentlemanly ease for a professional man with a wife and three adult children to his charge. Even during their son's years at Cambridge, the Marshalls' expenditure was not much above the mid-point of this scale. Complaining about being over-charged, at 11s. 9d. per head a day [£18 currently] for full board and lodging, in the hotel in Freshwater where they stayed in August 1876 and fed exclusively on mutton, Jeannette had written 'We have been living very simply, more so than at home . . .'; she clearly thought of their own fare as plain, and nothing she recorded in later years pointed to any improvement. In many other respects—only three indoor servants, the daughters' modest allowances—they continued to conform to the style set by the much lower income on which Ellen and John had managed while the children were still in the nursery. Even their contributions to charity were economical, usually in the form of labour-intensive efforts, embroidery for sales of work, simple home-made garments for distribution to orphans, rather than in cash. True, there was some regular assistance for one or two impoverished dependants of the

[3] See W. J. Reader, *Professional Men—The Rise of the Professional Classes in Nineteenth-Century England* (London, 1966), p. 200 (quoting T. H. S. Escott) and F. B. Smith, *The People's Health*, 1830–1915 (London, 1979).

[4] According to Harold J. Perkin, *The Origins of Modern English Society*, 1780–1880 (London, 1972), whose figures are based on those of the Victorian statistician R. D. Baxter (*The Taxation of the UK*, 1869), in the late 1860s some 30,000 families—or just less than 0.5 per cent of the total—had incomes of £1,000 or more. Of these about 4,500 families were in the £5,000 plus category. With Ellen's personal investment income added to John Marshall's professional one, the Savile Row Marshalls were in the early 1880s near the borderline of this top income group.

[5] See Peterson, op. cit., p. 222.

Williamses, and, occasionally, succour for a former domestic who had fallen on bad times; there were the shillings and half-crowns given to causes sponsored by neighbours and friends; but none of this amounted to very much. Sixpences were Jeannette's and Ada's usual contribution to the collection at St James's; they came out of their father's pocket, being additional to the regular issue of spending money (even when the plate went round on 'Hospital' Sunday, in mid-June, Jeannette's donation, raised to 2s. in aid of a charity of which she wholeheartedly approved, actually originated from Marshall).[6] The ten guineas which Marshall subscribed in 1887 to the Imperial Institute building fund in celebration of Victoria's Jubilee was about as high as his beneficence went during the years of real affluence.

Foreign travel was the one luxury the Marshalls allowed themselves regularly. Often they marvelled at the excellent value of hotels and meals abroad; at Macugnaga in 1875, the cost of full pension was only seven francs a day, though a few days later at Bellagio they paid twelve francs exclusive of wine. But some of their exploits were exorbitant by middle-class standards. In 1874 the estimated cost of hiring a horse carriage for an excursion to Italy through the Gotthard Pass was five pounds a day. The *train de luxe* they took from Calais to Cannes in December 1885 set them back £5 1s. 9d. per place, 'wh. I call very extravagant' commented Jeannette. Quite often they in fact travelled 2nd or even, on local runs in France, 3rd class, 'as carriages abroad are so good'.

Being careful in one's expenditure they saw as among the prime virtues, and considered profligacy as almost the paramount vice. They were certain that extravagance would in the end be invariably punished. Jeannette had been really shocked when in the late 1870s the Edwin Williamses spent at the rate of £5,000–£6,000 a year. The downfall, in 1887, with the Williams firm losing £6,000, she had already discounted; it provoked only a brief 'I am sorry for them' in the diary. But it was the Startins whom Jeannette regarded as really shiftless. She wrote of the widowed Aunt Sarah Startin who in 1887 still had three or four daughters and an epileptic son, Edward, to her charge: 'I do not think she is keeping within her £500 a year! She has not a notion of economy.' The Startins were removing to the West Country, and £500 was considered ample for provincial respectability. So when there was talk of cousin Connie Startin 'going out as "lady

[6] The church collections on 'Hospital' Sunday were destined for hospital funds.

help" ', Jeannette grumbled: 'Absurd idea! One wd. think they were paupers, when they are comfortably off, if they wd. only be careful . . . I really feel sorry for A.S. [Aunt Startin] when I see her, she is so helpless, but when I think of her, she riles me!' Despite his own easy way with money, Uncle Edwin joined the Marshalls in deploring that Sarah Startin had in fact spent £800–£900 in 1886, and saved only £200; he had good reason to lament, as his sister's shortfall had to be made good out of his pocket.

Some of Marshall's colleagues, either themselves rich or aping the rich to good effect, went in for conspicuous consumption. His exact contemporary Thomas Spencer Wells could be seen on fine days in his flashy phaeton, wearing a light-coloured coat and a tall white hat—ostentatious garb when the medical man's usual attire was a sober black frock-coat with a black topper. In the 1890s another acquaintance of the Marshalls, the successful chest specialist Edmund Symes-Thompson, with a house in Cavendish Square, kept seven indoor servants, beside nursery staff, gardener, groom and coachman. Both he and Wells acquired second homes, the former in Oxfordshire, the latter at Golders Green in particularly beautiful grounds. A few medical men accumulated excellent art collections. Henry Thompson collected contemporary paintings and Chinese ceramics. Ernest Hart and also William Anderson (who eventually succeeded Marshall in the chair of anatomy at the Royal Academy) specialized in Japanese art. But these were exceptions. Like Marshall, most medical men used the high surplus earnings of the peak years of their career to build up reserves for the lean years of retirement.

When Trollope wrote of Mortimer Gazebee, the flourishing solicitor who had married into the aristocracy, that 'no effort on his wife's part . . . could have forced him to spend more than two-thirds of his income',[7] it was not novelist's licence that made him fix on that figure, but close acquaintance with the habits and exigencies of professional life. Once the early years of upward struggle had been left behind, savings at something approaching Mr Gazebee's rate allowed a man to look forward to a secure old age for himself and his wife, with, perhaps, a trifle left over for the heirs. To lay aside £300 out of an income of £1,000 was not uncommon (see p. 195). Even out of a salary of £700 the economist Alfred Marshall (no relative of the surgeon),

---

[7] Anthony Trollope, *The Small House at Allington* (London, 1864), xlvi.

first Principal of Bristol's University College in the late 1870s, managed to save at the rate of £200 a year, and could still afford an annual holiday of two months abroad for himself and his wife.

Contributory pension schemes were virtually unknown in the nineteenth century. Moreover, the London professionals usually lived in rented accommodation, accumulating no capital in the form of appreciating freeholds or leaseholds. If at first sight their rates of saving appear enormously high, the successful professional who today buys future security, paying for it with his mortgage, his own and his employer's contributions to pension schemes and national insurance, plus life insurance and various other forms of voluntary savings, is almost certainly saving at a higher rate than his Victorian confrère, out of a much smaller income. That John Marshall chose to save not one-third but two-thirds of his peak income was in line with the prudence which had characterized the Marshalls' expenditure throughout their married life. It would have been unreasonable to change to more sumptuous ways now, when he was not certain how much longer he would be able to work a sixty- or seventy-hour week, with professional duties that spilled over into evenings and Sundays.

The chronic gout and the attacks of breathlessness that dogged his winters precluded long hours at the operating table, and surgery proper became by middle age a relatively minor side of his activities. Instead, he devoted an increasing proportion of his time to consultancy work, and was appointed consulting surgeon at the Brompton Consumption Hospital in 1876 and at his own University College Hospital, in 1884. And indeed, the private patients who came to consult him at Savile Row mostly sought out not the surgeon but the wise and tolerant general practitioner.

He had in any case never developed the sort of speciality which betokens the outstanding surgeon.[8] Medical historians report him to have been clever at the excision of varicose veins and to have been the first to introduce galvano-cautery to English surgical practice, but for neither achievement did he receive wider acclaim. In 1883 he attempted to promote his one contribution to surgical innovation, in

---

[8] Lister's nephew, Rickman Godlee, may have succumbed to a family bias when he wrote that Marshall's reputation was 'rather that of a scientific man with good business capacity than a distinguished surgeon' (see H. H. Bellot, *University College, London, 1826–1926*, London, 1929, p. 348). By contrast, among his Pre-Raphaelite friends Marshall's surgical skills stood in high renown, not least for having saved the life of the critic F. G. Stephens by a timely tracheotomy performed in 1878.

the Bradshaw Lecture on 'Neurectasy or nerve-stretching'. His daughter's diary records that in May 1884 he went to Bath to carry out a nerve-stretching operation. There may have been others. But by the time the lecture appeared in print it was 1887, too late to change the course of his career.

Twenty-odd years at Marlborough House and South Kensington, nearly two decades of lectures and demonstrations at the Royal Academy—proof, one would think, that Marshall was an inspired teacher. Jeannette once or twice wrote that, at the Academy, the students were 'wild' in their enthusiasm about her father's lectures. But at least one of his early medical students later admitted that he had slept through much of Marshall's course: 'He was a good friend to me, and I had a great respect and liking for him. But he was the most uninspiring teacher that I ever sat under.'

The voice that countered this assault spoke, moderately, of informative and thought-provoking teaching by the cultured, critical and scientific surgeon, ever ready to try paths of new knowledge; his talent for illustrating the subject-matter by blackboard drawings was not forgotten. But even this vindication did not deny that Marshall's delivery had been monotonous nor that chesty wheezing often impeded his enunciation.[9]

Where he shone was in the field of medical politics. Polite yet determined, he was a useful ally in the pursuit of institutional change. So there was never a time from 1872 on (when he began a two-year spell as dean of the medical school of University College Hospital) when his leisure was not eroded by university or professional committees 'that only squabble when they are called', and by 'wretched' meetings with 'horrible' discussions which went on till the early hours of the morning. At intervals Jeannette would mention the subject under discussion. In 1876 it was the 'horrid scheme of amalgamating Univ. Coll. and Middlesex Hospitals'. 'The medical staff is up in arms about it' she reported, and indeed the project fell through. Two years

9 Edward Sharpey Schafer (op. cit.) was once again the attacker; he had never quite forgiven Marshall for his victory over Lister in 1866; see also on p. 3, his derogatory remarks about Marshall's operating technique. Marshall's champion was John Tweedy, in a letter to the *Lancet*, 27 October 1923, pp. 1007–8; he contended that the views he expressed had also been those of the brilliant medical student James Stanton Cluff (1839–69), who had copied Marshall's lectures. But the biographer of Victor Horsley also referred to Marshall's lectures being 'dull in content' and 'delivered in an inaudible and feeble voice to a sleeping audience' (see J. B. Lyons, *The Citizen Surgeon*, London, 1966, p. 16).

later she grumbled about the 'everlasting conjoint scheme', the proposal to hold joint examinations of the two Royal Colleges, of Physicians and of Surgeons; another eight years went by before her father
'much rejoiced that the Conjoint Scheme had passed'. The most
radical and time-consuming of these campaigns started in the middle
1880s after Marshall had held two prestigious presidential offices, at
the Medico-Chirurgical Society and the Royal College of Surgeons. It
took several months of preliminaries till Marshall announced in March
1885 that he had agreed to become the Treasurer of the Committee of
the Teaching University. 'We are much interested in seeing the
subscriptions come in, for wh. M. sends out receipts.'[10] Eventually,
Jeannette too was co-opted, to help balance the Committee's accounts.
She enjoyed these small tasks she could carry out for her father. They
helped to put flesh on to the mysterious negotiations which went on
over the dining-room table and which banished the women into the
unheated drawing-room quarters. Using the new copier to reproduce
the committee's memoranda was also fun: 'I am quite mistress of the
"cyclostyle" now' she boasted in 1887. 'P. says my work is much better
than that done at the College!'

His achievement was not all to do with patients and students and
committee work. Marshall also sought longer-term fulfilment, apply-
ing his experience and common sense to the intricacies of hospital
architecture. The first sign of an interest in this field was an experiment in ward ventilation which he devised and successfully tried out at
UCH in the course of 1877. It must have been part of a more
ambitious programme, for in 1878 his daughter noted: 'P. is very busy
over plans for a new hospital. He thinks of having the wards in circular
towers, a very novel idea.' A few weeks later he summarized his
concept of the circular ward layout in a paper which was read at the
annual meeting of the Ladies' Sanitary Association in October 1878
and which, his daughter believed, excited a good deal of notice and
polemic: 'by each post he gets letters about it. Opinions vary much, but
some are very enthusiastic in its favor.' Two or three months later
came a setback: 'P. hears that some foreigner has had the idea of

[10] The idea of converting London University from an examining and degree-granting
body into a full-blown academic institution with direct control over a corpus of university
professors and lecturers had been mooted for many decades, with the historian George
Grote, a friend and neighbour of Marshall's, as one of its earliest promoters. The revival
of the scheme in the mid-1880s did not start bearing fruit until 1898, well after
Marshall's death.

Circular Hospitals too, & that one is actually being constructed at Antwerp. Rather tiresome.' By the autumn of 1884 when the Marshalls broke their return journey from a holiday in Germany and Austria to inspect the completed Antwerp project, they had forgotten their initial irritation. Marshall, especially, was 'enchanted' to see his 'pet idea' in operation. In England, meanwhile, the circular ward scheme had been taken up by the architect Henry Saxon Snell.[11] In time four hospital buildings utilized the circular ward idea. Marshall went to the openings of the first three, at Greenwich, Burnley and St Leonards, but did not attend the inauguration of the fourth, in Liverpool; it took place in 1890, by which time the seventy-two year-old surgeon had become distinctly less mobile.

When still young, John Marshall had given much of his leisure to forward-looking liberal causes, and had at times strayed on to bohemian byways. This, on top of his idiosyncratic career as the artists' anatomist, no doubt delayed his progress to the top. Distinctions, and the resulting affluence, came when he was already in his middle sixties and each winter brought warnings of failing health. The chain of high honours started in 1883 with the presidency of the Royal College of Surgeons and would finish in 1890 when he became an MD Honoris Causa of Trinity College, Dublin. In 1885 he was chosen to deliver the Hunterian Oration, of which Ford Madox Brown later ventured (with characteristic inability to get words to do his bidding) that it placed Marshall 'at the highest round' of his 'ambitious ladder'.[12]

As in his younger days, contemporaries and near-contemporaries had once again beaten him in the race for such prizes. Inevitably, John Erichsen, his past rival at University College Hospital, overtook Marshall, each time by three years, in becoming president of the Royal College of Surgeons and of the Medico-Chirurgical Society. Spencer Wells, another surgeon of the 1818 vintage, was chosen to deliver the Hunterian oration in 1883, two years before Marshall. As for the dignity of the summit of the combined medical establishments, that was blocked by Henry Acland, who, having become president of the General Medical Council in 1874, did not relinquish the post until 1887.

Marshall was not without some vanities and would have dearly liked the knighthood or baronetcy which was the manifest due of men who

---

[11] In *Charitable and Parochial Establishments* (London, 1881).
[12] Letter from Ford Madox Brown dated 2.5.1885, in the Marshall collection of autographs at Exeter University Library.

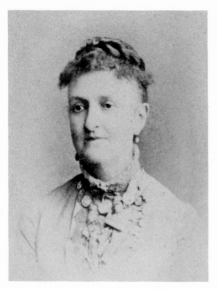

Ellen

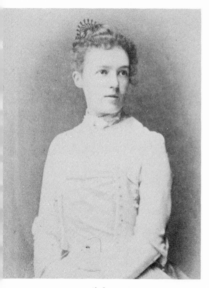

Ada

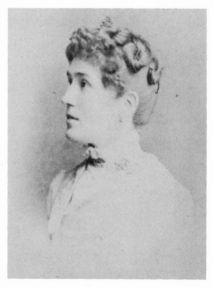

Jeannette

12. The Marshall ladies in Jubilee dress

Evening dresses, finished in May 1887. Ellen's was made by a dressmaker, Jeannette and Ada made theirs at home. 'The short skirt of cream alpaca edged with box-pleated flounce, with a long apron draped à la Marguerite one side, full back with pleated sides, and one side a panel of cream moiré & plush ribbon, on the other a knot & two long ends of the same tipped with pearl tassels, & with a row of pearl buttons below; the waistcoat is covered with a full front of cream satin. The sleeves are of ribbon up to the elbow, & thence of canvas fastened down with pearl buttons & with pearl tassels at the elbow. Collar of ribbon. Pink ribbon round neck & sleeves, finished with small bows. Tiny pink aigrette & comb in hair, cream silk gloves.'

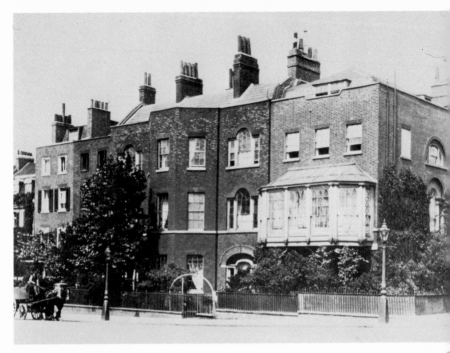

13. Belle Vue House; '. . . the Cheyne Walk house is ours at £850! So the deed is done!
I must say it is a great relief to all of us, and it is a very good bargain, as we all like it so.'

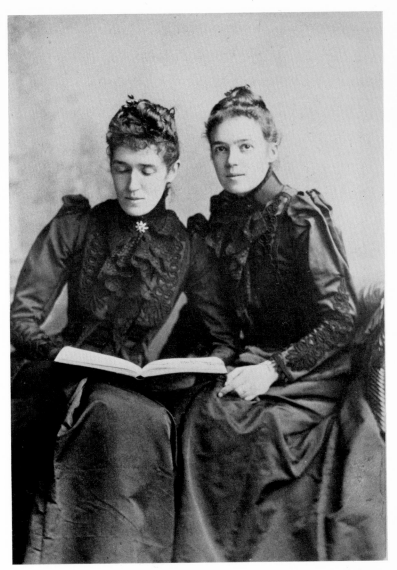

14. Jeannette and Ada, in second mourning for their father. The 'best' silk dresses were bought ready made, probably from Peter Robinson. 'Plain skirt with narrow passementerie on hem, coat bodice, tabbed behind, & long in front, edged same passementerie, & with long ornaments on the skirt, revers & sleeves, wh. are full above & tight below. Blk. silk waistcoat with full jabot of blk. guipure lace; quilled lace in neck & wrists . . .'

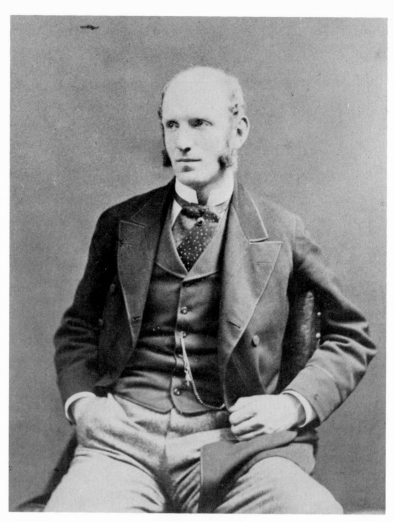

15. Dr Edward Seaton, 'kindness itself'.

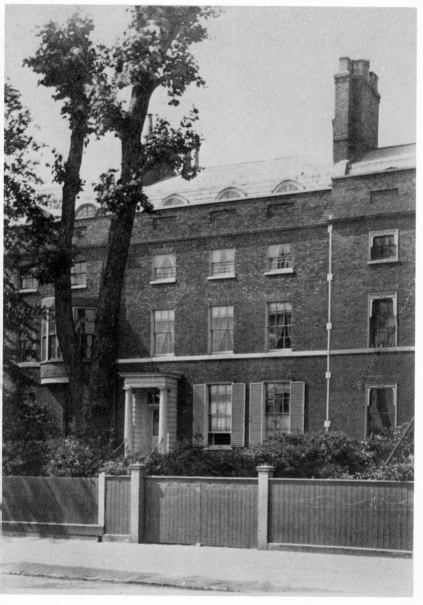

16. The Limes, Clapham Common: 'We were all fascinated by that dear old place, & I shd. like it most absolutely.'

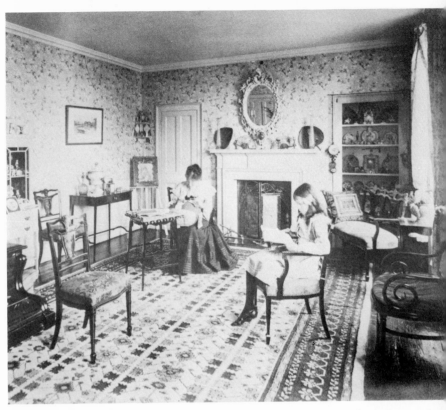

17. The drawing room at The Limes at the turn of the century, its furniture presaging Edwardian fashion.

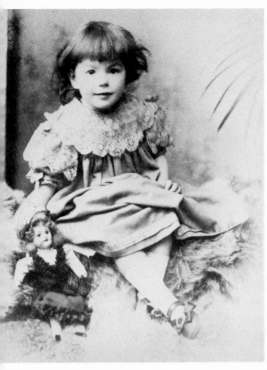

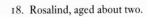
18. Rosalind, aged about two.

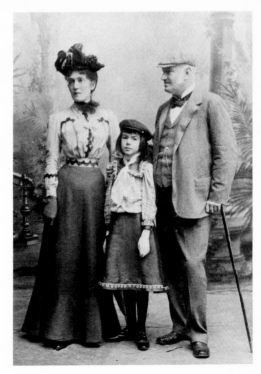

19. On holiday in Germany, *c.*1900.

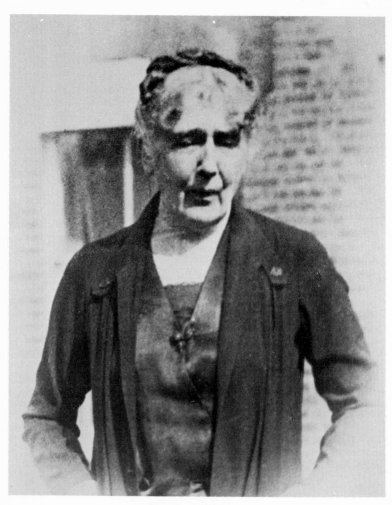

20. Jeannette in her seventies.

had reached high rank in the profession. But surgeons were relatively low down in the queue and some, with no useful strings to pull or just unlucky, waited for their title till the very end of their career. Of Marshall's exact contemporaries, Spencer Wells became a baronet in 1883, but Erichsen had to wait for his baronetcy till 1895. James Paget, who was four years older, had been appointed surgeon extraordinary to the Queen at the age of forty-four and was given a baronetcy at fifty-seven, in 1871. All three had been presidents of the Royal College of Surgeons before Marshall. There was clearly no rule about the granting of titles, though having the sort of speciality which recommended one for court appointments certainly helped.[13]

Marshall wanted a court appointment not only for the enhanced status that went with it, but also because it put a medical man within reach of the highest fees. Back in 1874, at the first signs of chronic ill-health, he had contemplated streamlining his hospital and College work to concentrate on the private practice and the professorship at the Royal Academy. However, on the advice that such a drastic change of direction would close the door to a royal appointment, he carried on with both hospital and College, only to find that the coveted title of royal surgeon continued to elude him. The nearest he got to court circles was to be introduced to the Prince of Wales and to attend two of his levées. The initial introduction—and the first of many handshakes from the Prince—took place at the Royal College of Surgeons' dinner following on Paget's Hunterian oration in 1877; it got no more than a couple of lines in the diary. By contrast, the first of the two levées was an event announced in advance in February 1881 with the news that Marshall had ordered from Poole's a 'Court suit of great gorgeousness'; on the appointed day Jeannette described her father's ceremonial preparations just as if it had been herself or Ada primping for a ball. He lunched and dressed in front of the specially lit bedroom fire, and then came downstairs, seeming 'rather nervous and amused at his appearance & yet rather gratified too'. She herself thought he looked 'remarkably well' in the sombre get-up, black silk stockings, shining shoes, with a sword at his side and a cocked hat under his arm. The servants, she added, had been 'vastly amused' by the unprecedented scene.

[13] Peterson, op. cit., p. 204, holds that knighthoods were in the main awarded to medical men for military service and baronetcies for professional services to the Queen and the royal family. W. J. Reader, op. cit., p. 150, points out that Lister's barony was recommended largely for his 'general scientific work'.

For one at the top of the ladder Marshall remained engagingly unspoilt, with some of the spontaneity which had endeared him to the young artists in the Mornington Crescent days. Such impulsiveness made him intervene when, in an alpine resort, 'two English girls (ladies they say) disgraced themselves by dancing with the common men, & letting them hand them about'; and allowed him to volunteer a cure (in the shape of a pot of oleate of mercury) for the defacing skin complaint of a railway guard at Amsterdam station. There was no swagger about him. When in Ely, in 1884, he put on the presidential gown of the Royal College of Surgeons with the hood of the Edinburgh LL D he had been awarded on the occasion of that University's quincentenary, it was not to parade his status, but to amuse his assembled relatives.

For all his lack of pretension, when the mid-1880s found him still without court appointment or title, John Marshall decided to prod those in authority. In early 1886 Jeannette reported that 'P. spoke to old Acland at the Medical Council, as he talks of resigning in P's favour, about some little handle to go with it. I shd. like a K.C.B. [Knight Companion of the Bath]'. He also found time for a little canvassing on the side. Eventually, in 1887, in a postscript to a letter announcing his impending resignation from the General Medical Council, Acland asked: 'Wd. you accept a Baronetcy? From what you said once, I imagine you wd.' 'Of course P. is crazed' wrote Jeannette, 'but I think Sir H. [Henry Acland] such a "woofly" old thing that it may come to nothing, though he is hand in glove with Lord Salisbury. P. wrote he shd. be delighted if it did not involve putting aside any money for his successor. I must say that's the rub to me.' A week or so later she recorded that her father had breakfasted with Acland and others from the Medical Council at Limmer's Hotel[14] and that the Prime Minister had been there. But she did not mention the matter of the honours list again till a year later when her father was having a 'mysterious confab' with a friend about, thought Jeannette, the 'rubbishing title'. He must have got discouraged, for in his letter of 21 May 1890 congratulating Acland on his baronetcy (Acland had previously been made Companion of the Order of the Bath in 1883 and KCB in 1884) he wrote that while he still hoped for eventual recognition, he did not 'intend to "fash" ' himself about the matter.

As early as February 1886, a few weeks after their return from the unaccustomed winter holiday in Cannes, Jeannette had noted a

---

[14] In George Street, Hanover Square.

marked decrease in the number of her father's patients: 'I regret to say that P. has scarcely anything to do just now! Whether it is the depression in trade, or the impression that he is still abroad, I don't know, but hope a change for the better will come soon.' The increasingly frequent bouts of bronchitis and gout meant that he was often not available to people who wished to consult him professionally, and that in turn discouraged some potential patients from trying to obtain his services. With the shrinking practice his income steadily decreased.

When in 1887 Marshall wrote to Acland that he would hesitate to accept a baronetcy if it entailed making special provision for his successor, the period of his peak earning had been too short to save a great capital sum, and while he had the reputation of being a shrewd man of business where the finances of University College Hospital or the Royal College of Surgeons were concerned, he was more casual about managing his own money matters. Occasionally, something he heard on his rounds would provoke him to action; for instance, in 1875 Jeannette reported that her father, concerned about the spate of bankruptcies that year, had been to his stockbrokers, Bragg Stockdale's, to confirm that his own investments were safe. Once reassured, he appeared to forget about them for a decade or more. Nor was there anyone in his circle whom he could usefully consult. His wife's brothers he considered as unreliable. His own brother William was himself a child when it came to money; he lost control over large sums he had lent out, and was careless even where the financial affairs of his clients were concerned; 1887 was in fact the year when his negligence landed him in jail and Marshall had to bail him out with a short-term loan of £1,000. The only sources of investment advice available to Marshall were either Mr Bartlett, his ultra-respectable solicitor, or his equally respectable stockbrokers. The options that came from them would certainly be on the cautious side, bringing 5 per cent in rents or mortgages, or if greater liquidity was preferred, 3 per cent from Consols or up to $4-4\frac{1}{2}$ per cent from reliable stocks. In the 1880s, a period of 'numbness in the industrial and commercial life of the country'[15] when the bank rate never rose above 6 per cent and sometimes hovered in the $2-2\frac{1}{2}$ per cent region, a greater return would have been seen as extremely risky. And when the period of high savings had been no more than five or six years, and the return, even if

[15] J. H. Clapham, *An Economic History of Modern Britain* (Cambridge, 1952), ii, p. 385.

practically tax-free, was no more than 3–5 per cent, no great fortune could be amassed.

In the event of Marshall's early death, his savings might have to support four people. His wife, thirteen years younger than himself, would most probably outlive him. He had as yet no proof that his son was capable of becoming entirely self-supporting. The problem would be resolved if either or both girls married, and launching them on to the road to matrimonial and financial independence had become urgent. It was important that they met and were seen by more and different people. Luckily 1887, the year when Marshall had reached the peak, was also the year of celebration and exceptional conviviality.

CHAPTER 12

THE YEAR OF THE JUBILEE

In tune with the prevailing mood of patriotic fervour, Jeannette opened the 1887 diary with the exclamation 'The Jubilee Year!' But then for a matter of several months her customary debunking style asserted itself. She appeared determined to spurn the festivities. When early in February the sisters were asked by Miss Paget, whose mother, Lady Paget (irreverently known to the Marshalls as the 'old Image'), was one of the organizers of the Women's Jubilee Offering to the Queen, to help with the door-to-door collection in Bond Street, Jeannette refused point-blank. 'To begin with, it is not our district, & to go on with I cd. not beg for myself, so why shd. I for the Queen? I think the whole thing a farce.'

'Everyone seems immensely disgusted with the Jubilee. No one has asked us for any money yet' she noted in March, after having remarked some two weeks previously that 'they are "Jubbing" away as hard as they can go, in India, releasing 23,000 prisoners, honours showered on blacks & whites, dinners, balls etc. etc.' Eventually the collecting card for the Women's Jubilee Offering reached No. 10, 'sent in from the Dalbys,[1] so we had to fork out. M. gave 5/-, A and I each 1/-, and Mars [the cook] -/6d; very handsome haul fr. one house!' On the Queen's birthday, four weeks before the Jubilee, she grumbled, as she did each year, about the 'horrid illumination' of the frontage of Poole, the tailors across the road from No. 10, and the 'depressing' roars of the crowds which came to view it.

Then, belatedly, the tone changed. The weather, after a wet cold spring, improved. With the warmer days the Season came into full swing; there were the usual invitations and a spate of others, as if all London had decided to join in the celebrations. Each time they went walking they saw carriages bearing celebrities, the Queen of the

---

[1] Probably the family of Sir William Bartlett Dalby (1840–1918), consulting aural surgeon at St George's Hospital.

Sandwich Islands—'such an ugly darkey'; the Crown Prince Sergius —'ugly & no mistake'; the King of Saxony—'who turned round to look at us'. The Park on the two mid-June Sundays was crowded and with the sunshine appeared the elegant toilettes made especially for the festivities. 'No end of nice dresses' commented Jeannette, whose own wardrobe had also been subjected to a thorough refurbishing to meet the requirements of Jubilee fashions. Vanity had prevailed over lack of enthusiasm. She and Ada had to have new dresses in which to 'Jub', and that year the cut and colour had to fall in with patriotic sentiment. So there was much white (or cream), and navy blue, with cardinal red trimmings, tight double-breasted bodices of a military cut above heavily draped bustles, lots of revers and epaulettes and fringes, and high casque-like hats. All of this added up, if not to the end of aesthetic influence in fashion,[2] then to a major hiatus which presaged its transmogrification into the styles of the *fin de siècle*.

In the mounting excitement on the afternoon of the Saturday which preceded the Jubilee, Jeanette and Ada went for a walk along an unaccustomed route, as far as Charing Cross; it was as if they had wandered back stage on to a gigantic, half-completed theatrical set: 'the streets are unrecognizable with the shops all filled with seats, skeletons of triumphal arches here & there, and sawing & planing of trees and planks going on by the roadside. The hammering of men putting up red cloth & decorations is deafening. Almost every house is preparing illuminations, and the streets are crowded with sightseers . . . Everyone seems gone crazy on the Jubilee . . .'

On Monday morning, the eve of the day, they got up to find their own decorations on display: 'a bouquet of flags was waving in front of each of our windows. The flags surmount 3 shields painted buff with gold-colored edge, the centre shield bearing 50, & the others V.R. These are painted white to show up the colored lights, wh. have not yet arrived. We look rather gay. The side windows have 5 Union Jacks each, the centre 4 & the Royal Standard.' Scarlet geraniums in the window-boxes of the first floor added to the festive aspect of the house. At this point, confessed Jeannette, they caught the Jubilee fever and

---

[2] 'The aesthetic revival itself will pass away, so far as mere accidentals are concerned; but the change which it has accomplished in all our artistic ideas will be permanent . . . the reds and blues of the reaction, even, are such colours as we never knew before the year One of the Aesthetic Revolution', predicted, as early as September 1881, an anonymous article, entitled 'Mr Cimabue Brown on the Defensive', in the London monthly *Belgravia*.

were impelled to go off on a tour of inspection: 'Went for a walk along
Piccadilly ... I crossed 5 lines of carriages by walking in & out, &
waiting in the intervening spaces. Everywhere is thronged, and the
houses are festooned & decorated, & hung with lamps, and the
Venetian masts with green garlands & wreaths are most festive.' She
bought a Jubilee brooch, one of several she, Ada and their mother
acquired that summer, and went home to lunch, after which they all
drove out in the carriage: 'I feel I can't rest indoors ... London has
gone wild, & no mistake.'

Towards nightfall, with the temperature dropping and a sharp east
wind blowing, anticipation turned into a rush of enthusiasm, and Ada
and she went out for the third time that day, again by carriage, to view
the illuminations in Bond Street, Grosvenor Square ('very little lit
there'), and down Park Lane; then to Buckingham Palace and the
Mall, and home by St James's Street:

Then our troubles began, as the place was a perfect block of carriages, cabs
and carts. The clubs were still putting up their stands, & the pavements were
crowded with planks & ladders. The street was alternatively bright as day, &
almost dark, and the traffic proceeded by inches. There seemed to be no
police, and the collisions were numerous, the women shrieked, the horses
backed, and the people crawled in & out, under the horses' heads. We took $\frac{3}{4}$
hour to get to Piccadilly fr. St James' Palace, and the whole time we seemed in
imminent danger of running into some one else or being run into ourselves.
The horse in the conveyance behind us all but came into our carriage, & we
took refuge on the back seat. Then we were addressed by some drunken man
in a cart, & at last determined to pull up half the carriage, & struggled with the
same till a gentleman came forward, & saying 'Allow me!' pulled it <u>down</u> agn! I
exclaimed 'We were trying to put it up! There is such a dreadful crowd!' Then
he responded cheerfully 'All right' & proceeded to pull it up, and tug & bang it
in proper style, so that it was up in no time. I said 'Thank you very much! I am
<u>so</u> much obliged'; he said 'All right! Not at all' and departed. We blessed him,
& were much more comfortable. Crossing Piccadilly was another phase in the
nightmare, & then we got home safely, and had some wine & water, & swore
we never wd. try <u>that</u> agn!

On the morning of Jubilee Day (21 June) they left home at 8.20 a.m.
carrying opera glasses and shawls against the east wind, and drove
across Piccadilly lined with masts tipped by gilded crowns, adorned
with sheaves of gay flags, and hung with inscriptions and loyal devices,
to the places from which they were to view the royal procession. Much
diplomatic manœuvring had gone into securing good seats for parents

and daughters (of John's whereabouts throughout the celebrations there is no mention). Eventually it was decided that Mrs Marshall and Jeannette would occupy the places allotted to Marshall at the Athenaeum, with Ada alone at Gwydyr House (now the Welsh Office) in Whitehall, in a seat sent by Sir George Young, a fellow-member of Marshall's on the Teaching University Committee. Jeannette had not been best pleased at this arrangement, which left her without any companion of her own age with whom to share her impressions: 'I am sorry, & wish M. were not such a baby, as then I cd. have gone with A.' Marshall himself, who had that spring at last taken over the presidency of the General Medical Council, was in his official capacity allotted a seat in Westminster Abbey.

Ellen's and Jeannette's seats in the second row on the Waterloo Place side of the Athenaeum were declared quite satisfactory, 'not so good as round the other (Pall Mall) side for the near view, though better for the general one'. Jeannette's immediate neighbour was an American woman who accepted a share of her opera glass and whose tremendous enjoyment of the scene and arrangements flattered her British companions. Before things got going they amused themselves in watching the crowd and the celebrities making their way to the Abbey. One of the first to pass was Buffalo Bill, 'a bold, impudent-looking man, but really rather handsome but for his hair' (too long for Jeannette's taste), with a girl on each arm and an escort of six Red Indians.

The account of the procession (which those at the Athenaeum saw twice over, on the way to the Abbey and on the return journey to Buckingham Palace) occupies four pages of the diary; the detailed description of the order and appearance of carriages and escorts differs little from contemporary newspaper reports. At the procession's head came a number of semi-state carriages bearing gorgeously attired Indian princes, who 'looked very pleased & delighted, and were well received. Two of them had their wives with them, in native costume with gold-bordered veils. It was rather a proud thought to feel all these sable potentates were our subjects, & had come in a way to do homage.' After commenting favourably on the Guards' escorts and on the demeanour and costume of the royal grandchildren, Jeannette went on, more caustically, about some of the older women members of the royal party: 'Louise looked sunburnt, Marie Alexandrovna haughty, & Bee I could not see', but gushed about the Guard of Honour of Princes:

Wales was enthusiastically received, & kept raising his hand in military salute. Next came Hesse (in dark uniform with helmet surmounted by an eagle & white plumes), Christian in I don't know what, & the Crown Prince of Germany looking like Siegfried! . . . in a white uniform, with the collar of the Garter, orders ad infinitum, and a silver helmet. He sat his big horse splendidly, and with his broad shoulders, and manly figure, and light beard he was absolutely 'too killing'.

In her enthusiasm she had borrowed the phrase 'too killing' from her American companion's vocabulary. And then at last came the carriage bearing Victoria, accompanied by the Crown Princess (Vicky) and the Princess of Wales: 'I used all my energies in looking at the Queen, who was in black as usual, but had a great deal of white in her bonnet, & they said diamonds, but those I did not see as she had mounted a parasol. The face looked pale, but she seemed very pleased, as well she might be, at the great reception she met with.' With unaccustomed empathy Jeannette added: 'I felt quite shaky myself, and wonder how she managed to keep up.'

In the interval between the end of the procession and its return journey in reverse order, they 'made for the hall and joined the queue for lunch' (the tickets, at what Jeannette had considered an exorbitant price of one guinea each, included refreshments). 'The crowd was considerable, & they pushed in a very unnecessary manner. A poor woman turned faint, and was very thankful for M's eau de cologne, and I saved a little girl from being crushed, & was thanked by her father, so we were both good "Smartans".' After Jeannette had helped them to 'some solid refreshments', they went back for the remainder of the show and were eventually reunited with Marshall and Ada, 'who had got on well, the Youngs having a private party & being very kind'. In the evening they went out once again, this time on foot, through Mayfair, as far as Grosvenor Square and Hyde Park Corner, moving with the great mass of people who had come to view the illuminations.

'I feel quite "brisée" ' she wrote on the morrow, 'and utterly disorganized. I cd. only brush my things, sit about, and talk about yesterday.' Nevertheless, as soon as lunch was over the carriage took the four of them to Westminster Abbey for a repeat of the Jubilee service. As was her wont, Jeannette was critical of much of the music, though Mme Nordica's singing of 'Let the bright seraphim' was a treat. 'It brought tears to my eyes; the pleasure was almost pain. I am fond of Handel.' After relatively unsuccessful attempts to see the Children's

Fête in Hyde Park (they only heard the cheering from afar), and to catch the royal carriages on their way to the station—this time they saw only the tip of the Queen's mauve parasol—they finished the day with another viewing of the illuminations. They drove up Regent Street (declaring 'Vanderweyd's: "All good Americans rejoice", in incandescent lamps, the best'[3]), and then eastward along Oxford Street and Holborn to the City and back. Then she summed up the experiences of several days' rejoicing: 'I must say the Jubilee is tiring. M. is quite knocked up. Still I have really enjoyed it, take it all round.'

By the following Sunday she had shaken off some of the loyal fervour and was her normal sharp self in her résumé of the sermon at St George's, Hanover Square, which in the 1880s competed with St James's as the Marshall sisters' habitual church: 'Mr Cure preached very prosily on the Jubilee, & tried to make out we were 50 yrs. better than in 1837. I rather doubt it.'

There were more Jubilee celebrations to come. On a sweltering day in early July they went to see the Queen lay the first stone of the Imperial Institute. They sat in the immense canvas pavilion erected for the occasion and had an excellent view of dignitaries and royalty. Jeannette singled out 'the Duchess of Teck, looming big as ever' and 'the Crown Princess, looking like a funny little Dutchwoman with a blk. & white striped silk, and oldfashioned white bonnet, & most absurd blk. satin basqued bodice ... Her three daughters were with her, looking very plain & heavy.' The Prince of Wales 'in a splendid uniform conducted his poor little Ma on his arm'. The Marshalls had never shown much reverence or liking for Victoria: 'feeble & as though she were not quite right in her head' was how Jeannette reported her father's impression of his monarch in March 1886; 'tiny & dowdy' summed up her usual view of the Queen. On the occasion of the 1887 stone-laying Jeannette did not think that the Queen looked fit to be inspected by her assembled subjects, estimated at some eleven thousand:

She was very dowdy, in a short black dress with her old blk. bonnet on agn., & some kind of round cape of an antedeluvian cut. The face was purple from the heat and she looked very much distressed, I thought. I really felt quite sorry for her. Wales supported her very carefully, & looked quite filial. The poor old girl was tremendously applauded, & bowed away no end when she got on the dais,

---

[3] Van der Weyde, a photographers' establishment at 182 Regent Street, used the slogans 'by the "Van der Weyde" light' and 'day light superseded by electricity'.

& kissed the Crown Princess. Then she subsided into a chair, & disappeared from sight, but I cd. see a large white fan waving, and someone offered her a smelling bottle.

The actual ceremony took place almost entirely out of Jeannette's sight: 'the big stone was raised, and some hocus-pocus went on with the coins etc, I presume, but the little Queen was so low down that I only caught sight of the top of her bonnet now & then.' Again, she summoned up some enthusiasm and finished the account of that day with: 'It was really a grand sight, scrumptious.'

Later that month the Marshall parents with Ada and Jeannette went down for two nights to Portsmouth, to see the Queen review her Navy. This time the preliminary arrangements which Marshall had set up in London proved quite inadequate; the two vantage-points to which they had hoped to gain admission were overcrowded and, true to character, their father did not insist on his rights. In the end they were reduced to watch the fleet sail by from an exposed ridge below Fort Gilkicker. 'We felt rather sold, but made the best of it.'

After five hours of parching sun and wind, with only rudimentary refreshments, they decided to call it a day. They got back to the hotel, soothed their sun-scarified faces with cold cream, dined, and then, too tired to face another expedition, watched the illuminated ships and the fireworks from the window of the girls' room: 'The most remarkable feature in the whole entertainment was however the search lights . . . To see the whole row of ships throwing out their dazzling beams, and flashing them right in our eyes, and then across the water & ships, the waves of light crossing & weaving in & out in the sky was most extraordinary, like a number of erratic comets.' The next morning in an annoying anti-climax they found that, after all, special places had been reserved for them at Gilkicker, to which they would have been admitted had Marshall not so easily abdicated the privileges of his status. 'I never felt more wild!' fumed Jeannette. 'It spoiled my break-fast.' And their return journey was if anything an even greater failure. At Portsmouth they had some difficulty in getting their box labelled: 'P. had to leave it with some other things far from the train, & all the way up was possessed with the idea that it was lost . . . on reaching Waterloo at about 10, no box was there, & P was frantic.' The next train did not bring the Marshalls' luggage either. 'P. was convinced the amateur porter had made off with it' and 'raged around all night . . .' Eventually, the trunk which contained their entire summer wardrobe,

as well as brushes, combs and other necessaries, was recovered by
Jeannette and Ada from the Lost Property Office and, after formal
identification, borne home by cab 'in great glee'.

Some three weeks later the sisters and their mother attended a long
Eisteddfod meeting at the Albert Hall. Jeannette mocked at the bards,
described the arch-druid as a 'very queer old codger' and pronounced
a great deal of the performance wearisome. The high point, as on
previous occasions that summer, was the arrival of the Royals, who
were three-quarters of an hour late:

They came down the side stairs to the platform, the Welshies cherring &
waving their hats like mad. The Prince is fatter than ever, the Princess looked
very thin & delicate, but very nice in a heliotrope & white foulard, with cream
brocade & lace waistcoat, and bonnet with sprays of lilac and a heliotrope veil,
wh. gave her a very made up look. The three girls are common & plain-looking
to the last degree, and were in neat but too tight dresses of blue foulard with
narrow white waistcoats & red hats. They have clumsy features & figures, &
are pulled in to a waist.

The Prince's reply to the President's address she thought very sensible. 'He certainly reads well enough, though he cannot pronounce an
R.' Mrs Marshall departed mid-way through the performance, while
the sisters stayed to the end, enjoying a great deal of the singing. After
five hours at the Hall they went home by cab, once again 'feeling rather
done up'.

As far as Jeannette was concerned, it was in fact the accelerated pace of
private entertaining that gave 1887 its special lure. The dull seasons of
mourning and semi-mourning were left behind. Right through that
year, against the background of loyal rejoicings, the Marshall sisters
had gone to more entertainments than at any time since 1880. In their
new Jubilee costumes they dined out and danced as much as in their
early twenties. Jeannette moreover flirted as much as ever, or perhaps
even more, for the objective of marriage as a means of escape from No.
10 was never far from the centre of her attention.

In the early part of the year two candidates were the chief objects of
her speculations. One was an acquaintance met on several occasions
earlier in the 1880s, the painter Edward Fahey. After a few casual
meetings with him and two episodes of mild flirtation, at a Boat Race
party and at a musical afternoon, she spent the great part of a February
evening dancing and sitting out with him on an 'agreeably secluded

sofa'. Undeterred by the knowledge that he was a widower with three children, she had let her imagination roam; when in April 1887 he sent the Marshalls an invitation to visit his studio, she became convinced (or perhaps pretended to herself that she was convinced) that he was seriously interested in her.

The other candidate in the running was the perennial Martin Pate. 'As far as money goes I might do worse, & I believe he is a good sort of creature, but I fancy I shd. prefer something a little more artistic' she wrote of the Ely farmer in mid-April; on the next day she was more specific: 'I would rather have Mr Fahey out & out!' Two days later her mind was again on Fahey: 'I really think I shd. like him, if he liked me well enough. Anyway I shd. not break my heart. "Shut my eyes & open my mouth & see what fortune will send me".'

Ada for her part considered the Ely option as viable, insisting, wrote Jeannette after a visit to Hill House over Easter, 'that I shd be very happy there, that Mr. P wd let me have my own way altogether'. Flippantly, she concluded: 'I will propose to him in Leap Year!! Happy thought!!'

As usual, there was no follow-up and, as usual, she became despondent: 'It is a week since I last saw Mr Pate & a month since I beheld Mr Fahey. It is rather like my fate! not to come across people agn! I verily believe if I had a fair chance with either I cd. "double them up", & both are not likely to cross my path agn. for a year or so! It was certainly written in the stars that I am to die an old maid!'

Why then did she not ask her aunt Wilkes to let her spend another week at Ely? Why did she not suggest to her mother that a hint to the Thornycrofts, in whose house she had once or twice met Edward Fahey, might result in some useful invitations? The conclusion must be that she did not care sufficiently for either Pate or Fahey to take the initiative into her own hands. That she was capable of doing so would soon become apparent.

The 1887 holiday abroad came as something of an anti-climax to the fun of the intensified Season. At the start Jeannette appeared less fit than usual. There were signs of excessive weariness after travel as well as shortage of breath on mountain excursions. She complained of primitive hotel arrangements, half-empty sitting rooms and uninteresting company, without 'pretence to style or even to neatness'. 'I am on friendly terms with 3 parsons!' she exclaimed on the third day at St Luc. 'Very dreadful, but the best there is.' It was only after they had transferred to the Riffel-Alp, high above Zermatt, that matters improved. Once again her fate, this time in the shape of Arthur Stone, the middle-aged barrister brother of Marshall's artist-acquaintance Marcus Stone, kept its alpine rendezvous.

CHAPTER 13

THRASHING AROUND

WHEN Jeannette had met Arthur Stone four years earlier, in the course of another holiday, at Lake Como, she had already thought him *empressé*. However, the handsome figure of Harry Brown had at the time been clear in her mind, and the looks of Stone had been against him. 'He is so frightful' she had scoffed in September 1883. Now she noted that he was 'clever & amusing, though most unfortunately plain!' But if his looks had not improved, her tolerance and her desire to find a husband had certainly made strides. He too appeared eager to strengthen the acquaintance, and made a bee-line for Jeannette. This time his attentions fell on fertile ground; they were soon inseparable.

But as her liking for Arthur Stone grew, so too did her sense of the relationship being doomed from the outset. Her parents, who at first had appeared to take to Stone, proved less than lukewarm about his possible candidature for Jeannette's hand. Mrs Marshall, in particular, perhaps alerted by the promptness with which he took up Marshall's half-hearted suggestion to visit them at Vevey, where the family moved after a fortnight of the Riffel-Alp, was distinctly cold. 'Why I don't know' worried Jeannette 'as he is most polite to her!' While her father behaved sensibly, her mother 'looked detestable' and comported herself with a lack of civility which still irked when Jeannette wrote about it two months later: 'she wd. not sit down in the chair he got for her, she marched in front with P., & never said a word to him, she never offered him a cup of tea after his journey & walk, and the moment we got to the Hotel door, said she must go & <u>dress</u>, though she sat in the hall for some time after he had gone. I never felt so uncomfortable, & so I told her. I was really ashamed.'

At the time there had been a 'most disagreeable scene' between mother and daughter: 'A. told me that M. had been raving about Mr Stone, so I tackled her on the subject and caught a Tartar. She has a most unreasoning dislike to him, and really was utterly absurd. I won't put down what she said for it was too insulting, and made me very angry. I shall not forget it for a good while. One wd. think that the man was a malefactor.'

Her regard for Stone increased in inverse proportion to Mrs Marshall's dislike of him. He was certainly not handsome, she reflected, '5ft. 10 by his own measurement, rather broad, but somewhat stooping shoulders. Very thick, <u>fine</u> & rather wavy red hair, light grey eyes, <u>very</u> good forehead, largish nose, and a plain mouth. Clean shaven but small whiskers, and a barrister cut . . . should give him 40–45'; but she saw so many advantages in him that she declared herself ready to put up with his appearance. It was in any event absurd that her parents should seriously object to his looks. 'I think he is clever & goodnatured, and in position & family is all one cd. wish, & I am certain I cd. make him devoted to me . . .'

Now, for the first time in three decades, Ada moved to the front of the stage. Presumably because she recognized that for her there was no hope of marrying unless Jeannette came off the shelf, she set out to sustain her sister's belief in Stone's devotion. It was Ada too who systematically spied out and reported to Jeannette the exact position of each parent *vis-à-vis* the unpopular suitor; what is more, she added fuel to Jeannette's anger and helped her to lay plans to defeat Mrs Marshall's opposition.

When they returned to London, it was Ada who tried to get things moving by suggesting that Stone be asked to the soirée in honour of the members of the General Medical Council which the Marshalls had fixed for 23 November. But Marshall, and in some measure Jeannette too, thought that the first move in London had to be made by the putative suitor. And Stone, whether offended by Ellen's 'black looks & inhospitable behaviour' at Vevey, or just shy (or even frightened by Jeannette's evident eagerness), did not call at Savile Row. This was upsetting to Jeannette, who had assumed that he would promptly want to follow up the Swiss flirtation. Taking his first move for granted, she had already speculated on what his second one would be: 'If he calls once, he can't [call] agn. If I meet him in the park, it is very unsatisfactory, & I don't think for a moment he will get asked here. To begin with, he is not liked, & to go on with, it is agnst. our traditions.' When they eventually ran into him at the distribution of prizes at the Royal Academy on 10 December, he appeared lukewarm. To add to Jeannette's chagrin, later that month he failed to be among the guests at a dinner given by their mutual acquaintance, Miss Williams of Vicarage Gate, though on a previous occasion that lady had testified to Arthur Stone being ' "the best creature" (her favourite phrase) & one of her best friends'.

What Jeannette resented most was the fact that her mother, and under her influence Marshall too, treated her as a child and did not trust her judgment sufficiently to disclose the objections to Stone's suit; that they might keep silent out of a regard for her feelings did not apparently strike her. Relations between mother and daughter were at an all-time low. Ellen was at this point of her life particularly given to fits of bad temper and to grouching. She was in her mid-fifties, possibly menopausal; also, a decade of strain over John was no doubt taking its toll. There were days on end with 'M. in the grumps as usual', when she picked quarrels even with Ada, who normally never gave offence: 'M is simply detestable, and her temper gets worse every day. I don't know what she is coming to, but existence is a misery . . . P. gave it to poor A. because M. made such a fuss over a babyish difference, & the whole day was a "supplice".'

It was Ada who reported Mrs Marshall's malicious remarks to which Jeannette (while claiming that scenes were not in her line) attached the worst possible interpretation: 'I hear M. says to A. that now I have gone half way, she hopes he will come the other! which is disgustingly coarse & moreover untrue. I do not feel I have gone any way at all, & am certain he doesn't, and to imply that I am crazy to marry him is really atrocious. M. is the most wrongheaded, narrow-minded woman in the world, when once she gets a bias.'

She now openly blamed her mother for Stone's failure to come forward. The atmosphere at home was further tested by a set-to between mother and daughter, with Jeannette accusing Mrs Marshall of deliberately sabotaging Arthur Stone's courtship. The row helped to clear the air. It confirmed that Jeannette was keen to continue the affair and that she could hope for no support from her mother.

Even though in her middle twenties Harry Brown had made her pulse beat faster than Arthur Stone now succeeded in doing, she had then not been desperate enough to subdue her pride and push the affair forward: 'I wd. not go a single step, out of my way, after him' she had declared at the time. The lessons of the Brown episode had not been wasted. Driven to distraction by Stone's apparent lack of interest and also by the questionings and taunts of certain maternal relatives who had come to hear of the Riffel-Alp affair, she decided to act.

Three times in the course of the winter of 1887–8 she took the initiative and tried to give Arthur Stone opportunities to resume his attentions. Two of these efforts met with a temporary success. To begin with, she wrote to ask him for admission to the New Year's Day service at the Temple. 'That neither pledges him nor me to anything further, but gives him an opening if he wants one, and is too shy to find it.' There was nothing clandestine about her letter; she had shown its draft to her mother, who was 'flabbergasted', but had raised no objections. The tickets came, and so on 1 January 1888 Jeannette and Ada went to the Temple Church, enjoyed the singing and after the service exchanged a few words with their host. This was Jeannette's cue for informing him that they were always 'at home' on Monday afternoons. When on the next Monday but one he called, she decided that she still liked him 'very much indeed! There!!' and kept the ball in play, asking him to look up some pieces by Russian composers in a catalogue in his sister's possession. However, after he had supplied the required information, her letter of warm thanks was not skilled enough to give him scope for further correspondence.

The way out of this new impasse was suggested to her by a chance remark of her Aunt Edwin Williams, reported on the bush telegraph via Aunt Eliza and Ada. 'Aunt B. said that he was so wonderfully attentive to me that everyone thought it was a "fait accompli". They evidently think it wd. be a good match, & have some impression that there is a hitch, as Aunt B. said that M. ought to invite him, adding it was very difficult for a gentleman to call unless he were asked to some entertainment!' For her part, Aunt Eliza had suggested to Ada that the most fit entertainment would be a dinner. Armed with this advice, Jeannette at once braved her mother's ill-temper, asking if Mr Stone could be invited to dine at No. 10 'in a quiet way'.

Ellen 'professed herself agreeable', though her daughter did not take the answer at its face value: 'I doubt if she means it, but will most likely work agnst. me with P. behind my back.' And on the next day she worded her animosity in even stronger terms: 'M. has not the slightest regard for my feelings, & puts things in a most revolting & brutal fashion. She will do for all my affection for her if she goes on in this way much longer.' Eventually however Stone was asked and came to dine *en famille* at very short notice. Jeannette resented this discourtesy, and also that the quest for advice about John's future career had been made the excuse for the invitation. She was apprehensive that her brother would make use of Stone, if only to cadge money from him. She was also disgruntled, on the evening of the dinner, because Stone had been 'anything but easy' and 'unusually calm & pompous'. After the meal, however, he followed her around 'à la doggie', politely conversed with Mrs Marshall and on leaving thanked them for a 'most delightful evening'.

A month or so later, when this initiative too had proved fruitless and further contact seemed all but impossible, she made her third—and final—attempt to add fuel to Mr Stone's ardour. This time, on meeting him accidentally in a friend's studio, she improvised a sudden enthusiasm for attending the distribution of Maundy Money. But Stone was unable (or did not try) to procure the desired tickets and moreover misunderstood the situation, addressing his reply to Ada, whom Jeannette had represented as being particularly keen to see the ceremony. This last failure proved too discouraging; it made her give up all hope of salvaging the relationship.

Three times she had failed, circumstances working against her. Was it that Stone had paid court to her in Switzerland in much the same spirit as one or two of her earlier alpine acquaintances had done, exercising his power to captivate without intending any follow-up action? Was he perhaps not of the marrying variety?[1] From what she had recorded about the twelve-day long Swiss episode, nothing very purposeful transpired. There had been the usual staring and sentimental whisperings and a great many *petits soins* of the most polite variety. She herself commented on her inability to note down exactly what had been going on: 'I find flirtations are difficult to do justice to, & take a great deal of room.' She used the term flirtation as she had used it at the time of the Thomas and the Brown affairs, and on several occasions since. To her it once again seemed less a holiday pastime than the serious preliminary to courtship proper.

She may not have been mistaken. After all, Stone circulated in much the same circles as Marshall, and at least one reliable friend, Miss

---

[1] With etiquette relaxed, Swiss hotels were a favourite venue for romantic dalliance. A. A. Milne, writing about a somewhat later period, asserted that 'Swiss engagements don't count' (*Once a Week*, London, 1914, p. 46). In reality this was not invariably so; see, for instance, George Adam Smith's lightning courtship of Lilian Buchanan, with only four months elapsing between their first meeting at Zermatt in 1889 and their wedding (in Lilian Adam Smith, *George Adam Smith, A Personal Memoir and Family Chronicle*, London, 1943, pp. 32–6).

Williams, gave him an excellent character. He was middle-aged and could be presumed to be aware of the consequences of leading a friend's daughter up the garden path; nothing she knew about him pointed to behaviour at once frivolous, discourteous and unkind.

There is an alternative explanation of his seeming volte-face. It has to do with Arthur Stone's antecedents and possibly throws some light on the puzzling reactions of Jeannette's parents. His father, Frank Stone, had been a painter of some renown and popularity (the *Dictionary of National Biography* comments that his most successful work was perhaps not his best). He had also been an intimate of Dickens, a friend of several other men of letters, including Thackeray, and an opponent of the Pre-Raphaelites. But Frank Stone's childhood and first youth had been less prestigious: up to the age of twenty-four he had followed the calling of his father who had been a cotton-spinner in Manchester. So that Arthur Stone and his brother Marcus were only half a generation away from the Lancashire mills.

This Jeannette presumably did not know when she remarked on his background being all that one could wish. Nor is it clear that Mrs Marshall's objections necessarily centred on Stone's origin, rather than on the ostensible reasons that she thought him too old and too plain for Jeannette. But if the parents were indeed aware of the spinner father and the spinner grandfather, this might have inhibited them from appearing too forward in seeking out the barrister as son-in-law. Stone for his part was perhaps extra touchy in his awareness that he might not be thought good enough for the daughter of an eminent professional man. If he had been waiting for a sign of clear encouragement from Jeannette's parents as they had been waiting for a clear commitment on his part, then the resulting deadlock needed more than the fumbling efforts of Jeannette to resolve it.

As a possible solution of the mystery of yet another aborted near-courtship this at least has the backing of solid genealogical fact, an advantage over the puzzles of Thomas and Brown. It leads one to ask whether the Marshalls would have come to terms with the idea of Stone as son-in-law, and whether Jeannette herself would have been so eager to pursue him had she been told about his family circumstances. As it was, the taboo about communicating on matters of origin and class may well have been the factor which completely obscured the issues.

For some months after the encounter at the studio Stone appeared to avoid direct contact when coming face to face with Jeannette unexpectedly, and she reciprocated by attempting to ignore him in the street and at picture shows. Her vanity had been dealt a blow from which she smarted for the remainder of that year and into 1889. It led her to muse, before she left for their annual holiday in August 1888: 'I don't suppose I shall have any flirtation, as I had one last year, and enjoyed it, though I had to pay dearly enough for it after. I must say I feel injured when I think of that time. It was a shame that I was made to pay because Mr Stone behaved so shabbily. I wish I cd. have that explained, as I think distinctly worse of human nature since & that is not a pleasant feeling. I shd. like to find <u>one</u> genuine person!' And, five months later, her bitterness still undiminished, she admitted that her mother might after all have been right.

The last two years of the 1880s brought changes into the Marshalls' lives which, though hardly perceptible in the detail of Jeannette's record, marked the beginning of an entirely new phase.

The most material difference was in the pattern of their social activities. Suddenly the Season, as far as Jeannette and Ada were concerned, was no longer a succession of opportunities for dancing. No longer had they to make time to renovate the flimsy ball dresses between one evening's entertainment and the next; indeed, in 1889 they owned only two ball dresses each and went dancing only twice.

Their theatre-going had also waned. In 1888 and 1889 Jeannette saw a total of six professional performances, a catholic choice ranging from *Macbeth* (with 'neither Irving nor Miss Terry . . . entirely satisfactory' but the witches 'simply perfect') and *The Taming of the Shrew* to *The Pirates of Penzance* and *Jack and the Beanstalk*. The number of concerts attended shrank to fewer than twenty a year. But Jeannette, who in girlhood had on occasion squeezed a couple of concerts into one day, continued to take concert-going seriously. In 1885 she started a systematic record of critical assessments of the music she listened to, in which the names of the newer composers, Berlioz, Brahms and Grieg, were now prominent. So was that of Wagner: after a concert of his music in 1886 she wrote 'I am a Wagnerian to the backbone'. Although after the middle 1870s opera had disappeared almost completely from the programme of the Marshalls' entertainments, parents and daughters went in 1882 to the *Ring* at Covent Garden, and in August 1889 took in Bayreuth as part of their continental tour. The visit proved a mixed pleasure, as within twenty-four hours of arrival Marshall had been robbed of a wallet containing the tickets to the

performances as well as all their holiday money, and much time had to
be spent on sorting out the resulting crisis. All the same they were
bowled over by the *Meistersinger*, and even more by *Parsifal*, to which
Jeannette devoted two-and-a-half pages in the diary, an amount of
space usually allotted only to major episodes of flirtation.

No doubt much of the change of style had to do with the reduction
in the flow of free tickets; the friends and patients who had been
responsible for such gifts in the past had either died or floated out of
the Marshalls' orbit. Most of the entertainments now had to be paid
for out of the family purse—and that purse was beginning to feel
distinctly lighter than when Marshall had been at the pinnacle of his
career as consultant. However, being at the top of the medical establishment was rewarded by a new category of perks. He and his family
got invited to numerous official functions, formal dinners, receptions
and conversaziones. With his wife becoming ever less sociable, he
liked to have his daughters accompany him on such outings and was
proud to have their handsome appearance and elegant turn-out
admired. Although fashion had lost much of its fascination for Jeannette, these were occasions for which she continued to prepare as
carefully and dress up as much as ever she had done in the years of her
prime.

The truth was that, however good a face she put on it, she and Ada
were no longer in their prime. And they increasingly frequented
families in which the daughters, like themselves, had failed to find
partners and were now on the shelf; or households consisting of older,
middle-aged, single women living with spinster sisters or women
friends, or even alone. At balls, fewer dancing partners now queued for
the pleasure of some turns with Miss Marshall. Those who did were
usually confirmed bachelors or middle-aged widowers.

Perhaps because she had come to terms with the fact that Ada was of
necessity her closest companion and support, Jeannette no longer
referred to her as poor Ada, except on the occasions when her sister
was indeed to be pitied because of ill-health (for Ada continued to be
subject to attacks of fainting and to what Jeannette called 'hysterical'
upsets). The sisters still dressed alike, though from time to time Ada
was daring enough to choose different headgear, so that she no longer
appeared as a clone of Jeannette.

However, the initiatives with which they furnished their daily existence were now no longer always generated by Jeannette alone.

Together they devised a plan to teach themselves Norwegian, for, since their Scandinavian tour in 1884, Nordic culture had fascinated them. Jeannette took the matter very seriously, reading and doing grammar exercises with Ada and also by herself. Within a month of starting she had become so concerned about her progress that on meeting (at Hamo Thornycroft's studio open day) Edmund Gosse with whom she was very slightly acquainted, she bearded him to get his views on a matter of pronunciation. Eventually the sisters engaged a teacher, 'funny little Fröken Hansen'; 'short & stout, 55, specs, smooth hair & quaint little phiz', in a matter of weeks Fröken Hansen had her two students reading and conversing in Norwegian with considerable gusto.[2]

Together, they walked in the Park, going further afield than they had ventured when accompanying their parents. And increasingly they went, the two of them alone, or with a spinster friend, to functions at which it was proper for women to appear unattended by men, to exhibitions, and above all, to lectures.

Public lectures were a new phenomenon in their timetable. Until the very end of the 1880s there had been no more than one or two of them a year. Now, in 1888 and 1889, they went to some fifteen, the subjects ranging from meteorites (by Lockyer) to Greenland (by Nansen) to photography (by Muybridge). The chief event was the cycle of talks arranged in connection with the newly launched Arts and Crafts initiatives. These were held in the elaborate setting of the New Gallery in Regent Street, about which Jeannette had gushed in the spring of 1888: 'it is most wonderfully got up, with beautiful marbles in the central hall, and the columns and balcony railings gilt, and the entablature covered with platinum leaf.' The gold-papered walls, the statuary and the 'dribbling little fountain' must have made a bizarre backcloth for the dedicated 'craftsmen' who lectured on their calling. According

[2] Jeannette, whose previous experience of Scandinavian authors was confined to Bjørnstjerne Bjørnson, in German and English translations, first attempted Carl Henrik Scharling (a Danish writer) and Jonas Lie (a Norwegian one) in the original and then embarked on Ibsen in December 1889. Reading Ibsen's plays in the original was probably the main object of the Marshall sisters' ambitious linguistic exercise. By the time her lessons with Fröken Hansen started, in 1890, Jeannette had already worked her way through seven of his plays: *A Doll's House*, *Peer Gynt*, *Brand*, *The Lady from the Sea*, *Rosmersholm*, *The Feast at Solhong*, and *Lady Inger of Østeraad*. In 1891 she went on to *Hedda Gabler* and to more works by minor Norwegian novelists. Between 1892 and 1895 (when the records of her readings cease) no Scandinavian authors appear in the reading lists.

to Jeannette, these, with the exception of Morris himself, looked excessively plain and dowdy. The first one she heard, Cobden-Sanderson, 'chétif, clean shaven, with scant & lank brown hair parted in the middle, & a nose like a sharp red chalk pencil', appeared for the practical part of his demonstration of book binding 'in shirt-sleeves, and a white apron tied under his arms . . .' The Jaeger shirt and the leather band [belt] in place of braces, 'which he was continually hitching', added to the unconventionality of his costume. Though she thought his manner affected and he turned his r's into w's, she had been both entertained and interested in what he had to say about his art. Holiday, who lectured on glass painting, also did not impress by his appearance, with the 'most distressing "champagne-bottle" shoulders' and a pince-nez; he was further handicapped by a weak voice and a cold, but again his subject-matter proved interesting and put over 'very sensibly'. Walter Crane's two talks on design and ornamentation impressed her less. His extempore draughtsmanship she thoroughly approved; already the first lecture made her a devotee of his art: 'Why don't the RAs do something of that sort' she wrote in January 1889, having just 'indulged in' a copy of his new picture book, *Flora's Feast*, 'instead of advertising Pears Soap!' The star turn however was Morris's talk on Gothic Architecture. Although she and Ada had set out 'in a profane & scoffing mood', afterwards she bordered on the enthusiastic:

Mr. Crane (with sad strands of hair on his brow) introduced the Lecturer in a few feeble words, and Mr M. (in a bright blue shirt & collar & no tie) stepped forth. He has a large, round head & face with fuzzy grey hair & beard, and a clever look. He sways from one foot to the other in the most ungraceful way, & has a bad way of speaking, wh. makes him rather difficult to catch. He read his Lecture, wh. was in most excellent & varied English, and well put together, though his views are wrongheaded, I think. He began by praising the Gothic style as the only one wh. seemed to be organic, & give an idea of growth. Then traced the development of architecture through the barbarous, the Greek, the Roman, the Byzantine, & the Gothic, & finally the Renaissance, wh. came in for many knocks. St. Peter's & St. Paul's were very harshly criticized. Of course Bureaucracy was to blame for everything, England is uglier now than 50 years ago, workmen are not allowed to think etc. Nothing will come right till all co-operate agn., and work for art, etc. Some of his phrases were epigrams, and some of them truly poetical in their suggestiveness, and his descriptions of the middle ages with their wealth of Art & Beauty very picturesque & telling, but after all may there not be something even better than Gothic, & why shd.

we go back to <u>that</u>, when he objects to our going back to anything else? The applause was great & deserved at the end.

The first Arts and Crafts Exhibition in the autumn of 1888 had also 'agreeably surprised' her; she had been particularly pleased by some of the embroideries and many examples of illuminated manuscript, bindings, wallpapers and the 'exquisite tiles': 'I think form is more regarded than colour, or rather more successful, as the colours are rather too much of the "greenery-yallery" kind. Morris is fond of a magenta tone of red, and a brownish puce, both of wh. are distinctly ugly. Burne Jones' window designs are grand, but weird, & somewhat crazy.' All in all, she was sufficiently stirred to apply to have three of her own embroideries, a screen and two smaller pieces, shown at the second Arts and Crafts Exhibition in 1889. This made her one of the 'craftswomen' and brought her compliments and praise from people whose opinion she valued; it was noticed by F. G. Stephens in the *Athenaeum* and honourably mentioned in the *Illustrated London News*. Crane himself, she was told, had admired her work. But there was nothing to convey that she recognized the importance of the groundswell of artistic innovation which would prove rather longer-lasting and at least as influential as the aesthetic movement which had been its origin. No excitement of such peripheral kind as a new direction in art was now strong enough to overcome, or even to dent, the sour disenchantment which eroded her outlook on what went on round her.

In 1890 her account of the third Arts and Crafts Exhibition was compressed into five sentences. The quality of the craftwork was uneven. She thought the furniture 'rather ugly than otherwise', the lustre-ware and glass good, and preferred the embroideries exhibited by the School of Arts to the 'coarse but effective' pieces from Morris's workshop; sour grapes perhaps, because some years earlier she had tried, and failed, to interest the supervisor of the Morris embroidery team, Miss Burden, in her own 'artistic' work. Her last words on the 1890 show were 'Nothing very new.'

CHAPTER 14

A FALSE START

DID Ada, in her own diaries which she prudently arranged to have destroyed by the executors of her will, ever refer to her sister as poor Jeannette? By the time they were both out of early womanhood she may well have done so, for Jeannette was now indeed a somewhat pitiable object. But the vital force which made her seek an escape route from permanent spinsterhood was not seriously impaired. By the late summer of 1889 this underlying buoyancy had made her forget all the fruitless frustration which had started in 1874 in the flirtation with Mr Thomas and culminated in the fiasco of the Stone affair, and embark on yet another emotional sequence resulting from a casual encounter in a Swiss resort. As if mesmerized by their desire to appease, and (in Ellen's case) to placate their foolhardy daughter, her parents did nothing effective to deflect her from this hazardous course.

The bare facts were as follows. On a cold, wet late-August day, after an exciting week at Bayreuth and in Munich, the Marshalls, parents and daughters, arrived in Pontresina and put up at the Hotel Roseg. On the third day there Jeannette's attention focused on a man who, she wrote, had 'begun to stare hard. He sat in the Salon, after dinner, & never took his eyes off me . . .' Next morning at breakfast he 'scraped acquaintance', and was declared 'not exciting, but better than nothing'. By the end of the first week Jeannette had decided that it was in her nature to flirt; she had indeed been dubbed a 'great flirt' by one of the fellow-guests at the hotel. The new acquaintance, Mr Gould, right from the start told her a great deal about his family affairs, 'wh. is always a bad sign'; she thought him 'most distinctly smitten'.

Gradually she recorded her impression of Mr Gould and also his confidences about 'his relatives, work and aspirations'. He was in his late thirties, 'rather above middle-height, stoutly made, dark hair with a little grey; moustache only, grey eyes, nice kind look'. Most of his family lived in Shropshire. It consisted of the widowed father, Philip Gould, two brothers (the elder, an invalid, lived at home, and the other, an ex-Indian army officer, had retired to Salisbury), a sister who was also an invalid, and, by his father's first marriage, a step-brother. Gould himself had been destined for the Bar, and had eaten his dinners at the Inner Temple and passed all the law exams, but had not yet been called. Instead, he had drifted into teaching and was at present a housemaster at Marlborough. He did not however intend to keep to schoolmastering, 'though he had got on well'; he hoped to retire within the next five years with, Jeannette understood, 'an eye on parliament'.

Soon she reported that the flirtation was flourishing. 'It is getting conspicuous, but he does it all, & I must say I don't object.' She also noted that their time together was running short. A day or two later the Marshalls transferred to Maloja (at the south-west end of the Lake of Sils) where Gould had preceded them twenty-four hours earlier. It was there that he made his strange declaration.

For once, Ada, perhaps at a hint from the parents, had discreetly withdrawn after dinner on the plea of wanting to get on with her book, and the older Marshalls, too, had gone to watch the dancing. This left Jeannette and Gould tête-à-tête. They sat on the terrace, with the dance music drifting out of the windows, and conversed haltingly on indifferent topics. Gould chain-smoked. There were 'awful pauses' and other signs of strain. At his peremptory request they then withdrew to the hall—'he was evidently struggling to keep calm.' Jeannette, sensing his agitation and guessing its cause, was also nervous and felt 'as cold as ice'. Then, as they paced up and down, she listened in silence to his declaration which came 'in fearful gasps, a word or two at a time':

he said that I had been so 'wonderfully kind' to him, and that he had most fully appreciated it; that no doubt I had a right to expect that he wd. make a request, which of course I shd. want time to consider . . . Then came another struggle, & he began a dozen different sentences in a dozen different ways, said he did not know how to say it, that he had seen very few women, had not cared about them, that he never dreamt when he came abroad of this happening, that nothing was further from his thoughts, that my character, talents, family, P's position etc. were all that he cd. possibly desire, that any man wd. jump at the chance but that he was not free at present to do so. That was not put half so clearly as I do, & then he said: 'Do you understand?', & I said, 'no, I don't, in the least', wh. was the plain truth.

His attempts at clarification, Jeannette complained retrospectively, only added to the confusion in her mind. He asked if she had perhaps wondered at his celibacy, and had tried to guess the reasons why he had not married: 'when I said "Perhaps you were not well enough off?", he said, no, that he was not rich, but comfortably off, & that he cd. offer me the position of the wife of a gentleman . . .' He then went on to say that he could not explain matters fully 'on such a short acquaintance, that it was a question of "conflicting duties".' Next, he repeated that he was not free 'at present' and went on trying to elucidate his position:

he perhaps was not so passionately in love with me as a young man, but 'when a man of my age' (he is 38, he says) likes a girl, it means a great deal more than a boy's affection, that he did not wish to tie me, but he wd. never marry anyone else but me, & that if I heard of his doing so, it wd. be entirely beyond his will or desire . . . Then he said he might have gone away without saying anything, & that I shd. then have thought it was a common flirtation, wh. he cd. not have endured, & he shd. not have felt he had behaved like a gentleman . . . I never heard such contradictions.

There were many more lengthy explanations from the peculiar suitor and laconic interpolations by Jeannette. There was nebulous talk of a visit at Christmas. To close the interview he asked if she intended to tell her parents about what had passed between them. When she replied she would decidedly do so, he expressed his approval: 'he wished me to do so, & if P. thought he had said or done anything wrong that he wd. write to him. I did not fall in with this as I cd. not see what P. was to write, when he suddenly suggested "or shall I write to your Father?" I said "If you don't mind, I think that wd. be best", feeling that was tangible at all events.'

A moment or two later Ada came to announce 'that P. & M. had gone to bed, & it was time for us to go, and then seeing our "boule-versé" appearance, she withdrew.' However, the signal had been understood and nothing much more passed that evening.

The drive she had shown in the later stages of the Stone affair was a thing of the past; now she was once again passive, but this time her passivity had to do with her concern about Gould's predicament, new empathy, which resulted from her growing maturity. Both the candour and the unaccustomed sober tone of what she wrote testified to her involvement:

Of course this is not all he said, but the best idea I can give of it. He had a most difficult task, as he had to avoid seeming to think I wanted him, & yet at the same time to justify himself in my eyes. I don't think I let it appear if I liked him or not, & yet I certainly do. I must say for a man to put himself in such a position, & go through so much suffering as he did to explain, shows he has **some moral** courage, & is in earnest. Then I said as I offered my hand, wh. he held indefinitely 'Then you will write to Papa', & he said 'Yes! when I have seen my people'. Then he said 'If you think over what I have said, I think you will understand it better', & I replied 'I will try!' & looked at him as he looked down at me. His eyes were as honest and straightforward as ever, but looked quite strained & bloodshot, & his lip visibly quivered under his moustache. I never saw a man look more wretched.

The interview convinced Jeannette he was a gentleman; her instinct told her he was to be trusted. But it also made her feel completely at sea. She told Ada about it, 'because I felt I must tell some one, or go cracked. I never felt so completely bothered about anything, or so powerless to understand the situation.'

The events of the following days did nothing to explain matters. She did not see Gould again before he left for Cadenabbia early on the next morning, but found out later that he had after all at once sent her father a note to announce he would shortly be writing at greater length, unless in the intervening period he heard from Marshall. After Jeannette had explained what had passed between her and Gould, Marshall wrote by return of post 'a very kind note' to say that they, the parents, viewed Gould's feelings with sympathy and that he looked forward to hearing from Gould after the consultation with Gould senior. The kind regards with which this reply closed and the Savile Row address at the head of the letter made it abundantly clear that the Marshalls regarded Gould's move as a first step in a sustained courtship; this gave his suit a stamp of approval. The letter was dispatched to Cadenabbia and three days later Marshall received Gould's reply, which they discussed at length and which added to Jeannette's perplexity. 'I think it must have been written with a view of excusing himself & me, but does not throw any light on the mystery & therefore has aggravated the situation instead of improving it. In a PS he acknowledges P's letter, wh. "adds to his regret", tho' he agn. repeats he is not free to marry, & he promises to write agn. from England.'

For the first time in the development of this particular affair Jeannette found herself at variance with her father. Marshall, having read Gould's second letter, believed he was 'backing out' and was angry about it, while she thought that the only thing to do was to wait.

The third letter, the one Gould promised to send from England, never materialized. There were no further developments for a whole year. Jeannette filled pages of her diary with speculation about various matters pertaining to the affair, from his Christian names to his changing family situation. In early February she saw his father's death announced in the paper and remembered that Mr Gould had said such an event 'wd. make a great difference to him, & he shd. at once give up his position at Marlborough. Wd. this affect his inability to enter the "Holy Estate"? It might, I fancy.' She accordingly scanned the lists of those called to the Bar, and on not seeing his name, decided that he would have postponed such a drastic change till some future date. And gradually, the trust she had put in him waned and with it her hope of a happy outcome: 'I suppose Mr Gould was "very much married" —more than I shall ever be.'

For one yet again disappointed, she was at intervals surprisingly sprightly. 'I want a change & a little society & flirtation! I have been good a whole year, & can't keep it up any longer' she wrote in August, looking forward to their annual trip abroad. But she lacked true enthusiasm for this prospect: 'As I shall not meet Mr Gould I don't much care where I go.'

That year they tried new ground in Switzerland, choosing Grindelwald for their first alpine stop. On the fourth day there Marshall's bronchial condition gave cause for anxiety, so they decided to move to the altogether gentler and milder climate of Lake Como. Their choice fell on the Hotel Bellevue at Cadenabbia.

Reality now took on some of the obviousness of third-rate fiction. Within minutes of arrival, Jeannette espied Gould at the evening table d'hôte. She thought he, too, noticed her; at any rate, 'he wandered about like an unquiet spirit outside all the evening'. The next morning, 'he made the plunge, looking extremely agitated, & when he had shaken hands, not having a word to say.' But by the afternoon her hope had revived. 'He simply joins on from last year, & I believe likes me as much as ever.'

It is not clear that any of the four Marshalls, or indeed Gould himself, were particularly taken aback by the coincidence of their overlapping visits to the same resort and the same hotel. Jeannette did not even bother to declare herself innocent of having sent out signals (deliberate or inadvertent) of her family's plans for that year's holiday. For four days she was kept in suspense, expecting Gould to refer to the state of affairs between them. 'If he goes away without any further

explanation, the parents will rage, and I don't know whatever I shall do'
she wrote on the morning of the fourth day. As at Maloja, he postponed the crucial interview till the eve of his departure. It was getting
late, when he suddenly began, in an agitated voice:

'I scarcely expected to meet you agn., though I hoped I might do so'. He then
proceeded to tell me that for years he had not been his own master, that his
father's invalid condition, his sister & elder brother (who is delicate & does
nothing but live at home etc.) hampered him a good deal. I said 'Then things
are not changed from last year?', & he replied they were better, but not yet
satisfactory.

He went on to say that he had tried to draft an explanation of the
position to send to her father, but that he had destroyed the letter,
judging it better to leave matters as they stood.

But face to face with her, that evening, he must have been aware of
her challenge to his reticence, for he attempted to clarify his position:

he solemnly assured me agn. & agn. that there had never been, & never wd. be
anyone else, and that I might ask anyone who knew him as to the absolute truth
of the first part of his statement. He added 'You believe me, don't you', & I
said 'Of course, I do'. I must say it relieved me 'some'. Then he said he might
explain all fully, but he felt that [he] was not called upon to do it, as evidently it
is some family affair, & I acquiesced, as nothing is in worse taste than to appear
to want to know what others don't want to tell you. I said 'then you mean it cd.
never be', & he said 'No!' but the prospect was too remote to justify him in
trying to bind me, that if anyone else whom I cd. like appeared, he wd. feel
grieved to think he stood in my way . . . He feared his speaking agn. to me was
troubling me, but he cd. not bear me to think that he had forgotten last year,
and regarded himself as a mere acquaintance. He said 'You wd. rather I spoke
agn?', & I said 'Yes, certainly'. As last year I was the calmer of the two, and he
was dreadfully miserable-looking & agitated, but I really felt miserable enough
too.

Many more words were spoken, mostly by Mr Gould, but nothing
essential added to what Jeannette had understood at Maloja. He did
however leave her with the feeling that he cared more than ever. In a
fleeting bout of optimism she concluded 'I hope as we both feel the
same, we may be happy yet.'

The 1889 affair had lasted a matter of eleven days; this second (and
last) episode was shorter still, from the first sighting on Wednesday
evening to a snatched farewell first thing on the following Monday,
prior to Gould's departure for England. Before parting, Jeannette

made sure that he had their correct London address. Also, after coyly enquiring whether he cared to have it, she gave him a tiny likeness of herself, a postage-stamp-sized photograph, of which there is a copy in her scrapbook.

She probably never discovered more about Gould than he had told her in the sixteen days of their acquaintance. Even after their second meeting, she still did not know his Christian names: they were Marius Herbert. At Cadenabbia he must have referred to a change of plan with regard to his career. The idea of the Bar and going into politics was apparently abandoned in favour of continuing at schoolmastering. Two days after he had left Cadenabbia she wrote: 'He still has the notion that I shd. not like his position, but I don't think I shd. mind it for a time. Of course I should prefer it if he wd. get a good Headmastership.' That he continued teaching is known from an extraneous source, the memoirs of Siegfried Sassoon; Marius Gould was his housemaster at Marlborough in the years 1902–4.[1] Sassoon's view of him further blurs the impression which comes from Jeannette's account; he drew an eccentric, not uncharming bachelor, looking 'like an easy-going clubman who had put away a great deal of port in his day.' Gould in fact stayed on at the school till his retirement in 1910. At the time of his second meeting with Jeannette, in 1890, he was still only an In-College housemaster, condemned to a bachelor existence until some future date (in his case, 1895) when promotion to an Out-College housemastership, with a residence 'down the Bath Road', would provide him with married quarters. To marry earlier would have meant either giving up the housemastership and with it the chances of eventual promotion to Out-College housemaster status, or establishing one's wife, as if she were a concubine, in rented (or purchased) accommodation in Marlborough town and joining her only for the vacations. There was, of course, another solution which Gould could have put to Jeannette: that of postponing marriage until his turn for an Out-College appointment came round. But prospects of promotion were hazy, and to delay might have condemned the bride-to-be to give up the hope of bearing children, an obstacle which Gould may have been too delicate to spell out.

All this would of course have been known to Gould at the time of his original declaration at Maloja. It must be assumed that in 1889 he

[1] Cf. *The Old Century* (London, 1968), pp. 208, 210, 216–24, 232, 243–4.

indeed thought he had a chance of circumventing the Marlborough College impasse altogether, by switching to another career. Here the complex family situation at which he had hinted on first meeting Jeannette may have proved an insurmountable obstacle. Perhaps his daydream of a seat in the House of Commons had depended on expectations, which after his father's death had proved inadequate to free him from the shackles of Marlborough.[2]

Having at the second meeting told her something of his prospects at Marlborough, could he not have discussed all options with Jeannette or her father or both? It must be supposed that in the very short time available to them he was incapable of laying bare complicated and delicate matters, some of which might well have been confidential to the Gould family. And it cannot be excluded that Jeannette herself, for all her eagerness to understand, and for all her down-to-earth evaluation of other people's financial problems, may have in this instance steered clear of explanations centred on money matters. It must have been obvious to her that to face reality would have been tantamount to allowing this particular dream to shatter.

A fortnight later the Marshalls made their way back to London. Jeannette was gradually coming to terms with the thought that once again fate had let her down. But while from the Brown and the Stone fiascos she had emerged depressed and disillusioned, she now remained relatively unscathed, as if she found compensation in the certainty of Gould's emotional involvement. Moreover this time the excitement of recent important changes in her family's domestic set-up softened the impact of the collapse.

The first inklings of these changes had come a year or so earlier, when the lease of No. 10 was about to end: 'P. is rather worried about the diminution of his professional income, people thinking he has retired, & says we must leave this house & give up the carriage. Of course we wd. much rather do this, than be worried, but it is rather distressing to think of leaving here . . .' she wrote in June 1889. So it was with relief that she recorded, five weeks later, that on looking

---

[2] Philip Gould's estate amounted to less than £40,000. After a token legacy to the son from the first marriage, who was 'otherwise sufficiently provided for', the bulk of the inheritance became a trust, the income of which was divided, in unequal shares, between the three sons and the daughter of the second marriage. It is unlikely that Marius Gould's annual share of this would have been sufficient to tempt him to give up a housemaster's salary, emoluments and prospects.

through his accounts to determine what income he would have if he retired from practice, her father had found that it would be 'comfortable, very'. Providing he kept the Royal Academy professorship as well as the Medical Council and College of Surgeons appointments, it would amount to £1,430 a year, and even without the emoluments from the public bodies, it would still be around £1,200. The smaller sum was in fact also adequate for their needs, so she concluded: 'This discovery is a great comfort to us.'

Now came the business of the house. To renew the lease would have meant facing a substantial increase, amounting to one quarter's rent, from £200 a year to £250. They therefore decided to make use of the stay of execution granted them for one year by the landlords' agents to look for alternative accommodation. As there was no enthusiasm for leaving Savile Row, they house-hunted in fairly desultory fashion: Jeannette and Ada were delegated to inspect one or two Kensington houses, which they declared unsuitable. That was all.

The indolence paid off. On the Pre-Raphaelite grapevine Marshall heard that the Chelsea home of the painter William Bell Scott was on the market. Belle Vue House (fate had destined that it should share the name of the hotel in Cadenabbia) stood, and still stands, at the western end of the Chelsea Embankment, just beyond Battersea Bridge, on land belonging to the Cadogan Estate; its postal address is 92 Cheyne Walk. It is a fine ample structure some 40 ft. wide, built in 1771 reputedly to designs by Robert Adam.[3] The central windows are part of the deep bay which rises up all four levels of the house, from basement to second floor. On the first and second floor, the bay window is flanked on either side by elegant Venetian windows. On the ground floor, below these Venetians, the doorway (on the right), and (on the left) the entrance of what is now a garage but what was originally stables, are crowned by two generous 'depressed' arches.

In the autumn of 1889 parents and daughters were shown round Belle Vue by the quaint Mrs Bell Scott (her husband had long since transferred his easel, and his affections, to Scotland, where he died in 1890), and declared themselves 'rather fascinated' by 92 Cheyne Walk. 'It is rather far, and the neighborhood not nice at present,

[3] Nikolaus Pevsner, *The Buildings of England—London: Volume Two* (Harmondsworth, 1974), p. 102, cautiously calls them 'worthy of Adam'. Its original owner was John Hatchett, a coach-builder from Long Acre, father of the FRS chemist Charles Hatchett, who lived at Belle Vue until his death in 1847. The William Bell Scotts had moved to Belle Vue House in 1870.

though it is improving . . .[4] The garden is a desolation, everything in the sitting rooms dirty, & the bedrooms most poverty-stricken, but the place contains great possibilities.' The unanimous verdict was that once put in repair, cleaned and decorated, the Scotts' house would suit the Marshalls 'down to the ground'.

The negotiations over the lease took three months; eventually they got it for £850,[5] 'a very good bargain, as we all like it so.'

The impending move and the preparations for it now became paramount in their thoughts and conversations. In the diaries, Jean-nette's growing excitement about Belle Vue displaced even the specu-lations on whether Mr Gould would or would not press his suit. As if to mark the start of a new era, she abandoned a custom which had lasted ever since her mid-teens: when in December 1889 she came to purchase a new diary, she replaced the usual olive-green Pettitt's Diary, with its almanac and long pages of information about the ramifications of the royal family, by a more elegant notebook bound in dark red morocco and free from the constraint of date-numbered pages. This, and an identically bound but slimmer version, would eventually contain the remainder of her record of youth and young womanhood.

For a week or two they were distracted by bad news from Ely. On 3 February 1890 a card from Aunt Wilkes announced Uncle William Marshall's illness; two days later they heard of his death; he was buried, sharing Aunt Julia's grave, on the 8th. Two wreaths and a special bunch of Riviera flowers—'these Ada insisted on paying for,— Poor Uncle was so devoted to flowers!'—were sent to the funeral, which in view of the cold weather none of the Savile Row Marshalls attended. Mourning was procured. This time Jeannette and Ada made even their vigogne (vicuña) 'best' dresses without the help of a dressmaker; with mourning etiquette increasingly relaxed, their recently remodelled 1888 travelling dresses, brown with a white hair-line, were sufficiently sombre for everyday use. Uncle William's will

---

[4] Access, whether from the north, via Beaufort Street, or from the east, along the Embankment, was through slums. The effect was compounded by the fact that until the middle of 1890, the building of the Embankment round the north end of Battersea Bridge, and the conversion of the bridge itself from timber to iron, made the whole area into a vast builders' yard.

[5] The original lease was very short; the sum paid suggests expiry within no more than twelve years. The Cadogan Estate issued 'a concurrent lease of 21 years fr. Lady Day next [25 March 1890] at £70 per annum'. It was presumably extended in 1911, as Ada lived in the house up to the time of her death in 1936.

and financial affairs ranked some attention from Jeannette, but by mid-February she was once again engrossed in Belle Vue matters.

The repairs and decorations in the new house were not completed until March 1890. To refurbish the bargain cost £980, almost double the original estimate. The fact was that their ideas grew in grandeur as the work progressed. All four, and the daughters in particular, were carried away by the charm of their new possession. With so much elegant space at their disposal, they determined to make it into a showpiece.

For Ada and Jeannette it became an exciting challenge. The parents gave them almost complete *carte blanche* over the choice of colour schemes and designs; for a month or so the two young women wallowed in pattern books and swatches of curtain and loose cover materials, and were delighted when the parents (and the foreman of Curtiss, the builders) approved their taste. It was not unlike the planning of an entire Season's wardrobe which had occupied so much of their time some ten or twelve years back. The sisters worked well as a team; together, they measured and matched colours ('looked at different shades of paint till I did not feel as if I had any "eye" left'); together they shopped and presented their choices to Mr and Mrs Marshall; the task of instructing and arguing with the foreman was usually Jeannette's. And to her, besides proving a welcome distraction, the planning and contriving connected with the move was a gratifying test of what could be achieved without professional advice.

Not that such help was unavailable; it was rather that they themselves, besides being very careful in their spending, set greater store on comfort than on interior decorators' 'stylishness'. Uncle Edwin Williams had early on suggested commissioning an architect to draw up plans for the conversion; indeed there was one in his immediate family, his son-in-law, cousin Leila's husband, Walter Stokes. And while they were still at Savile Row, Marshall received a visit from a budding architect, Randall Davies (the son of the incumbent of Chelsea Old Church), who wished to be put in charge of the work at Belle Vue, which he gratifyingly called 'one of the most beautiful old homes in Chelsea'. Both offers were rejected. 'We are going to trust to Curtiss' & our own taste.'

Starting from scratch gave them much more scope than they had had when refurbishing No. 10 in the late 1870s. The four drawing-rooms alone required two separate colour schemes and turned out 'sweetly pretty', the main ones with pale yellow and white wallpaper, pale chocolate and white woodwork, fawn and blue chintz curtains and light Indian carpets to set off the exquisite designs of the cream and white ceilings; dark-blue velvet chair seats contrasted with all these pastel hues. The side drawing-rooms were in the fashionable grey-green, with pink and white papers and light cream curtains. The generous stairway, the landings and the double hall were all papered in cream with a formal buff flower and vase design, very highly varnished; cardinal and black were the colours chosen for balusters, door and window frames, and also for the swing doors which divided the inner from the outer hall. Downstairs, the central suite of dining-room, on to the river, and Marshall's study, on the garden side, looked dignified with deep blue-green walls and golden brown highly varnished paint and green curtains. The Turkey carpet and the oak furniture of the dining-room came from No. 10. On the western side of the ground floor there had originally been stabling space. This now became a large library, 34 ft. deep and some 12 or 13 ft. wide, with an arched, full-length window on to the Embankment and a vaulted ceiling. For this room they chose an Indian red for the woodwork, lightened by the terracotta-on-cream ground of the wallpaper. The red curtains had previously hung in Hill House; the carpet, with a black ground, also came from Ely; there was enough of it to cover Marshall's study too. Perhaps because the three main bedrooms on the second floor faced fully south on to the river, they cooled them down with blue paintwork and artistic blue and white paper. The soft furnishings on this floor were also predominantly blue. Even the servants' bedroom became a matter of pride; Jeannette thought it looked sweet, with its pale brown paintwork, and yellow and white floral paper.

The final effect was more self-conscious, more calculated to impress, than what they had lived with at Savile Row. It was as if they intended Belle Vue to become material proof to the world at large that the Marshalls, despite the move, despite the father's semi-retirement, despite the fact that they were about to give up the carriage, were still going strong. They had imbibed over a score of years the artistry of their aesthetic circle; having modified it with their own good sense, they were now ready to exude the Marshallic version of the high-art style.

Under his brother's will Marshall inherited Hill House and its contents; Charles Bidwell, a remote kinsman of the family, was charged with arranging an early sale. In the middle of March, with what the Marshall aunts regarded as unbecoming haste, Jeannette and Ada were dispatched to Ely to pick out any pieces which would come in useful for their new abode.

The Ely heirlooms, mostly eighteenth-century pieces, a little glazed cabinet thought to be a genuine Chippendale, a tiny tulip-wood table of the same style, two or three small armchairs, an oak writing-table, a bedstead and a picture or two, came in useful in supplementing the Savile Row furniture when they allocated them to their new positions in Cheyne Walk. After the 'rather salt' builders' bills and the purchase of huge quantities of curtaining, floor coverings and chintzes for loose covers, very little else was spent on equipping the new home. One or two objects had been renovated; two large wardrobes, out of Mrs Marshall's and Jeannette's rooms, were divided to fit their allocated spaces. There was the usual long bill for small items, from curtain rods to door mats; they bought oil cloth, a set of kitchen chairs from Harrod's, and a new range; they acquired a folding bedstead for the manservant (who, as it happens, gave notice five weeks after the removal; his successor, a drunkard, was eventually replaced by a parlour-maid). They also splashed out on a large number of lamps for the four drawing-rooms and a green bronze and brass chandelier to hang over the dining-room table. But the bulk of the furniture were pieces familiar from Savile Row.

As a preliminary to moving, Jeannette and Ada packed all the plate, including the costly salvers, epergnes, and salts from grateful patients, into crates for removal into the safekeeping of Marshall's bank. The move itself, entirely orchestrated by Jeannette, followed a week after their raid on Hill House, and extended over six days. On 20 March (a Thursday) the parents were dispatched for several nights to Bailey's Hotel, Gloucester Road, dropping Jeannette at Belle Vue. Ada and Harriet, the housemaid, followed with a cab-full of essentials and a cold pie for their first lunch at the new house; cook came later with more parcels. The removal men (from the Army and Navy Stores—'the real article') had been packing since the morning of the Wednesday, and by the evening of what Jeannette later described as a 'nightmare day' delivered the first three van-loads. Later that evening the sisters called on the parents in their 'very comfortable quarters. They took all very cooly, & cannot imagine what a state we are in.' Back in Belle Vue, they retired to bed, with cook and housemaid to support them, for the first night in their new home. Exhausted and over-excited, Jeannette next morning complained of having slept 'so badly'. 'Such queer noises. We hear several clocks strike, wh. I am glad of, & the river looks like Venice.' Two more van-loads arrived that day and also the grand (which Aunt Eliza had bought for Jeannette ten years earlier), brought over by three giants from Broadwood's. And so on for another four chaotic days, till Jeannette was glad to see the last of the 'dreadful army of removers . . . quite 20 of them', though she admitted that to a man they had been very civil and respectable. On Monday 24 March the parents came at tea-time for a first look at what had been accomplished. And still the sisters went on: blinds went up; they unpacked the wine, the china and the glass; they arranged trophies of ornaments on overmantels and supervised the hanging of pictures. In the midst of it all, on Day Six of the move, they received the visit of Sir Henry Acland. In his search for Marshall, he found his way through the kitchen, '& wd. have come up to the bedrooms if Harriet had not stopped him!' 'My poor feet feel quite battered' she wrote that evening. Day Seven brought another visitor, Mr Justice Denman, also looking for his old friend Marshall; he 'cd. scarcely believe that P. was going to live here altogether'. When later that day the parents moved in, they all had their first dinner in the new dining-room. 'It was a treat to have a meal in Christian style.'

It took them another five weeks to get quite straight. On Monday 5 May, their first 'at home' day at Belle Vue, with a spirea on the landing, a genista on the tea-table and jonquils all over the drawing rooms, they received their first accolade. Jeannette later noted that those who came had been 'in raptures, pure & simple. We had our fill of compliments, & no mistake.' And it was altogether gratifying, to them who had never before had their full measure of callers, to receive on this and the following Mondays of the Season (barring afternoons of catastrophic weather) up to a dozen or fifteen visitors, all exclaiming in delight over the beauties of the house and the taste of its amateur interior decorators. 'Mrs Edis was particularly delighted, & said so'; this praise from the wife of the fashionable authority on the furnishing of town houses was indeed flattering. At the end of May they were hosts to some hundred and twenty guests, mainly 'medical cows' and artist-friends; some were however only vague acquaintants, a few of them unknown to Jeannette. The soirée was a success: 'We had a certain number of lions, including Surgeon Parke (of the Stanley expedition) who was

unexpectedly goodlooking & young & nice. He came early & stayed to
the last. Had also Mr Justice Denman, Sir Henry Acland, the Justin
MacCarthys, the Holman Hunts, the Hamo Thornycrofts, nearly all
the Medical Council, the Wakleys & Ernest Hart!' As on the afternoons 'at home', compliments abounded: 'our taste was pronounced
perfect . . . Many folks declared they wd. die of envy.' She especially
appreciated the fact that Theodore Watts-Dunton, a member of the
Rossetti (and Bell Scott) coterie whom she usually met only at the
Royal Academy, had come to inspect what had been done to Belle Vue
House. He was 'enchanted with our decorations, & said that we
deserved the house. The two rooms thrown together astonished him,
he exclaimed agn. & agn. "What a noble room". The pink rooms were
declared "perfect".' Jeannette's cup brimmed over.

Belatedly the Marshalls had turned over a new leaf. It was as though
acquiring a house worthy of being shown off had bestowed on them
the self-assurance and warmth of born hosts. Or was it that with
retirement Marshall sloughed off large numbers of boring patients
(including many from his wife's family) and equally boring colleagues,
so that they could confine their hospitality to the more entertaining in
the medical, scientific and artistic coteries? There was, moreover, an
element of reinforcement in the self-selected assortment of callers;
news of the charm of Belle Vue spread in the Kensington and Chelsea
circles sufficiently to draw to their soirée and their Mondays 'at home'
a few who would not have dreamt of visiting Savile Row unless it was to
consult Marshall himself. Friends and acquaintances brought their
families and friends to see this latest addition to the number of show
houses. Some of the visitors were people to whose receptions the
Marshalls had been in the past, but who had been too grand to return
the compliment. The 'magnificent' Mrs William Priestley now came,
and so did Mrs William Crookes; the Wakleys of the *Lancet* joined the
throng and so did the wife of another influential journalist, Mrs
Leonard Courtney. The seventy-five year-old Sir James Paget did
them the honour of a visit, though usually only his wife (the Image) and
his daughters called on the Marshalls. He had known the house when
Bell Scott's predecessor, Mr Slocock, had occupied it; 'curiosity at the
bottom of the compliment' commented Jeannette. Another doyen, Sir
John Simon, also came to congratulate Marshall on the house, 'wh. he
said emphatically was a gentleman's'. Mrs John Westlake called, 'by
Mrs Garrett-Anderson's desire'. She, and several others, never came

again; it had been a formal courtesy to new neighbours who also happened to be friends of friends. Proximity was in fact one of the clues to the influx of new acquaintances; many of them lived in Chelsea or Kensington, south or west of the Park, within walking distance of Cheyne Walk.

These West Londoners were part of the evidence that the Marshalls' focus had now shifted. Their map was no longer that fan-shaped segment, radiating from Piccadilly Circus. The new map, at least for Mrs Marshall and her daughters (for Marshall himself continued to visit most of his old haunts), now covered a smaller area, with Park Lane to the east, the Bayswater Road and a little of Notting Hill as northern confines, continuing southwards through Holland Park and the Earl's Court area into Chelsea, and eastwards again, along the Embankment and Royal Hospital Road, to turn up Sloane Street and zigzag back to Hyde Park Corner. Having relinquished the carriage (except when they hired one for special evening occasions), they paid their calls by public transport or on foot. Even their church attendance changed; they abandoned St James's, Piccadilly and St George's, Hanover Square, for the newly consecrated, artistic Holy Trinity, Sloane Street. However they also occasionally ventured as far as Vere Street, north of Oxford Street and more distant than St George's. St Peter's, Vere Street, abutting on London's main medical enclave, was regarded as the church of the profession, and it may have been this that attracted the Marshall sisters. Eventually they also modified some of their shopping habits, patronizing Oetzman's and Tully's in the Fulham Road rather than Shoolbred's in Tottenham Court Road when buying for the house. For their personal needs they remained faithful to the Regent Street shops, but their fashion purchases took on the form of organized sorties rather than casual visits, and the old mainstay, John Lewis, was now no longer on their regular route.

Later in 1890, as the novelty of the nine-day wonder that was Belle Vue House wore off, there was a noticeable reduction in the number of callers; but then the pace of autumn sociability had never equalled that of the spring and early summer. For the moment they continued to be well-pleased with their achievement. And for all her anxiety about the unsatisfactory development of the affair with Mr Gould and the underlying conviction that she was doomed to stay at home indefinitely, with her parents and her fellow-sufferer Ada, Jeannette was on the whole less dissatisfied with life than she had been for the past ten years, ever since Harry Brown had so disappointed her.

Her end-of-year budget was bitter-sweet; the bitter predominated, with good reason as her father's ill-health caused them great anxiety. Under these circumstances, the beautiful new house and the boon of not having to share it with John did not receive a mention; nor did she remember the pride of achievement she and Ada had shared when the compliments had rained down on them last spring and summer. 'Here is the end of the year, & I can't say it ends well, & it has brought us many sad sad times' (this referred presumably to Uncle William Marshall's death, for the other deaths in the family, of uncle-by-marriage, Mr Yate, and a cousin-by-marriage, Mrs Gerald Williams, hardly elicited the equivalent of a sigh when she noted them earlier in the year):

I see that poor old Mr Cropley died on Boxing Day. Wd. have been 93 in January (31st). The only bright spot in this year was meeting Mr Gould agn., and of course I don't know if that will lead to anything, or if it would be for my happiness if it did. I cannot help thinking him a true & honorable man, & liking him despite his mysteries, & he seems certainly to like me as much as ever. I do hope & trust the next year may bring us happy days, and a favorable solution to all these puzzles. I wish <u>first</u> for P.'s recovery however. Goodbye to 1890.

She herself had felt unwell on Christmas Eve; by the evening she lay back in the easy chair, convinced she was 'going to be ill'. By Christmas morning she was covered by a 'full-blown & painful' rash, which spread alarmingly. 'Eat scrap of turkey somehow, but pudding impossible.' Her father's dismal expression, on Boxing Day, made her think that her own diagnosis of smallpox must be correct; and when she was told that Marshall had decided to call in Dr Seaton, 'the greatest authority on smallpox', she resigned herself to all this perilous disease implied.

When the specialist, after a very thorough examination of the rash, told her she was suffering from a mild attack of chicken-pox, she was much relieved, though she 'did not think it particularly nice either'. Three days later Ada too had come out in a rash and Mrs Marshall now had her hands really full, with two daughters in bed and her husband suffering from a violent recurrence of his usual winter bronchitis. On New Year's Eve, Marshall's doctor, Thomas Barlow, brought a nurse to help with the routines and Jeannette, feeling much better, saw Dr Seaton, who had been in daily to check on her progress, and now had another patient in Ada. She also wrote some letters and the annual budget, quoted above.

At 7 a.m. on 1 January Ellen came into the room which her daughters were sharing since the inception of Ada's rash. 'We both started up, & asked how Papa was, & when she said "Very bad", I knew all was over. He died at 5.30.'

CHAPTER 15

REVERSALS OF FORTUNE

IT took Jeannette a full day to overcome her reluctance to look at her father's body. When she did, she found it consoling that he was so 'majestic and beautiful', at rest in the inner coffin.

After the initial hours of abandonment to total pain, she was too busy to give way to despair. The Marshall aunts had to be notified of the death of their only surviving brother; so she wrote letters to Aunt Yate (with whom Aunt Wilkes was staying) and to Aunt Dix; she also dispatched a note to Aunt Eliza who could be relied upon to broadcast the news to the other Williamses. There were decisions to be made about the funeral arrangements and mourning for the three of them. Within a matter of hours of Marshall's death Mr Bartlett, their lawyer, had summoned two saleswomen from Peter Robinson who brought samples and took measure. In all this activity Mrs Marshall was of little use and Ada of no use at all; she had given way to hysterics on hearing of their father's death, and had to be sedated by a soothing draught prescribed by Dr Barlow. Constant vigilance was then required to keep her calm. Jeannette and the nurse (a sensible German woman who stayed on for a week after the death) had their work cut out to manœuvre things so that neither Ada nor Mrs Marshall would hear the undertakers' men tramp up and down stairs and hammer down the lid of the oak coffin.

The first test of Jeannette's decisiveness and competence came on the eve of the funeral, when she countermanded Bartlett's arrangements to have the coffin transferred to Ely on the 7.20 a.m. train from Liverpool Street, which would have entailed sending the hearse from Chelsea at 5.30. Telegrams buzzed backward and forward till the train of departure was changed to the 11 o'clock[1] 'wh. is respectable & reverent. Really I was completely crazed until it was settled.'

In the days preceding the funeral the three women had gone

---

[1] A slow train, hearses not being accepted on fast trains.

through a few spontaneous rituals, much as they had all done, Marshall himself and young John included, seventeen years back on taking leave of Reggie. Before the coffin was nailed down, Ellen had placed a ring of hers on her husband's finger. Later they had all three put their hands on the lid of the coffin and kissed it and asked forgiveness for any wrongs that might have hurt or offended the deceased in his lifetime. Jeannette reverently bent a knee 'as to a Saint' each time she passed the door of the room that housed the coffin. And they each took a flower for remembrance out of their own wreath, and kissed it before affixing an envelope which bore a last message in which they had included John: 'To the dearest Husband and Father from his grieving wife and children.' 'We have not that foolish prejudice agnst. flowers' wrote Jeannette, reflecting a more general change in funeral fashions; at Reggie's funeral there had still not been any flowers other than the little white bouquet contributed anonymously and the few blossoms which Ada had cast into the grave. This time over a dozen wreaths, besides their own, were placed on or around the coffin.

Neither the wife nor the children followed the coffin. John, of course, was still in St Petersburg; his letter, expressing (Jeannette thought) remorse, did not reach them till a week later. Ada was only just beginning to get up after the chicken pox. Jeannette had developed one of her bad colds, and Mrs Marshall was 'so hysterical that she would not go herself' nor let Jeannette attend the funeral or even accompany the coffin as far as Liverpool Street station. So the coffin went off, flower-bedecked but followed only by a few empty carriages. Dr Barlow was late, but eventually caught up with the sad cortège; a carriage, bearing another lovely wreath from a patient, was also sent on to Liverpool Street.

That evening they received a telegram from Dr Barlow 'to say all went well. My darling "Pappy" as I used to call him is with dear Reggie & poor Uncle. God let them rest peacefully, & mercifully grant we may meet agn!' It was Barlow, too, who two evenings later made time to bring them a more detailed report on the proceedings at Ely: 'He & Mr Bartlett & Mr Tweedie at Liverpool St, Prof. Macalister at Cambs. & Mr Dix, Mr Cross & Mr Coates at Ely. Mr Lowe read the service, and our wreath was put in the grave, & the others on it'; a sparse account—could it really be that distance and the January weather reduced the attendance of friends and professional associates to a handful, and of relatives to only two?

Perhaps because he sensed their disappointment—they would not have expressed it, having themselves stayed away—Barlow went on to tell them that the medical journals were 'taking the greatest pains with the obituary notices' and that he had been told by Sir Andrew Clark 'that Papa would have had the refusal of a K.C.B. almost directly! How pleased he wd. have been, & how empty it seems now! I like him better as he was than with all the titles in the world!'

Within a week of the funeral, the feeling of having been anaesthetized, which had protected Jeannette from sensing the implications of her father's death and the intensity of pain it had left behind, wore off. 'I am beginning to realise our loss, & I am so wretched!' Little melancholy tasks and little dispiriting miseries confronted her. Their wardrobe of coloured dresses and bonnets had to be dispersed among deserving connections. A replacement had to be found for the 'little wretch of a cook' who drank and did not send up anything fit to eat. The people who came to value the contents of Belle Vue for probate had proved over-zealous, poking their noses everywhere and demanding to know every detail, down to the number of dusters; a complaint in Jeannette's hand went off to Mr Bartlett.

They had money worries also. Their longer-term financial outlook was satisfactory: 'Our income (with M's money) will be fully £1,100. How we wish Papa cd. have lived to enjoy it.' But for the present they were seriously embarrassed by cash-flow problems. Huge amounts had to be paid out, £872 in death duty, representing 4 per cent of the probate valuation of £21,800, and later another £120 to meet lawyers' bills and disbursements. 'We are in a great muddle & uncertain as to what we can afford' Jeannette wrote in February, and again, seven weeks later: 'That disgusting tax has nearly beggared us. We feel we must be most careful, & live from hand to mouth.'

In the early weeks of bereavement Dr Seaton was particularly attentive and kind. Indeed his calls were so frequent and so prolonged that both Jeannette and her mother once again started the usual speculations about the causes of this special courtesy. However, after mid-February a medical complication gave Seaton ample excuse for some weeks of regular visits. On 16 February he inoculated Mrs Marshall, Jeannette and Ada against smallpox, a routine precaution if further panics were to be avoided, as their previous inoculation dated back to the epidemic of May 1881. Jeannette's inoculation proved only too effective: within three days her arm swelled and turned septic, requiring daily dressings. Seaton, who blamed himself for excessive zeal in wielding the lancet, seemed to appreciate the opportunity of these sessions for relatively informal chats. By late February Aunt Eliza, at Cheyne Walk for a few days' stay, was led to ask if it was her niece's arm or her niece herself that were the object of the doctor's visits. So that when her arm at last healed the incorrigibly speculative Jeannette had for once good grounds to wonder in what way Seaton would justify his future calls.

Right from the early days of their acquaintance, when he had set her mind at rest and gently teased her for having apprehended the dire diagnosis of smallpox she had detected a resemblance to her last-but-one admirer: 'He ... beams on me most graciously, & looks appallingly like Mr Stone!' This referred more to his manner than to his appearance, that of 'a red-faced, clean shaven, fair man of about 44, with a disgustingly healthy aspect'. And once she had equated him with Stone, it was natural that she should fear a recurrence of the familiar pattern of early enthusiasm, followed by some shilly-shallying and ending in frustration.

She was underestimating Seaton. A middle-aged, successful professional (his speciality was public health; shortly after meeting Jeannette he was appointed first Medical Officer of Health for Surrey), a widower of some seven years' standing, he was too busy and took his work too seriously to engage in aimless dalliance. Because of the peculiar circumstances he happened to be the only eligible man with regular access to Belle Vue. Once he had decided that Jeannette attracted him, time would be on his side; no holiday arrangements would snatch her from his reach after only a few days' acquaintance. All this made him quite relaxed about allowing the relationship to develop at an unhurried pace.

She could also not have known how exposed she must have appeared to any reasonably self-confident suitor, now that she was no longer the privileged daughter of the privileged surgeon at the top of the establishment, but a captive prey in her mother's drawing-room immobilized by the recent bereavement. It must have been evident that she was ready to snatch at the lifeline presented by marriage to get out of what she saw as a dismal predicament. Throughout that spring and for most of the summer she speculated about the strength of Seaton's involvement, pretending that even if she were to decide that she preferred the single state, to bring him to the point of proposal would be to add yet another scalp to those already hanging from her belt. 'I feel that if I had him for myself, I cd. finish him now. Curious how one knows that, & rather amusing feeling too ... ' she wrote in early

March, and again, after six weeks had passed: 'had I a proper chance, he is a "gone coon", but flirtation in the proper sense is impossible before witnesses.' At other times, however, she was less sure: 'I wonder if he is in love with me?'; she did not appear to realize that the very fact that she now used the term 'in love', where in earlier affairs she had written of being liked or admired, put Seaton's attentions in a special category.

The lessons of the past seemed altogether forgotten: '<u>Does</u> he or not? . . . My experience rather points to <u>yes</u>' she conjectured, as if her intuition had never let her down on previous occasions. In fact not many weeks passed before her position started to change from one of faint amusement to the less detached one of expectant acquiescence. 'I have no doubt of his worth, but don't think I could' she had written in mid-January. Three months later she speculated that his age, which she now knew to be forty-three, would suit hers well enough. Then it was: 'I like him & respect him. Is that enough?' till, by mid-July, she was ready to give him the benefit of any remaining doubt: 'I cannot help thinking he is épris, & I might do worse!'

Despite his undisputed seriousness, Seaton appears to have been quite accomplished at flirting. Whether fortuitously or by design, his non-professional visits were sufficiently irregular to keep Jeannette guessing; he would call several times in a single week and then be absent for up to three weeks, leaving her to speculate about the cooling of his attentions. He flattered her by listening closely and retaining what she told him of her interests and preferences yet she soon discovered that he did not take her views altogether seriously: 'I take the opportunity of differing from him on most points, particularly matrimonial ones, whereat he chuckles.' He kept the few notes she sent him, and brought them out ostentatiously from his left breast-pocket. He sent her roses because she let it fall that of all flowers she liked roses best. And, very cleverly, he put himself under obligation to her. He consulted her about the choice of a wedding present for a relative and made her feel good when he followed her advice. Better still, he availed himself of the skill Jeannette (and Ada) had recently acquired and asked her to help with the typing of a paper; he was then unstinting in his praise for the neatness she and her sister had achieved.

It was this help which provoked his most adroit (though not necessarily deliberate) move. This was to misunderstand a letter in which Jeannette parried his thanks with a rather clumsy though well-intentioned message to say she had been glad 'to balance accounts a little'; he took it as evidence of having caused her offence, for which he apologized by return of post. 'He must have had a sunstroke!' she wrote on perceiving what havoc she had caused by her riposte. 'What stupid creatures men are!' But she wrote an 'ultra-amiable answer' explaining that he had misread her meaning. 'Still, I am amused, for it is the worst sign yet. I suppose he thought I was sarcastic, when I was in earnest, & has been fashing himself. It is too funny!!' At this stage of their relationship her speedy and placatory response must have convinced him that she was not indifferent to his feelings.

His own reply was in the form of a wooden box full of roses, honeysuckle and ferns which arrived by post from Guildford on 20 July. 'What does the good man want in exchange? M. & A. both grin; I can't help it. I suppose it is a sign I am forgiven.' At their next meeting there were further explanations after which they 'made it up' for good. 'When he leaves, he holds my hand a very long time, & with a very tight pressure. It is interesting, but I don't see how he is to get on, when I am always c. M. & A!' This was the third or fourth time this year that she complained of being excessively chaperoned. In the seven months since she had first met Seaton, they had been left alone in a room only a very few times. One Thursday in April he happened to call when Mrs Marshall had left for Holloway and Ada was changing dresses upstairs; in tête-à-tête with Jeannette his conversation had inclined towards the 'personal & complimentary'. But he was aware that the intimacy would soon be interrupted, and left without in any way attempting to press his suit.

As a personal approach was out of question, some other way had to be found. At the end of July Seaton went to Bournemouth to deliver the address—the one Jeannette (and Ada) had typed earlier that month—to the annual meeting of the British Medical Association; on Bank Holiday Monday Jeannette was 'very pleased' to discover that the paper (on the evolution of sanitary administration in England) had been the subject of a leader in *The Times*. On the following day, 4 August, came the communication she had been eagerly expecting for some weeks past:

When I came down, there seemed to be no letters, so I went to look at the 'glass', & there in the outer hall lay one for me from Dr Seaton, sealed with a big seal. My heart went into my shoes there & then; I opened & read what I expected. He has been wishing for an opportunity of speaking for some weeks, that he admired me, & when he saw my 'loveable character', became 'deeply

attached to me'. 'Indeed I love you very sincerely.' Can I care for him? etc.
Really very nicely expressed, no flummery, but straightforward & manly, & I
shd. say genuine. I felt distinctly queer, but went back & made the breakfast &
endured Aunt Anne's commonplaces, with the fatal document in my pocket.
After breakfast I told M, who says I must decide if I like him well enough. Poor
me! Went to town c. A. & told her en route. She does not think him good
enough, but then she wd. not think anyone <u>that</u>.

They went to the bank to check a box of Marshall's securities,
and carried on with the rest of the day's business, shopping, avoiding
a downpour, and then returned home to lunch, needlework and some
urgent letter-writing. This did not include replying to the one
Jeannette had received earlier in the day: 'Dr Seaton must really wait
for his answer, as I must have time to think it out.'

She retired to bed without having come to a conclusion. 'I had a
wretchedly bad night, awake till 2.30, and then snoozed till 5, & from
then broad awake agn! Really the man is too great a bother!' Nevertheless, by mid-morning on 5 August she had 'hammered out' (on the
typewriter?) her answer to Seaton's offer:

After my sleepless night I felt as stupid as an owl, but had come to the
conclusion that if I refused him I shd. regret it, & being superstitious I cannot
forget that the last letter my dear Papa wrote was to ask him to come to see me.
But I felt I cd. not accept there & then, so managed to frame an answer to that
effect, saying that I had reflected on his letter, that I was flattered etc., that his
kindness had made a deep impression on me, & that I thought I cd. feel
towards him as he wished, but as his letter had come on me a little suddenly, I
shd. prefer delaying my final answer. In the P.S. I mentioned Aunt Anne's
presence, & said she knew nothing of his letter etc., and finished by saying fr.
M. we shd. be pleased to see him when his engagements wd. allow him to
come. Shut up this, and then wrote a correspondence card to say I was going to
Hol. tomorrow, & Aunt Anne's friends coming on Fri, so offered him
Thursday, Sat. or Sun. for dinner.

Having posted the letter and the postcard to Seaton's George Street
home,[2] she felt relieved. But the respite she believed to have gained
was cut short by the suitor's impatience. Soon after tea there came a
knock on the door, announcing Dr Seaton:

I cd. have expired on the spot, but didn't. A. fled, but M. & I had to stand our

[2] The coincidence of George Street, Hanover Square, having in 1854 been her
father's temporary abode, after Crescent Place and before he married and moved to
Savile Row, did not elicit any comment from Jeannette, perhaps because this part of
Mayfair provided accommodation for so many other medical men.

ground. He entered looking so solemn that I thought he had not had my letter, & felt worse than before. However he gave me a most <u>meaning</u> clasp of the hand, & said 'I was so very pleased to get your letter!' I <u>gave</u> him some tea, & we talked on commonplaces tant bien que mal. I shook <u>inside</u>, but was pretty calm <u>out</u>. He said he feared he 'shd. give M. a great deal of trouble' (I'm sure I hope not), 'but you mustn't mind that!' After ¼hr. or so M. most treacherously withdrew, saying she wd. see what A. was doing. Her back was scarcely turned when he moved to her chair, wh. was close by my easy one, took possession of my hand, & said how happy my letter had made him. I was afraid what was coming next, so hastened to say 'You understood what I meant', & he said 'Yes; I won't hurry you or press you', for which I was thankful. He wd. not let my hand go, so I had to leave it where it was, while he said 'Yesterday was a frightfully anxious day; he did not know what to do with himself'. I said 'You did not expect to hear yesterday, did you?' and he replied 'No! I rather hoped not; as I feared it wd. be bad news if I did.' Then he proceeded to say that when he found nothing this morning, he thought it best to 'go about his business', and rushed to Haslemere, did his work, & tore back by 3. Nothing but a wretched Congress letter awaited him, but by the next post my 2 letters came. As luck wd. have it a horrid man from Minnesota had called, and wd. not go, and he had to put my letters in his pocket, & remain in agonized suspense, & doubly intrigué at there being <u>two</u>, till the Yank took his departure. I really cd. not help laughing. The minute he had read the fatal epistle, he came & le voilà. He spoke next of Scotland later, & said 'You'll let me come', and asked if he might fetch me fr. A.E's tomorrow afternoon. I had to say 'Yes', but felt appalled. He does not let the grass grow under his feet. I said I wd. fetch him V. Horsley's letter, & escaped for a moment. He read & approved, & the rest of the interview was conducted standing. He got my hand agn, & said how happy he felt, but added 'but I am very impatient!' & tightened his grasp so that he quite hurt me. I trembled for consequences, so said hastily, 'but you will wait, won't you'. & he said he wd, & that he wd. take the 'greatest care of me', wh. was not exactly pertinent. He then kissed my hand, said 'Goodbye', and departed. I was thankful I had managed him so well, for I was really afraid of him twice, & I <u>do</u> want a little time.

The delay was a token of the customary hesitation which younger women, who could be expected to have many irons in the fire, regarded as becoming. As luck had it, on her way back from Holloway the following afternoon (Ada and she were coming back unescorted, after all, as on learning that there might be other Williamses at Aunt Eliza's, she had countermanded Dr Seaton), she saw Mr Gould 'solemnly stalking' along Regent Street. However, this made no difference to the present situation. She had long since given up hope of a resumption of Gould's attentions; he had in any case queered his pitch by his 'heartless' failure to condole after her father's death. So she noted briefly: 'A. says there must be a duel, but I don't think he is likely to make any move', and then went on to record another letter from Dr Seaton, who declared he would wait to hear from her when he could come again, but suggested a time two days ahead, adding that he would hope to have the opportunity of an interview with Mrs Marshall after he had spoken to Jeannette; 'another awful prospect! Really I shall be a threadpaper, and I am so tired, and have such a headache.'

She assented to Seaton's suggestions ('I suppose I must "get it over" ') and on the afternoon of the appointed day changed her dress and 'endured existence somehow', waiting for the interview:

I never felt in such a fright in my life. I managed to get Aunt Anne to lie down & rest about 4, wh. was somewhat of a relief to all of us. When Dr Seaton came (about 5.30) he was asked into the dining-room, & I had to go down to him. I nearly died en route, but managed to get in, & shake hands. He said he had thought of me so much, that it seemed such an age since he had seen me etc., and asked if M. wd. see him. I said 'Yes, certainly', & after a little ordinary sensible talk I went to call her, & she took my place. It was not dreadful at all, & I felt quite relieved and light-hearted. He is really a kind, good creature, & has mercy on me. I heard he told M. how fond he was of me, that he wd. take the greatest care of me, & be all she cd. wish. I hope he will. His appointments bring him in £1000 a yr., and this income can be augmented, so this is comfortable, & he is perfectly satisfied with what M. can do for me, viz: £1000, or the interest fr. it. We must consult Mr Bartlett. He was to stay to dinner, so came up into the drawingroom, and we were all talking when the 'inky' arose fr. slumber, and appeared in our midst. She was agreeable, & not so suspicious as I feared. Dinner was as usual, & while A. was making the coffee, the talk turned on Ely, & Aunt wanted Jeremy Bentham[3] got, so I had to offer to get it, tho' I felt it was dangerous. He asked if he might come to carry them as they were heavy, & followed me to the Library. He lit the gas, & I got the big vols., and a duster, & rubbed them vigorously, but the fatal issue was not to be avoided. He came quite close as I stood by the table, got hold of my hand & said: 'I had such a nice talk with your mother; she quite approves.' I responded 'I know she likes you', & he said 'You will say Yes! won't you?' I felt driven up a corner, so meekly responded 'If you really wish it', & the next instant he had me in his arms, & was kissing me. I was so astonished at the rapid & irresistible nature of the assault that I did not resist, but when he put my head on his shoulder, & proceeded to spoil the set of my fringe by resting his cheek on it, I feebly protested that we must go back, they wd. wonder what had become of me. He let me go for a moment, but said 'Oh! I shd. like to keep you here; I

---

[3] The correct name of the historian of Ely, who inhabited Hill House in the eighteenth century, is James Bentham (1708–94).

have so much to say to you', but I was firm & said that must be postponed till later. Thereupon he put his arms round me agn, inflicted half a dozen more kisses, & whispered 'I will make you so happy; I will take such care of you' etc., all interspersed with many dearests & darlings, and then shouldered the fatal volumes, & returned to civilized society. I flatter myself I carried it off better than he did, as I believe I was quite natural, while he got hold of some engraving or other, & pored over it without saying a word.

Before leaving that evening, he told Mrs Marshall that Jeannette had 'made him very happy'. Before closing the record for that day, Jeannette herself added: 'M is glad, I think, but A. is frantic at present. I do hope & trust I have done right. I really like him, and he is a good, kind man, and I think & hope will be a comfort to all of us. He certainly appears devoted to me, and I do trust him, and believe in him. Anyhow I have "cast my lot", and will do my best.'

The months that followed put this determination to the proof. Some of the business arrangements which normally followed on engagement proved in this case unexpectedly intractable. To begin with, there was an immediate conflict of interests about the date for the wedding. Mrs Marshall insisted that proprieties were to be observed; the strictest mourning etiquette laid down a minimum of twelve months in deepest mourning after the death of a parent, followed by another few months in full black; the ceremony could therefore not take place before March 1892. This was totally unacceptable to Seaton, who felt he would be making a generous act of patient forbearance in allowing Jeannette three months for the preparations; he opted for November. Jeannette quite early on decided that direct negotiations between mother and husband-to-be would lead to trouble. She therefore undertook the task of mediating, and eventually got both parties to agree on late January as a compromise date. When in mid-December the time for sending out wedding invitations had almost run out, she at last managed to get Mrs Marshall to fix a day; reluctantly, Ellen agreed to 19 January.

Also, for all Jeannette's diplomacy, relations between her mother and Dr Seaton were bound to come to grief over money matters. The doctor had taken 'something very much like a dislike' to his future mother-in-law; 'I can't wonder either' wrote Jeannette towards the end of the engagement, 'as she really behaves like a child . . . He told me about his first interview with M [hitherto she had known only her mother's version of what had been said about financial matters] & was evidently surprised that I had nothing in my own right. Of course poor Papa wd. have left us something if it had not been for M. However he is satisfied as it is, and says he wants me for myself alone. He certainly won't get much more.' Marshall's will, dating from 1885, with a codicil added soon after the move the Cheyne Walk, allowed his wife to enjoy the house and the income from what he left in the way of cash and investments for the duration of her life; on her death the remaining lease of Belle Vue, and its furniture, were to be divided between the daughters (or their issue), and the remainder of the estate including such valuables as plate, jewellery, pictures and the like would go in equal shares to all three children. There was no provision for marriage settlements, perhaps because the eventuality of either daughter marrying had been discounted; on the other hand, it may have been a deliberate decision of Marshall's to leave the matter of dowries to the mother. Nevertheless, the will included a clause which empowered the trustees to advance to any one of the residual heirs up to £1,000 against his or her future entitlement. In the case of Jeannette, Mrs Marshall not only did not supplement this sum with a more substantial dowry, but argued—persuasively enough to convince her brothers Edwin and John (her co-executors and co-trustees)—that Jeannette's immediate rights were not to the capital sum of £1,000, but to the income thereof. The actual settlement was delayed till 30 December. Then, three weeks before the date set for the wedding, Mr Bartlett explained that Jeannette was to have this interest, £50 a year, in quarterly instalments, and that the principal would stay in trust until after Mrs Marshall's death; to add to the injury, the trust was to be settled not on Seaton, but on Jeannette, and administered by a cousin on the Williams side of the family.

To argue might have endangered the match or at least delayed the wedding. So the settlement was drawn up according to Mrs Marshall's wishes, and Jeannette signed it four days before the ceremony. But despite the compliance of the Seaton interest, the atmosphere remained charged. By the day of the wedding not only Mrs Marshall, but also Ada, whose animosity against her sister's fiancé had strengthened as the months had passed, could hardly bring themselves to speak to the bridegroom.

Meanwhile Jeannette revealed a great deal of aptitude at handling delicate situations. In contrast to her mother, she showed herself far from grasping. Right from the start, when Seaton consulted her about the sort of engagement ring she would prefer, she specified something 'pretty, not heavy and not too expensive'; three days later, when he put the ring of his choice, set with diamonds and pearls, on the third finger of her left hand, she declared it perfect, 'only far too good'. She insisted on contributing her savings, or a substantial part of them, to the furnishing of their future home; to share the cost was her way of repaying him—within the means at her disposal—for her mother's stinginess; it also gave her a chance to replace discreetly some of Seaton's own pieces which were not to her liking.

Then, having established a reputation for restraint and common sense, she carried off an easy victory in the important matter of their future home. For a very few days she allowed her imagination to aspire to Orange House, a fine though dilapidated building dating back to the turn of the seventeenth century, at the top of Cheyne Row.[4] But she was easily persuaded that this was unrealistic, and fell in with Seaton's wish to settle within easy distance of the Surrey line, south of the river, to simplify his journey to and from work. However, once they had fixed on the area round Clapham Common, she steered him gently away from several properties in indifferent locations and towards a fascinating, 'highly respectable' Georgian house, 'with big trees at the gate' and 'a nice portico', on the north side of the Common. She took Mrs Marshall and Ada to see this, The Limes, in late August, and they were all three charmed by the 'dear old place', with its 'too–too' garden front and back. Within two days she returned with Seaton to show him over The Limes, and to reject yet another Clapham house. Her mind was made up.

What remained to be settled was the financial side of the transaction. Seaton hoped to save £300 out of his regular income from the Surrey appointment as Medical Officer of Health. What this left for their annual budget was £700, augmented by any windfalls such as fees for articles or lectures. It was at this point in the calculations that Jeannette almost casually let it slip that £50, equivalent to the annual income wrung from Mrs Marshall, would amply suffice for her own needs: 'that would dress me, & leave something over to buy things for the house. He exclaimed & I said "Why I have never had more than £30, & have never spent that on my clothes alone". To see his face was

---

[4] William de Morgan, who lived a few doors away, rented Orange House from 1876 till 1882, to extend his studio space. In 1895 it was replaced by the RC church of the Holy Redeemer.

a study; I cd. not help laughing. He said that was one thing wh. he had been worrying about, wondering if I shd. be satisfied with £75!' This evidence of her frugality decided Seaton to risk committing himself to a repairing lease for The Limes at an annual rental of £110. In addition to the rent the lease stipulated that he was to spend at once at least £100 on essential repairs; the sellers for their part would contribute £250 to the builders' bills, in the form of an allowance out of rent. The contractor's first estimate (Jeannette had again plumped for Curtiss, with herself as 'clerk of works') exceeded the sum allowed for by the lease by £150 to allow for decoration as well as repairs. By 5 November the lease had been signed; it then took only nine weeks and seven supervisory visits by Jeannette (and Ada) before the caretaker, who was to watch over the contents until after the honeymoon, moved in and the first van-load of furniture was delivered. The final bill from the builders' amounted to £376, only a very little more than the sum set down in the lease.

So much for the business side of the engagement. Jeannette had in the meantime to unlearn, in a five months' apprenticeship, half a lifetime's habits of Marshallic reserve. Lessons in warmth and spontaneity could be had for the asking in Seaton's immediate circle. His relatives were both more closely knit and more demonstrative than she was accustomed to in her own family. His two sisters called within days of being told of the engagement, and insistently brought their young to inspect the new aunt-to-be; they expected her to call back and to come to family meals. In contrast with the barriers which Marshalls and Williamses alike erected against physical contact ('I do not like kissing' was Jeannette's regular complaint on meeting effusive friends or distant connections), the Seaton family went in for cordial handshakes and kisses and hugs. Jeannette was surprised and slightly shocked to hear a niece refer to 'dear old Uncle Ted', when she herself had only just overcome her reluctance to write of him as 'Edward'. She was even more astonished when his sister Alice Buchanan greeted her with a 'hearty smack' or his other sister, Mrs Soden, wrote to her as 'My dear Jeannette' and finished the letter with love and 'Yours affectionately', styles which the Marshalls reserved for their most intimate correspondence. Indeed, when her fiancé headed an early letter to her 'My dearest Jeannette', she thought it 'rather cool'.

Entering a new family also brought entirely new demands on her tolerance of the irregular. Of Seaton's two surviving brothers, the younger, Frederick, was in the tea business in China; the other, William Sharpey Seaton (whose second name was a homage to the same Dr Sharpey who had been Marshall's patron at University College Hospital), lived in Cornwall. A month or so before Dr Seaton's offer Jeannette had chanced on an announcement in *The Times* to the effect that 'a person "known" as Charity Thomas was henceforth to be called Catherine Seaton'; 'evidently the person in question lives with Dr Seaton's brother, at least Wm Sharpey are his names, & he is an electrical engineer.'[5] At the time she had made a note to 'demand an explanation' of the mystery, but the subject did not arise again till late in the year, when the lists of people to attend the wedding were being drawn up. It was then that Seaton explained that his brother William was 'a good sort, but wrong-headed, and that he wd. not marry the woman fr. some high filutin notions, but gave her his name in that unusual style.' True to precedent Jeannette was ready to accept an irregularity which did not threaten her own interest; she took a 'sensible view' of the matter, and a wedding invitation went to William Seaton, though Catherine Seaton, alias Charity (or Cherry) Thomas, was apparently not included.[6]

With Mrs Marshall 'absurdly starchy' in her notions about chaperoning, unhelpful about equipping the new home, and stubborn about fixing the day of the wedding, and Ada touchy and huffy by turns, Jeannette was in the mood to appreciate the Seaton connection; a day or two before her gesture towards William Seaton she set her seal of approval on all of them: 'My new relations are most amiable.'

When after a month's engagement Seaton asked if anyone else had ever kissed her, he 'was enchanted to hear they hadn't'. She had everything to learn, from hesitantly referring to him as Edward in the diary to actually calling him by his first name to his face, from being kissed to (occasionally) kissing back. The first time she took the initiative and kissed him of her own volition was when he gave her a special Christmas present, 'a little gold bar tipped with diamonds, & with 2 rings entwined of diamonds & pinkish rubies in the centre', bought, 'to show his devotion', with the £10 which his mother had given him in her last illness twenty years earlier. 'It quite touched me, & he was quite affected too.'

[5] He *inter alia* laid the cable between Oran and Marseille.
[6] She eventually married William in 1893; of their five children, the four daughters are believed to have been born before that date; the fifth, a son, was legitimate.

Five months was a short time in which to learn her role in the sexual partnership. She was, it will be remembered, thirty-six. Seaton, whose birthday was in the summer, was now forty-four. During the seven months' courtship which preceded the engagement he had his libido well under control; a prolonged handshake or a tender touch when dressing Jeannette's sore arm was all the gratification he claimed from her. But as soon as her acceptance legitimized his suit, physical demands asserted themselves.

He was a persevering, and on the whole considerate, teacher, aware no doubt that her nerves would be on edge and her dignity at its most fragile. And Jeannette, for all her protestations of passive endurance of his advances, enjoyed the process of learning as if it were a sport. She played at counting kisses and lapped up the endearments and declarations of devotion. It did not take her long to discover that 'anything flirty' or even one look from her made 'his eyes regularly gleam'; 'I am fully aware of the effect I can produce when I like.'

Mrs Marshall and her daughters spent most of September at Shanklin on the Isle of Wight, where Seaton joined them for weekends. As always, chaperoning arrangements were less efficient on holiday, so that Seaton could be sure of a few sessions alone with Jeannette, or with only Ada as escort. On his first visit he and Jeannette excursed *à deux* to Ventnor, with the train passing through a long tunnel soon after Wroxall. 'No lamp, & I read mischief in Edward's eye. The sequel showed I was right, as he put up the window, and returning just as we entered the tunnel, caught me in his arms, and began to kiss me. He fumbled at my veil, & turning it up, pressed his lips on mine & kept them there until we came out agn, about 2 minutes I shd. think. It was really too bad, but he declares it was "delicious".' This rail journey was such a success that they repeated it the following weekend, and again, with Ada, towards the end of the holiday. After this last excursion Jeannette noted: 'Lamp in tunnel, wh. was disappointing.' She had progressed quite far in the four weeks' holiday.

That autumn she reported her encounters with Edward Seaton, detailing every endearment and each new embrace, just as years ago she had described the making of a new dress or bonnet. On occasion, she noted, he 'half-frightened' her. 'Just before he left he had one of his savage fits; & I really tried to get away, but it is a hopeless business as his grasp is like iron, & if he wants to kiss me madly, he does, that's all . . .' At other times, 'quite alarmed at the conflagration' she had raised, she would succeed in repulsing his kisses. He then held her tight in his arms, which calmed her and gave him time to get over the passionate paroxysm. He would later explain, half-apologetically, that his immoderate outbursts were due to her power over him, that she 'made him feel so bad and then reproved him'; 'if only he cd. walk or row 50 miles a day, & tire himself' he would, he maintained, cope more easily with the strains of waiting; 'but he is so strong he can't tire himself (more lucky me!)'

She learnt quite quickly about the dangers of precedent. From kissing her standing up—she was just the right height for kissing, he declared—he went down to a kneeling position; later, he would wrap her in the wings of his greatcoat, to make escape virtually impossible. As her shyness gave way and the engagement drew to a close, she allowed him greater liberties. 'He has worried me agn. & agn. to sit on his lap, & I have refused agn. & agn, but today he represented we were to be married so soon, & besought me so long that I consented for a minute or two, tho' I warned him I was very heavy. He exclaimed "Heavy! I cd. nurse you all day!" He kissed me, & declared I had the most beautiful figure, & whispered a fair amount of nonsense.' Just as other privileges the 'nursing' became an established right; within a fortnight, on the occasion of his Christmas gift, she wrote: 'I cd. not refuse to sit on his lap after this, & indeed he makes me now. That is the worst of giving in once.'

Most of the love-making took place in the short moments which they snatched out of the routines at Belle Vue House, moving from dining-room to drawing-room, going to the library on the pretext of consulting a dictionary or atlas, or into the hall for leave-taking. Jeannette found these stolen moments very inhibiting and tried to avoid such passionate clinches, with doors never closed and her mother and Ada within earshot. Poor Seaton, who no doubt was at least equally ill at ease, was inclined to bluster through these situations. On one occasion, as she tried to escape from his embrace in the hall, he challenged her direct: ' "You are afraid of the kisses sounding?" ' and, when she admitted this was so, remarked: ' "Why shd. you mind my darling?" ' On her reply ' "Because it's shocking!" ', he laughed and kissed her harder than ever; 'I can't keep him in order now!'

As the wedding drew closer, Mrs Marshall increased her vigilance; she scarcely allowed Jeannette out of her sight, when Seaton called at Belle Vue: 'About 11.15 Edward came, intending to sit with me. So he did—with me & M. It was really pretty disagreeable of her, & I cd. see

he was bored. I hate (& so does he) discussing things before her.'
There were rows whenever they were late returning from a visit or
walk. Jeannette was remarkably philosophical about her mother's rant-
ing: 'after supper we stayed down some time. Of course I was blown
up, but I am used to it. It makes me rather long for matrimony too!'

Seaton resented Mrs Marshall's attitude on Jeannette's behalf as
well as on his own. Throughout the months of courtship and engagement he had tried to do 'the polite' and so gain approval in Ellen's
eyes. But neither the calls to enquire after her health, nor the time-
consuming semi-professional visits to Edwin Williams or Aunt Eliza,
to reassure Mrs Marshall about their illnesses, appeared to mollify her.
And while courting Jeannette by the clock, with furtive embraces in the
hall or on the drawing-room floor landing, might have added spice to
his ardour, it also increased the strain of keeping his passion under
control. This showed in tense sessions of complaint:

I fancy M's perpetual presence tried him a little, as when at last she withdrew
& left us together after supper, he was rather worrying . . . complaining that he
never 'had me to himself' now, that I 'docked him off his kisses', & that he felt
so not being allowed to kiss me at 'the Limes' the other day [when Ada had
accompanied Jeannette on a tour of inspection] . . . he thought at one time that
I was a Diana, but now he thought me more like Venus! He really ought not,
but I can't stop him . . . He is a crazy man! He says he feels as though he had
waited all his life for me! that I am the crowning point of his existence . . .

At times it was Jeannette who herself added to the tension, occasions
of devilment, when Ada mischievously reminisced about her sister's
earlier romances and Jeannette found the opportunity to tease irresistible. Seaton's self-esteem, undermined by the strains of semi-public
love-making, was very vulnerable to such attacks:

He was very nice at first, but then began to worry and ask if I had ever liked
anyone else etc. He bothered me so that I said Yes, thinking of Mr Brown, but
of course said it was years ago, & never came to anything. Then he did worry
so that I wished I had not told him. He is so frantically jealous . . . Then he got
the notion that I did not love him, and that the French saying about 'un qui
aime, et un qui se laisse aimer' was illustrated in our case. I cannot go on as he
does, of course, but I do like him, or I never wd. have accepted him. This I
tried to explain, but not very successfully . . . After coffee we had another 'go'
at the same subject, and he drove me up a corner, & in my feeble condition
[she was suffering from influenza symptoms] I told him a little more. I fear
agn. the result was not good, but I really can't go in for a full report till I am
married. I hate talking about those things. At last I said he might be sure no

one cd. say anything about me, & that I thought he might trust me, wh. melted him.

A week later it was Edward's turn to talk about his past:

He showed me a portrait of his wife, who had a nice, sweet face & good features, and gave it me. He evidently liked her very much, & was happy in a calm fashion. But he is anything but calm with me. He says . . . that he feels as if he had never known what it was to <u>live</u> before! That the combination of sentiment & passion wh. he feels for me is the most perfectly exquisite feeling anyone cd. have, that I have changed his entire nature. He raves too much, but declares that we are so near being married that he may express his feelings a little more freely.

On one occasion he exceeded the limits of what she regarded as permissible. Early in December the engaged couple attended a dinner in their honour at the Edwin Williamses. After the meal at which there once again had been some teasing about Jeannette's past conquests, in the hired coupé which carried them back to Cheyne Row, his love-making was at its wildest:

He caught me in his arms, & went on in the craziest way. I really was quite frightened, tho' I remained outwardly calm. He scarcely seemed to know where he was, & what he was about. He was a perfect savage! I really had to expostulate & resist, when he put one hand down the nape of my neck & the other arm right round me, & covered my face with burning kisses. He let me go, & put down the window for a few minutes, then took my hand, & sat & looked at me. I felt pale & agitated, but sat still & did not look at him. I hope he was ashamed. He really should not behave like that . . . I had a bad night. Worried.

The following day, instead of showing contrition, he added to her dismay by harping on the previous evening's gossip about her past flirtations: 'Feeling aggrieved as I did, to be taken to task was <u>too</u> much, & I gave him a slight 'set down', wh. had a salutary effect, in making him a little more reasonable. A worm will turn, & I thought it time <u>I</u> shd. . . . After supper we had a longish talk, and had it out.' On his remarking that she had looked pale towards the end of the previous evening, she gradually let out the cause of her indignation:

I smiled sadly; he asked me to sit closer, I shook my head, & said 'I wd. rather not, after last night'. Then he understood, and was most repentant. He made me own I had slept badly in consequence, & that he had hurt my feelings . . . he was so grieved to think what he had done, saying: 'What a brute I was! Do forgive me my darling! You know I worship you, and would do anything for you'. He seemed sufficiently miserable & sorry, so I forgave him, & he begged me to <u>trust</u> him, that he wd. never offend again etc., & was altogether nice & kind & good agn.

He did however once again repeat that some more freedom was permissible now that they were so close to becoming man and wife. And though she had made her point about being treated with proper respect, she knew that keeping his ardour within what she considered as permissible limits would from now on depend on her: 'It is a good thing that I can keep cool! I had to let him nurse me agn. nolens volens, and hear his mad speeches. He behaves respectfully, "because he promised, on his honour", but says very shocking things, in low whispers, as "I want you so badly! No woman was ever longed for as I long for you! I adore you! I have a <u>desperate</u> passion for you!" . . . He does go on like a maniac.' A week later, there was one of the rare references to her own feelings: 'Whatever will he be like when we are married? He declares he loves me now much more than I do him, but that then he will <u>make</u> me love him, and I <u>shall</u> love him. I think I do now, well enough.'

He tried to obtain the promise of a special Christmas treat, whispering various 'more or less shocking' suggestions in her ear; 'the least so that I shd. let him kiss the back of my neck! It made me feel quite warm as I did not know what was coming next.' He was once again playing with fire for several days later she complained: 'He still recurs in a disgusting manner to his Christmas privileges. I don't quite see it.'

None too soon, the period of their probation was drawing to an end. They still had to face a series of trials. Each of them was sufficiently catastrophic to jeopardize the wedding. Just after Christmas news came of Aunt Dix's death; unexpectedly, Mrs Marshall decided against a postponement of the ceremony. Early in January, the marriage settlement threatened to come to grief; this was avoided only because Seaton, who saw it as an attempt by Mrs Marshall to make him back out, decided not to contest its wording. At mid-January, on two doom-laden days, they heard in turn that Uncle Edwin's health had deteriorated dramatically, that Aunt Startin was critically ill with influenza, and that Uncle John Williams who had been entrusted with the privilege of giving Jeannette away was now far too ill to come up from Brighton for the ceremony. The fact that Mr Blunt, the vicar of Chelsea, whom Jeannette had asked to officiate at the wedding, happened also to be on the sick list was a relatively minor contretemps.

Their own health also showed signs of breaking under the strain. Ten days before the wedding Jeannette caught a nasty cold; Seaton's trouble was a gumboil, bad enough to require poulticing and to restrict his diet to 'spoonmeat'.

In these last weeks of her life as a single woman Jeannette as usual behaved as if nothing could knock her off-balance. One by one she chalked off the tasks which had to be accomplished before her wedding day. In the first eighteen days of January she wrote and sent the wedding invitations, unpacked and acknowledged over seventy wedding gifts, arranged them (with Ada's help) in the library on three tables covered with pink sateen cloths, fitted her wedding dress and veil at Allison's, finished making her 'best' dress, trimmed a hat and a bonnet, ran blue ribbon through the insets of her undergarments, and appointed a caretaker for The Limes. She shopped for the new home and for her trousseau, bought a beautiful going-away cloak, chose the field-glasses intended to be her wedding gift to Edward; all this, besides the usual duties of receiving callers, dealing with post-Christmas and New Year correspondence and supervising the arrangement of furniture in the new house.

She also managed to steer a perilous course, soothing Edward (who had vacated George Street and was now billeted in the providential Bailey's Hotel) and keeping his ardour 'within bounds'. On 6 January, to 'his supreme satisfaction', she instructed him to order their joint visiting cards, as well as her own in her married name. 'He says he can scarcely believe he is going to have me at last.' Four days later, on the plea that they would hardly be allowed to see one another without witnesses on the days preceding the wedding, he 'was more familiar than I approve . . . He is so tremendously in love with me, and so strong that I feel I have to be on my guard . . .' But she found his embrace consoling when he called on the evening of 16 January, at the end of the two disastrous days: 'After all that worry & misery, it was a real comfort to feel his arms round me, and hear him say "My darling!" agn. & agn.'

The following day was a Sunday, most of which Seaton spent at Cheyne Walk, walking over from Bailey's for dinner, for tea and again for supper. That evening Ada did not come down, feeling too low-spirited. 'I was so sorry, but what am I to do?'

On the Monday, the eve of the wedding, things looked up a little. The news of two of the invalid relatives, Uncle John and Aunt Startin, was distinctly better.[7] Mr John Thornycroft wrote to say he would give Jeannette away 'with pride & pleasure'. Canon Chapman had earlier agreed to replace the vicar and officiate at the ceremony at St Luke's, Sydney Street. Edward came to Belle Vue at tea-time: 'He is longing for tomorrow more than I do. I rather dread the whole affair. Still here goes! I believe he loves me very much, and I like him sincerely, and trust we shall be happy together. Good luck to us both! Amen.'

Of the practical arrangements for the wedding there was relatively little in the diary, for all the world as if Jeannette had been indifferent to as well as apprehensive about the proceedings of the day, and interested only in its outcome. There were to be three bridesmaids: Ethel Topham, a friend of Jeannette's, and Edward's niece, Florence Buchanan, in addition to the baleful Ada. The costumes prepared for them were of pale grey crépon with white ribbon trim, with hats of grey felt adorned with white ostrich tips and white velvet bows. The bridesmaids' bouquets of pink tulips and tinted foliage and her own spray of orange-blossom had been chosen by Jeannette, but paid for by the bridegroom. Seaton also gave each bridesmaid a small ribbon-shaped brooch of gold and pearls to wear on the 19th and to keep in remembrance of the day. Jeannette's dress had been ready for some days. She declared it 'just perfect', of cream-coloured brocade woven with a pattern of lilies of the valley tied into sprays with true-lovers' knots, and trimmed with cream chiffon, satin ribbons and pearl passe-menterie. The veil was of plain white tulle. The 50lb. cake from Buszard's, surmounted by a basket of lovely fresh white flowers, was pronounced a 'wopper'.

Jeannette's account of Tuesday 19 January, 1891 is laconic: 'Slept frightfully badly of course. I wept before & during breakfast. Edward came very early, and took away my box. I did not see him, as it [is] not the "right thing", & my eyes were very red.' She went on to describe two more presents and then closed the entry quite abruptly: 'We finished doing the flowers, and got my things out, and now I feel things are getting on. I hope all may go off well, and that Edward & I may be happy. I feel nervous, but suppose most brides do. Good luck!!!!'

---

[7] Aunt Startin subsequently had a relapse and died on the day of Jeannette's wedding. Jeannette was not told of her death until she returned from the honeymoon.

CHAPTER 16

AFTER THE HONEYMOON

THE honeymoon logged a single paragraph in the diary; this referred to the morning after the day of the wedding, with Edward and Jeannette no further than the south coast: 'We made up our minds to go by the later boat, as the early one wd. have been a scramble, so we had breakfast at something nearer 10 than 9. Most lovely sunny morning, and we sat by the fire with the window open to our meal.'

They had discussed their travel plans as far back as September 1891, rejecting the Riviera in favour of Biarritz. One of the magnets that attracted them there was its proximity to Pau, still the domicile of Mme Canut, Jeannette's former tutor. The encounter with Madame took place, though whether the Seatons went to Pau or she came to meet them on the coast is not clear. What is certain is that besides Biarritz they visited St Jean de Luz and Bayonne, and also spent some days in Paris. At Biarritz itself Jeannette recognized some acquaintances from Ely, whom she later accused of being stuck up because they had affected not to know her; that they might have pretended to ignore her out of tact did not apparently strike her.

They returned to London on Saturday, 20 February. The diary record resumed the next day. Edward was immediately drawn into the routines of his Surrey duties; on most weekdays Jeannette now had long clear mornings on which to get things straight at home. It was as if the clocks had been turned back two years to when she and Ada had created order and beauty out of the chaos at Belle Vue House. Ada was once again her assistant and together they shopped, measured, sewed and wielded paint-brushes to embellish The Limes. It took a fortnight to get the main rooms straight; on 4 March Ada came over to inspect the total effect, including the placement of several house-plants Jeannette had instructed her to buy. She approved what she saw; and yet the visit was not a complete success: 'I can't help feeling she is rather "pokery".'

A week later Ada returned with Mrs Marshall to lunch and tea and a formal visit of inspection. 'M. was personally conducted over the ground floor by E, I showed her the next one, & after lunch the remainder, & she was very pleased, & admired all very much. I must say I think the rooms are getting to be pictures.'

Although Ellen's guided tour suggests long vistas of public rooms and a maze of bedchambers, The Limes was not a grand house on the scale of Belle Vue or 10 Savile Row. Built on the standard Georgian plan, it consisted of a hall, four reception rooms and as many bedrooms; in addition there were good attics and the usual conveniences, a bathroom on the second floor, and the kitchen with its sculleries, larders and pantries in the basement. These lower regions held little interest for Jeannette; her mother's example had stuck and she stayed out of the kitchen quarters. But from the ground floor up to the attics the house was very much her pride and joy, with Edward, who shortly before the wedding had declared himself a convert to aestheticism, as an acquiescent though appreciative partner.

Not that The Limes was much influenced by her earlier aesthetic notions; it was much more up-to-date than that. She had done wonders, on a relatively small budget, to achieve a feeling of lightness and modernity. The beds and bedding were of course bought new. But the bulk of the other furniture she bought second-hand, mainly in the Fulham Road where a patient shopper, with time and appetite for frequent exploratory expeditions, could pick up wonderful treasures for next to nothing. She paid £3 5s. for a 'real old' rosewood side-table; a seven-piece suite of inlaid, Sheraton-style, drawing-room seating, 'delightfully pretty', cost £16 10s.; the dignified dining-room set in carved walnut came to £14 10s. The more heterogeneous these bargains, the better did they conform with the new feeling for eclecticism; all that was needed to fit them into a harmonious modern whole was a sure eye for colour, reflected in the choice of papers and paintwork, of carpets, curtains and other soft furnishings.

For the new house Jeannette settled on two main colour schemes. In the chief one blue was dominant; blue carpeting with buff walls for hall and stairway; blue and red Turkey carpet, blue Utrecht velvet upholstery setting off Middle Eastern saddle-backs, and many other blue accents to go with the walnut of the dining-room furniture; pale greenish-blue as background to the pattern of white feathers on the wallpaper in all the bedrooms, with deep cream paintwork and plenty of cream and pink in the curtaining. The second scheme was warmer. It went into Edward's study, with its pinky Axminster (a wedding present from Edward's relatives, the Sodens), the red and cream cretonne of the sofa, the crimson curtains, transferred from George Street, and several other pink and red and gold highlights. It dominated the drawing-room, first-floor front, 'sweetly pretty' with pale apricot and ivory walls, old gold upholstery and light-coloured Indian carpet; its small anteroom was decorated to match. The two schemes merged on the attic floor where the servants' rooms had turned out 'very quaint & Japanese-looking with pale brown paint & peacock & cream paper with a daisy pattern'.

Did all of it, the attenuated Victorian dignity of the dining-room, the light-hearted presage of Edwardian frivolity in the drawing-room, the vestiges of aestheticism in the hall, add up to something resembling a comfortable, welcoming home? A set of eight photographs taken just after the turn of the century supplements the copious entries in the 1892 diary, giving an almost complete view of the interiors at The Limes; even individual wedding presents and the paintings and prints on the walls can be clearly identified. Only the study is entirely convincing, a business-like workroom of a man too busy and too serious to strive after effect. The rest of the house seems self-consciously static, a showpiece for the delectation of Jeannette's friends.

Early in April 1892 Jeannette sent out cards to inform that she intended to be at home on Sundays and Tuesdays 'à perpetuité'. Friends, relatives and acquaintances came in a steady trickle, but not in the great droves which two years earlier had invaded Belle Vue, to exclaim and wonder at the beauty of the transmogrified house. Praise from people regarded as the originators of the fashionable interior was of course particularly gratifying. When first Mrs Eastlake, 'who congratulated me on all, including my husband', and later Colonel and Mrs Edis, who 'went into details as only artistics do', were most appreciative of the house and of the furniture in particular, Jeannette knew her efforts were well rewarded.

Most of the visitors were not (or no longer) carriage folk, though they might occasionally hire a brougham for a round of afternoon calls; and for many of them, to reach Clapham Common without a carriage was to undertake a complicated journey, by train, or by tram and boat, with several changes and some walking in unfamiliar streets before they got to The Limes. A similar problem arose whenever Jeannette went to pay calls north of the river, or indeed to visit her mother and sister at Cheyne Walk or to shop in any but the most casual fashion. It was not that at Clapham she was entirely deprived of shopping facilities. Within easy walking distance there was the Pavement, the curved parade at the junction at which Clapham High Street meets the Common, where chemist, hardware and china shops supplied her most urgent needs; this was also where the butcher and fishmonger whom she favoured with her custom were located. Occasionally she ventured a little further afield, to 'prowl' along Lavender Hill and replenish 'after a fashion' her supplies of other simple items such as curtain hooks, ribbon or postcards. But for more ambitious purchases of hardware, ironmongery and dry groceries she went or sent orders to Harrod's, or to 'the Stores' where she had opened an account by depositing £5.[1] Much of her shopping for fabrics and other dressmaking materials was now transferred to the relatively accessible region round Sloane Square, with Munro's, Wakeford's and Peter Jones, 'a goodish shop but slow', as some of the suppliers. Though going to Regent Street or Oxford Street entailed quite an expedition, she remained faithful to Liberty's for soft furnishings, and went to Peter Robinson's for outer garments and to Evans' and Swan and Edgar's for millinery and odds and ends.

Going to Cheyne Walk usually meant a tram journey and crossing the river by boat to Cadogan Pier; if there were parcels to carry on the return journey she often took a cab. Trams and buses were in any case overcrowded during rush hours, so that she had an excuse for that extravagance. Her chief objection to public transport was its tedious slowness: 'we are both sick of the tram & omnibus route [which took them to Piccadilly to exhibitions or the theatre, and also to Victoria, to visit Edward's relatives in Belgravia] but there is no other.'

All of this meant that social calls north of the Park became a rare, hired-brougham, occasion, which required careful planning. If people on whom the Seatons intended to call happened to be out, it took but a minute to leave cards, so that with luck six or eight or even as many as a dozen calls could be achieved in an afternoon. As for visiting Aunt Eliza in Holloway, the alternatives now were 'a long, horrid journey' by train with a change at Aldersgate, or to take five different buses, a

[1] It is not clear whether she took her custom to the Army and Navy Stores in Victoria or preferred the stores in Waterloo Place where they had mainly shopped for household items during the Savile Row days. The practice of paying an annual subscription or of putting down a deposit to open an account was common in stores run on a co-operative basis.

round trip of anything from three-and-a-half to four-and-a-half hours. The record for an inconvenient journey was achieved when she excursed to Uncle William Williams in Highbury; to get there she took a tram to the station, changed on to a train which got her as far as Camden Road, and continued north-eastward first by train and then by cab—all for a twenty-minute formal call on uncle and cousins. No wonder that even the visits to Aunt Eliza were all but cut out. In the seven months from March to the end of September she went to Holloway only four times. However, Jeannette took care to maintain contact with Eliza, the only close relative on her own side of the family with whom she remained on excellent terms throughout. She made a point of going to Cheyne Walk when her aunt was visiting there, and twice during that summer Eliza came to stay with her niece at Clapham Common.

For Edward, the house on the Common was ideally situated. The proximity of the Junction gave him fast access to most places in Surrey. St Thomas's Hospital where he lectured on Wednesday morning throughout the late spring and summer months of 1892[2] was reached by a short rail journey to Vauxhall and a few minutes' walk along the Albert Embankment.

The problems connected with suburban living were soon to be modified by radical developments in Jeannette's life. The first of these was the not entirely unexpected cooling-down of relations between The Limes and Belle Vue. Visits to her mother and Ada became less frequent and were matters of duty rather than pleasure. The second change, one that did catch her unawares, was pregnancy.

The first signs of change in her condition appeared almost as soon as Edward and she returned from Biarritz. From 22 February on she noted unusual tiredness but for two or three weeks ascribed it to the effort that went with getting the house into ship-shape order. On 10 March, when one of Edward's periodic fits of jealousy reduced her to tears, she had a first inkling of some unknown process which made her excessively vulnerable. 'I never was a crybaby, so there must be some reason for it. I must have more rest . . . I cannot stand living at high pressure all the time.' And throughout the remainder of March she continued to complain of unaccustomed lassitude and other

---

[2] These lectures, which he was to continue to give year after year, were 'almost honorary' (*British Medical Journal*, 27 August 1910, p. 562). He also examined in State Medicine at the Universities of London, Oxford and Cambridge, as well as for the Diploma in Public Health at the Royal Colleges of Physicians and Surgeons.

disturbances. 'Wonder if there can be any reason for my feeling like this . . .' she noted on 15 March after she had felt 'horridly sick & queer all day'. She took a pill that evening which settled her stomach, but three days later she returned to her speculations: 'I feel better the last few days, but cannot help thinking there may be something.'

Perhaps in response to Jeannette's concealed discomforts, Edward too was showing signs of strain. The subject of Jeannette's past admirers was aired repeatedly and evidently preyed on his mind. It became Jeannette's turn to suffer when in a moment of misguided frankness, he admitted to having 'known something of' a Gaiety "super" whom he pointed out to his wife at a Saturday matinée; he then went on to make a clean breast of some other distressing trans-gressions. The discord which ensued lasted the best part of a week. Edward's bouts of penitence and tender apology alternated with further fits of jealous harping on her own past behaviour. Jeannette felt vexed and offended.

It was against the background of this first episode of marital strain that she intimated her conjectures to Edward. He had once again returned to the subject of her earlier flirtations and was demanding to be shown her diaries when she decided to break the news: 'I said to him at last "You really must not worry me!", he said "Why", & I said "You know:" very meaningly, whereupon he looked unutterable things & said "I wd. do anything you ask on that plea"; whereon I responded "I think the plea is a real one!" with he said such a lovely expression that he was completely melted, & caught me in his arms, & went half crazy.' 'I really & truly believe what I said' she continued, as if reassuring herself that she had not used her surmise to get out of a tight spot, and went on: 'He is nearly wild with joy at the very idea. My feeling is a mixed one. However I won't go into that just now.' She did not, at any later time, explain exactly what her thoughts had been on that occasion. As for Edward, within twenty-four hours of her announcement he had succumbed to toothache—a standard couvade symptom.

Later evidence supports the hypothesis that she conceived at some point between her wedding and 9 February and that by the time of her announcement on 30 March she had already missed two periods. Edward's evident enthusiasm now helped her to accept this latest shift in her destiny, so that on her next visit to Cheyne Walk, three days later, she felt able to share her conjectures with her mother, and hence also with Ada: 'I told M. what I believe. I think she was pleased, but she is so depressed that she does not seem to take interest in anything.

A. was more startled than anything else. She is getting very much soured & altered. She accuses me of changing, but really I think it is that she & M. react on each other. I am very sorry, & it quite worries me.' This last sentiment became a formula. In the months to come she would often use it to close her description of a visit to Belle Vue.

Some days later Ada came over to The Limes bearing two pairs of infants' socks, evidently in redress for the cold reception of her sister's news. She stayed to lunch, helped to cut out the sofa-cover for the study and consulted with Jeannette about her maternity wardrobe needs. For a matter of three hours it was as if old times had come back. But the harmony did not last. Next time Jeannette went to spend the evening at her mother's, she found Ellen 'pretty well and cheerful, but A. poorly & grumpy, & as cross as possible. She is getting so sour, & is so frightfully jealous. I had to steer my way with great circumspection, & was not sorry when E. came for me at 10 o'clk.'

The indifference with which her news had been met at Cheyne Walk discouraged Jeannette from broadcasting it elsewhere. But Edward did not share her reserve. By his desire she took the next opportunity to tell his sister Alice Buchanan of the 'coming event'. 'She was evidently very pleased, & was sure "Ted" was, wh. I cd. honestly assure her of.' Lady Buchanan (her husband had been knighted a few weeks previously, on his retirement from the post of chief medical officer to the Local Government Board) then promised to let the news go no further. Late in May Seaton himself used his auspicious tidings in an attempt to restore good relations with his younger sister Bella Soden, who with her husband Thomas was among the chief protagonists in yet another of the standard Victorian quarrels about a family trust. 'I hope she will reply properly' wrote Jeannette; when the reply came, she remarked that it had been more friendly than previous letters from the Sodens. She added: 'E. troubled about our mutual relatives, who are distinctly trying.'

For all its engaging, relaxed ways, Edward's family must have found Jeannette difficult to integrate. Her stiff-necked formality came under attack when first Bella Soden and next Alice Buchanan suggested that she should call them by their first names. 'I wrote to Mrs Soden about what to call each other. Cannot "Christian name" strangers!' she recorded on 3 March and followed up her letter (which to her secret relief had not made Mrs Soden 'huffy') by a verbal explanation when the Sodens called at The Limes: 'Had it out about the name, & made her understand the difficulties. I can't dub them all alike, so must keep the formalities.' 'Put it all right' she hopefully concluded. But the exchange with Bella Soden had made a breach in her resistance; when Alice Buchanan asked to be called by her Christian name (this followed within three weeks of George Buchanan's elevation to the knighthood and was presumably intended to avoid being addressed as Lady Buchanan by a sister-in-law), Jeannette gave in, with a grudging 'so be it'. This concession to familiarity also had the effect of making her eventually switch to 'Bella' for Mrs Soden. That the matter of correct appellation could create misunderstandings even among close family members is evinced by the fact that later that year Jeannette herself, to her manifest amusement, was addressed by her first name, Ellen, in a letter from her new sister-in-law, 'Mrs Fred' Seaton. Even the problem of how her husband's nephews and nieces would address her gave rise to formal decisions: after discussion with Alice Buchanan, the solution reached with regard to the Buchanan tribe was that henceforth she was Mrs Seaton to the elder ones, and Aunt to the younger children. Whether Florence Buchanan, who was adult by the time her uncle married his second wife, and who became a great favourite at The Limes, was exempted from this arrangement and allowed to call her Jeannette is not on record.

After their early meetings Jeannette had described Bella Soden, a tall, dark, good-looking woman of 'no figure', as 'very excitable' and 'too all-pervading'. Alice Buchanan, handsome in a different way, with bright auburn hair, grey eyes and fair complexion,[3] also appeared in the diary as rather larger than life. Compared with Jeannette's own connections, her expansive good-nature seemed to verge on heartiness. After they had known each other for a few months, Jeannette became privy to some of Alice's 'tales of woe', but cannot at this point have guessed that this sister-in-law's high spirits had from her early youth hidden a diffidence which would in later life change into a state of habitual depression.[4]

Edward, too, was a creature of moods. It must have come as a shock to Jeannette to discover, even before they were married, that this rational, dependable man would suddenly turn desperately anxious. Once a minor-key mood prevailed, he would be at the mercy of fits of jealousy, which in turn gave rise to irrational quarrelling and unhappiness. In the first few months of their marriage there were two or three

---

[3] Cf. Lilian Adam Smith (1977), op. cit., p. 14.   [4] Ibid., p. 15.

such unhappy episodes, each of several days' duration, when he harassed her by harping on earlier admirers, and made her, in the vulnerable condition of early pregnancy, profoundly uncomfortable.

On occasion he also inflicted on her, in retaliatory attempts to arouse her own jealousy, confidences about his own past. This may have been the case when at one or two points in their engagement he had volunteered explanations about his relationship with his first wife and mentioned a subsequent fruitless attachment. The confession about his acquaintance with the Gaiety girl which preceded Jeannette's disclosure about her presumed pregnancy had left a 'nasty taste' in her mouth: 'I cd. not help crying & was <u>so</u> miserable. E. asked me to forgive him, & I said I was not angry but sorry, wh. rather touched him I think, & was the absolute truth. Bad night!' And on the next two days she carried on the account:

I felt quite ill . . . He was so distressed at my grief that he told me something else wh. made a great difference, & showed I had thought him (as he put it) 'worse than he was'. I feel certain now that I am the one woman he ever loved in a complete sense, & after breakfast I sat with him in his room, & he told me his whole life. Truly fact is stranger than fiction, & many things wh. I found puzzles are explained. His extraordinary & passionate devotion to me is explained. He says he worships & adores me, & that the love he had for me before we were married was nothing to what he feels now . . . I must say I feel <u>much</u> happier.

None the less she had another bad night. 'All the excitements & agitations are very bad for me.' Edward too had worn himself out by three days of such scenes; he felt so 'sick and queer' that he had to take a day off from work. But he still returned to the subject of his wife's past and it was not until on the next day she closed the argument, by distracting him with hopes of future parenthood, that this particular exchange of miserable charges and counter-charges was interrupted.

Within forty-eight hours he was once more on the offensive; in a late-evening conversation 'on very private & personal matters', he harped in very worrying fashion on her relationship with Mr Brown whose existence, it will be remembered, she had revealed to him shortly before marriage:

really I have forgotten all about him ages ago, & shd. not think anything whatever of him now. I cd. not help saying that what he had told me about himself still pained me, but I tried not to think of them. He endeavoured to justify himself, but sees my & his points of view are [as?] utterly different. When he expresses his sorrow etc. I feel more satisfied, but I cannot help feeling that he does not stand quite where I thought, & it <u>does</u> hurt me to think it, & I can't help showing it. The questions of 'discretion' & 'expediency' into which he enters do not touch the matter in the least.

All through the next day she felt very depressed: 'I . . . cd. not get it out of my head that I shd. die with this baby, & when we went to bed, I surprised him by a good fit of crying. He made me explain, & then went into a transport of tenderness, reproached himself no end, smothered me with kisses, & I verily believe cried too! There is no doubt of his devotion.'

But this was still not the absolute end of the matter. They were both on edge about other things, Jeannette about the pregnancy and the worsening conflict with her mother and Ada, Edward about problems connected with his work. The tension may have been what caused him to return over and over again to the theme of Jeannette's comportment towards other men. 'He . . . says he has no objection to my flirting, & wd. like me to be admired. He has perfect faith in my knowing how to take care of myself, wh. is quite right of him' she wrote, adding sanctimoniously: 'I think dignity shd. be one's first idea in these matters.' Regardless of these sentiments, within hours they were back at square one, with 'E. very worrying in the morning, in a jealous mood. I know it is in a way a proof of his devotion, but it is very trying.' When he then called her the most charming of women, she concluded a trifle spitefully: 'He is competent to judge, I am afraid!' And there the matter rested, till five days later Edward and she went to a couple of Boat Race parties given by the Thornycrofts and their relatives, the Donaldsons. In the informal setting of the Chiswick riverside two of Jeannette's past admirers in turn made a beeline for her without realizing that she was now married and beyond their reach. Their blunders amused Jeannette but not Edward, whose dormant anxiety was once again aroused.

'He took it pretty well at first, but turned grumpy after, & is most furiously jealous.' He then, perhaps in jest, withdrew his earlier permission for Jeannette to engage in flirting and 'was very cross about nothing at dinner, sulked all the evening, & kept me awake all night. His only excuse is that he is half crazy with love of me, but really I cannot stand such worry. I stayed in bed till 12, and had a violent headache all day Sunday.' On Monday he calmed down, declaring that he felt safer seeing her in workaday clothes: 'I sat with him in the morning, with the fatal result that he did little else but look at me, and assure me how he worshipped me. He says he is my slave & that he **has** not a bit of will left but I assure him it is nonsense. Still there is no doubt that somehow or other I have "done for him" most thoroughly. He is ever so much worse than when we were abroad.' Declarations were not her strong point; instead that afternoon she went shopping on the Pavement and brought back a tobacco jar of Flemish ware as a peace offering for Edward; it later stood in a place of honour on the mantelpiece in the study.

The matrimonial crisis had lasted seventeen days, from 26 March until 11 April. For a while it rumbled on, Edward's moods bringing on waves of demonstrative affection which preceded or followed scenes of unwarranted jealousy. Jeannette had bouts of depression connected with the unknown adventure which faced her in the autumn. She now knew that Edward was an inveterate worrier; 'I suppose it is his temperament, but I am sorry on both our accounts.' She had still to find out whether he could be prevented from making mountains out of almost imperceptible molehills. That he may have reaped gratification from this habit of dramatization did not occur to her.

At the end of May came another outburst, when Edward demanded to see her diary (this time the current one) and to her chagrin disapproved of its tone: 'I suppose I write in a "whatever comes first" style, & tho' I understand it, other people mayn't. He declared I did not care about him etc. till he made me perfectly wretched. Of course he must know that I do, & some day will understand me, I hope.' Next day she reflected: 'He says I write this still as "Miss Marshall", & I think I do. Habit is an odd thing. Anyway the storm has blown over, & we are very happy agn. I suppose the "course of true love" does not run smooth after marriage any more than before, at any rate until people have got to know each other thoroughly.' After this there appeared to be no more matrimonial discord for the rest of the year. She not only had learnt to take his moods more philosophically, but also had other, more pressing things to occupy her mind. For one thing, a few days before the complaint about the style of her diary entries, the child in her womb had quickened,[5] and now developed an emotional reality as well as a physiological presence.

It would be entirely wrong to see this amount of matrimonial strain out of proportion; to offset some twenty-odd days of misery and conflict,

[5] She did not refer to the quickening in so many words, but wrote on 25 May: 'v. faint & queer the other evening—had to lie down'; this coincided with what most probably was the end of the sixteenth week of pregnancy.

there were, that year, over three hundred days of conjugal harmony, if not of bliss. And although Edward complained that Jeannette had not succeeded in shedding the Miss Marshall image, the wonder is that she had adjusted so rapidly and over such a wide spectrum to being Mrs Edward Seaton. It must have seemed to her as if, alongside the marriage and the move to Clapham Common, everything (with the signal exception of the entries in her diary) had shifted, as if her eyes had been provided with an entirely new focus.

To begin with, the timetable of her life was now completely different: this applied to the whole range of activities, to the annual calendar as well as to the shape of the week and, above all, to the contents of each individual day. The weekday mornings which in her single state had been devoted to the making and care of clothes, followed by a regular walk, were now filled with more varied pursuits. Shopping expeditions ranged in scale from local ones which could be fitted into the odd half-hour to major occasions, north of the river, requiring two to three hours from beginning to end. Edward's work made its own demands: on days when he had to travel to remote parts of Surrey, they breakfasted at 8 a.m. and she would then see him off, with lunch in his pocket, at about 8.30. At other times he worked at home, dealing with correspondence, preparing a lecture or writing one of the many reports and letters to the press required of an ambitious MOH. She still typed for him occasionally, and in all events he enjoyed having her with him while he was in his study. Quite often, the work sessions then ended with Jeannette on Edward's lap or perched on the arm of the armchair, while she listened to litanies of endearments and protestations of love. If they stayed at home in the evening, it was to sit, 'very Darby & Joan'y', with Edward reading aloud some pages out of Dickens, while Jeannette plied her needle. On days when he lunched at home, they sometimes made time for a stroll across the Common in the early afternoon. These outings, plus supervising the jobbing gardener and the brief sorties to the Pavement shops, were her only exercise on days when she did not travel across the river, but she did not appear to miss the long walks of her Savile Row or Chelsea years.

After the first few weeks at The Limes when she made curtains and arranged books and ornaments, household duties claimed relatively little of her time. The servants—cook, parlour-maid and under-maid —were given a free hand, and they appeared in the diaries no more frequently than when she had been single and the running of the household reposed in her mother's hands. All the same, she could no longer fit regular sessions of three or four hours' dress- and millinery-making, plus afternoons and evenings of fancy needlework, into her timetable. Fortunately her trousseau had been planned on a generous scale, so that until the pregnancy made it necessary to alter garments for herself and prepare for the baby, she could afford to cut down on this part of her daily life.

The weekends, too, took on a new shape. On Saturdays, Edward often arranged to have the afternoon free, so that at least some calls, to members of his family or of his own medical circle, could be undertaken together. It was also the day when they would fit in a visit to an exhibition or the theatre. Unlike the theatrical fare of her girlhood, the plays they now went to were chosen purely for their entertainment value and their humour at times bordered on the 'broad'. As a married woman Jeannette could afford to be seen at burlesques and risqué farces, which propriety had previously put out of bounds. It was the stuff which Edward preferred; but while she enjoyed a good laugh, squeamishness which in her girlhood had made her squirm at the nudes at the Royal Academy, was still to the fore; 'too "kicky" for my taste' she wrote of the dancing at the Gaiety; and 'the tights are certainly most unbecoming to women with fat legs & somewhat of corporations. I cannot see why the fact of the becomingness of skirts is not recognized.'

It was a pleasure to dress up in her trousseau finery and to have Edward, when not in one of his jealous moods, glad to see her stared at and admired: 'in Piccadilly a man stared at me much, & then found to his amazement that he knew E, who was amused' she reported; when three weeks later, for a soirée at St Thomas's, she put on her cream brocade wedding dress, now cut low for evening wear and let out a trifle to accommodate her spreading girth, she boasted: 'Looked very well, E. declared the handsomest woman there, & certainly people stared at me & my dress.' This was the occasion when she caught sight of an elderly couple who proved to be her erstwhile beau, H. P. Thomas, with his 'plain & insignificant, & likewise dowdy' wife on his arm. 'I flatter myself I wear better than he does' she reflected, but did not tell Edward, who was on nodding terms with Thomas, about this apparition from the past. This allowed her husband to reflect serenely on the new sensation of taking her out among a crowd where she was so well known and knew so many, and of his pride in her, 'wh. of course I am glad of'.

She must have been altogether prepared to set her own preferences aside, for concerts are never once mentioned in the 1892 diary. Edward's musical tastes cannot have been highly developed and during the engagement she did nothing to cultivate them. Two weeks after their return from the honeymoon, she at last found time to sit down to the Broadwood; 'I played him some Grieg & Valey de Paz, & he was enchanted! Fancy him never having heard me play before! He believes I can, now, & says he shall enjoy listening to me.' 'He likes characteristic music' she added in a slightly patronizing afterthought, and that year confined most of her performances to what she labelled 'national' music.

When they stayed at home, dinner on Sunday would invariably be 1.30 p.m.; on occasion a friend or two were invited to join them at this informal meal. The rest of the day would generally be a leisurely catching up with reading, correspondence, gentle exercise or just relaxation.

Church-going now all but disappeared from the regular Sunday timetable. Late rising was almost invariably the excuse; Sunday breakfast at or after 10 a.m. became a feature of life at The Limes. At other times it was the weather that was too wet or too thundery, or too dark and foggy to encourage the walk to church. If she now went to a Sunday service it was usually for a special reason, to hear a fashionable preacher (as her father had done before her), to accompany Aunt Eliza, or to see the medical crowds on 'Hospital' Sunday. It was not until July that Edward and she attended the old parish church on Clapham Common; they found the experience unrewarding, though the service, 'a dingy & slow affair . . . seemed to attract the "rank & fashion" of Clapham, such as it is. Very dull sermon.' Only on out-of-town weekends did their zeal return; during their four days at Ely they attended the cathedral service five times.

By calling at Belle Vue on Mrs Marshall's afternoons 'at home' on Monday, Jeannette could be sure to find both her mother and Ada; with visitors present, intimate conversation would be impossible, and this often suited Jeannette. But she also often dropped in on a Saturday with or without her husband, and visits on other days were not uncommon. All this was in the spring and the summer of 1892; the time was approaching when relations between the two households, The Limes and Belle Vue, would deteriorate to the point of excluding regular visits.

To help trace the rights and wrongs of the estrangement the testimony of only one witness is available, and this witness, Jeannette herself, naturally emerged unsullied from the account of the conflict. Her sister was cast as its chief instigator and the terms which Jeannette chose to describe Ada's behaviour and moods illustrate the deteriorating relationship: 'highty-toighty', 'fit to turn the milk sour', 'cross as two stiches', 'aigre-douce', 'meddlesome & cross', 'riling'—a whole vocabulary of resentment and hostility. Jeannette also wrote of Ada's depression and hypochondria, which she ascribed to jealousy.

Mrs Marshall, by contrast, was for a while positively warm towards her newly married daughter (though, noted Jeannette, 'not cordial' towards Edward). But the appeasing mood did not last; by the time Jeannette told her mother of her pregnancy, Ellen's reaction was uncertain. Jeannette, it will be remembered, diagnosed depression. Depression about ageing, about widowhood, may indeed have been what set off Ellen's ambivalence *vis-à-vis* her elder daughter's condition. Within three weeks of the announcement, Jeannette accused her mother of being distinctly unpleasant, and she voiced her own complaint: 'M. takes but a faint interest in my affairs, & has forgotten all she knew about clothes etc. . . . She gave me one or two little gowns etc, et voilà tout!'

Once or twice things appeared to improve. Ada, noted Jeannette on the point of announcing her pregnancy, had sent her an affectionate note, to which she had responded with equal warmth. 'I cannot afford to quarrel with her, & do not want'; after two successive meetings in the first half of June, she declared Ada to be 'better than usual' and pleasant. In May and until mid-June her mother, too, seemed in a better, more co-operative mood. In spite of her initial reluctance to take part in the preparations for the birth of her grandchild, she offered to sew some of its outfit, and she also made the first approaches to Mrs Workman, a trusted nurse, who had in the past looked after Marshall's special cases (including, it will be remembered, Rossetti), and who now was to act as monthly nurse to Jeannette. All seemed set for *détente*. Edward shouldered his share of the effort: he was being extra polite to Mrs Marshall whenever they met and made all sorts of small conciliatory gestures.

The remission did not last. On 19 June, 'Hospital' Sunday and therefore the occasion for one of their infrequent church attendances, the Seatons met Ada at Holy Trinity, and after the service walked up Sloane Street for a short stroll in Hyde Park: 'There was a little shower, wh. frightened A. home, but we went on, & sat down, and saw a big crowd. No one particular, but it was amusing. Cab home. The afternoon turned out so wet that we cd. not go to Belle Vue as we intended. Wrote.' The monosyllable which closed Jeannette's account of that Sunday referred presumably to a note of apology which she sent her mother to explain the change of plans. It may have been the wording of that note or something that had been said on the walk that caused offence (Jeannette had remarked that in church Ada had seemed very pale and queer, perhaps a sign of tension of which the elder sister took insufficient notice). In any event, when Jeannette called at her mother's after shopping next day, she found that hostilities had resumed:

They were all right at first, but all wrong after, and M. blew me up so that I quite broke down, and was all but hysterical. The result was that I had to stay till 4.30, have tea, eau de Cologne & go home in a cab. I felt absolutely fit for nothing, & had a splitting headache. It is really very unkind of M, & I cannot see that I deserve it, or that I am so utterly selfish & bad as she makes out. Anyway I cannot stand being made ill like this, & wd. much rather not go than have scenes wh. knock me up. Soon after I got home E. returned, & saw at once how upset I was. He comforted me, & was very kind, and quite indignant over my treatment. Really it was a treat to feel someone loved me, & was sorry for me. He feels now that I love him too.

From then on relations were on a slippery slope and their deterioration was only halted, once or twice, for a matter of days. Somehow the news of the estrangement got around; perhaps Jeannette herself in her bitterness sought to gain allies for her position. In the very first week after the scene which had brought on such an attack of self-pity, she recorded that both Dr Garrett Anderson and Miss Williams (their old friend from Vicarage Gate) were decidedly on her side in the quarrel with her mother. Elizabeth Garrett Anderson, met late in June at a dinner at their mutual friends, the Donkins, may have been told that Ada had been particularly 'stiff & starchy' with Edward when she called at The Limes earlier that day to help with Jeannette's dressmaking. But Dr Anderson's comments referred specifically to Ellen: 'She evidently thinks M.'s behaviour a pity & rather morbid. I am afraid it is getting to be the general view.' This was confirmed when on the following evening, at another dinner party, Miss Williams expressed herself 'quite indignant with M., & her pessimistic views of my marriage, & begged me not to worry myself about it; it was quite refreshing to hear a sensible outsider's view.'

On Edward's first free Saturday the Seatons called at Cheyne Walk at tea-time. 'Really it has come to this, that I am glad of E's protection chez ma mère! She was all right, but A. gave it me well in the hall just before we left.' Two days later, Jeannette, armed with a bunch of red roses as a peace offering for her mother, dared to go alone, and repeated the visit on the following Saturday. Both these occasions were relatively free from strife. Mrs Marshall was consulted about the probable date of delivery (which she calculated to be late October) and asked to suggest a suitable doctor. Next, Edward and Jeannette dropped in on Sunday 10 July to take pot luck at supper-time. This made four visits in eight days—a determined effort on the part of the Seatons to set things right. And in the short term the effort paid off. When the four of them met at dinner at The Limes nine days later on the occasion of Jeannette's birthday, 'M. enjoyed it thoroughly ...', but, added Jeannette, 'A. looks pale, & was dismal.'

It was Ada who then set off the resumption of conflict. The occasion came late in July, when Aunt Eliza was staying at Clapham, and Ellen and Ada came over one afternoon, carrying some of the completed baby clothes and a pot of musk for Jeannette, and very hot after their journey from Chelsea. Edward was at home but did not join them at tea, a Williams reunion, for Aunt Bessie and one of her daughters had also happened to call. Later, in recording the events of the afternoon, Jeannette expressed her regret at having told Edward when her 'amiable Ma & Sister' were about to leave. Dutifully, he had come upstairs to pay his respects, at which Ada 'received him so brusquely that he was much annoyed & declares he must have it out with her.'

As usual in times of crisis all sorts of circumstances had built up to make a clash inevitable. Edward was very worried about the 'Soden affair' and about his thorny relations with the Surrey authorities; he also happened to be suffering from an inflamed eye, and from stomach trouble which that very evening ended in violent sickness. Ada had a distressing cough, and both she and Mrs Marshall had just then a specific focus for their depression: earlier in July Jeannette had heard that her brother John had been 'very worrying lately, & bleeding M. as usual'. This was her first mention of John since she had responded in March to his decent but belated congratulations on her marriage, and he would not figure in her record again that year; but to the women at Cheyne Walk his erratic behaviour must have been a source of constant anxiety. As for Jeannette, she was now, in the seventh month of pregnancy, perhaps not at her most alert and less fit than usual to steer her tense relatives through troubled waters.

Her immediate reaction to Ada's hostile behaviour was to express loyalty with Edward: 'I have spoken to her several times and can do no good. She is half cracked on the subject, & impossible to reason with.' After a 'Council of War' Edward drafted a letter of remonstrance on Ada's conduct and addressed it to his mother-in-law; both Jeannette and Aunt Eliza thought it 'moderate in tone', so it was copied and dispatched on Saturday, 30 July. Ellen's reply, received on the Monday, struck them as far from moderate: 'It is very illogical & violent, & I am afraid means something like an open breach. I wish they (M & A.) were not such explosives. Letter fr. A. to me, affectionate but wild. I am very sorry. E. comforted me, & does everything he can to show how he loves me, & we must stick to each other closer than ever.'

Jeannette's own letter to Ada, 'of a remonstrative but affectionate order', brought her a summons to Belle Vue, where on 5 August she was interviewed by her mother in the dining-room, while the friend whom Jeannette had brought over to act as 'buffer' was being entertained upstairs by Ada. Though Ellen was kind and affectonate, their discussion of the 'unfortunate business' led to no satisfactory outcome: 'I am rather hopeless of its ever coming right. Both M. & A. are ill & warped in their views, and it is impossible to do much good by arguing with them. I stuck to my guns, insisting on A's rudeness to my husband, but the whole thing makes me very sad & unhappy.'

Six days later she returned to Cheyne Walk for a final meeting with her mother and Ada on the eve of their departure for the Continent. In response to a note from Jeannette advising her mother to consult Dr Russell Reynolds, a physician friendly both with the Marshalls and with the Seatons, Mrs Marshall now enlarged on her ill-health which she attributed to angina pectoris. It was altogether a very uneasy leave-taking: 'They both look wretchedly ill, and A. cried all lunch time, & seems all but brokenhearted over this affair. She declares she never meant to give offense, & begs me to make it up with E. . . . These sorts of unpleasantnesses are most difficult to patch up.'

Mrs Marshall and Ada did not return until 13 October. Their travels took them first to Ouchy, and thence to Florence via the Italian lakes; on their return journey they spent a week at Montreux. Regularly once a week one of them wrote to Jeannette. Ada's letters were not always calculated to please; in early October she suggested 'in a very meddle-some & offensive way' that Jeannette should consult a doctor. Jean-nette thought this unnecessarily officious; 'E. much put out about it, & it worries us both very much. I cried and we both of us had a bad night.' In the last weeks of her pregnancy the strain between Edward and her mother and sister had been a source of constant preoccupa-tion: 'Of course I feel with E., but cannot help worrying over a split at such a time as this . . . A moderate apology wd. satisfy E., who really has right on his side . . .' But, with both sides intransigent, she was at a loss for a solution.

CHAPTER 17

ROSALIND

'IN the time wh. is coming I seem to <u>want</u> a woman belonging to me!' wrote Jeannette on 22 September, a month or five weeks before the date of her expected delivery. Dr Jeaffreson whom they had chosen to attend her, largely because he lived no further than the south side of the Common, had after his second interview in early September (the term consultation hardly applies, as no medical examination took place either then or at any point before she went into labour)[1] assured her that she was one of 'Fortune's favorites'. After the first two months of pregnancy she had flourished, with no more than an odd few hours of discomfort. Her resilience was so marked that even the St Thomas's soirée, followed by a round of eleven formal dinner parties plus a wedding, which she and Edward attended in the nine weeks from mid-May did not exhaust her unduly. When in the second half of June they went to four dinners in five days, she did on one occasion succumb to the heat of the unventilated dining-room and had to be revived with eau de Cologne and fanning; two days later, dining at the Donkins, she again felt 'queer' but this time not even her husband (nor apparently Dr Garrett Anderson) noticed that there was anything amiss. It was all a challenge, part of the game of not letting outsiders in on the privacy of one's bodily functions. With it went another game, that of efficiently disguising her spreading waistline.

Because in the months of engagement she had somehow avoided connecting marriage with the possibility of motherhood, her trousseau had not included any of the versatile garments, teagowns or semi-fitted indoor jackets, which brides of greater foresight usually acquired against the eventuality of an early pregnancy. Most of what she now wore in the daytime or for going out in the evening were trousseau (and pre-trousseau) dresses, slightly modified to allow for her chang-

[1] The avoidance of obstetric examination in home deliveries was almost certainly common practice and, in view of the danger of cross-infection, perhaps the only safe way.

ing shape. It will be remembered that even her wedding dress had been so altered, when by the fourteenth week of pregnancy its bodice became much too tight to be comfortable. In true bridal fashion she then wore it to several dinner parties, and again at the last stages before her confinement to sit for a miniature.[2] Another dinner dress, a black net and velvet affair, made to wear during her engagement, she altered by lowering its *décolleté* and adding a bow with long streamers in front, and wore from mid-April on; 'I am wonderfully stouter, & un peu decolleté suits me' she wrote; 'E. would like me to wear it very much so.'

With her customary thrift, she acquired only four new garments, of which two, a silk Garibaldi bodice and a salmon-and-blue shot silk maternity jacket with a guipure lace jabot and great loops of baby ribbon, were made at home for wear during the hottest summer days. But the foundation of her maternity wardrobe was a black alpaca dress ordered from Allison's early in pregnancy and regarded as something of a luxury ('I was extravagant & ordered another dress, as I must be carefully arrayed now') and a long black lace cloak bought at Stedall's in Brompton Road, ideal camouflage modelled on a current Worth design from Paris. Until the eighth month this veiled her figure adequately; but even this cloak, over the black alpaca, no longer hid the reality of spreading waist and heavy hips when she wore them in August to visit an old Ely connection, Mrs Luddington. 'Mrs L. "twigged" my condition, but said how well it suited me, and agn. & agn. remarked she had never seen me look so well. She considers my costume a great success fr. the hiding point of view.'[3] Edward also approved, especially as his favourite bonnet topped the outfit, a small

---

[2] For the custom of recently married brides wearing their wedding dresses at evening parties, see Margaret Blunden, *The Countess of Warwick* (London, 1967), p. 39, and Gwen Raverat's *Period Piece* (London, 1952), p. 78. Having one's portrait painted or a photograph taken in late pregnancy was not unusual; Alexandra, Princess of Wales, did so six weeks before the birth of her fifth child; Kate Amberley—in the sixteenth week of her first pregnancy (see *The Amberley papers—The Letters and Diaries of Lord and Lady Amberley*, Bertrand and Patricia Russell eds., London, 1937, i, p. 378). Jeannette had a photograph taken in the seventh month of pregnancy; as this was not a success, Edward commissioned a young miniaturist, Miss Collyer, to paint his wife at a cost of £10 10s. 0d. The idea may have dated from an earlier era of high maternal mortality and have been designed to leave a likeness in legacy for one's family in case of death. Another, even more morbid, custom was for the mother-to-be to make a will; Jeannette in fact instructed her solicitor to draft a new will in early October and signed it ten days before her delivery, with two of the domestics as witnesses.

[3] For more about Mrs Seaton's and other late-Victorian maternity wear see Zuzanna Shonfield, 'The Expectant Victorian', *Costume* (Journal of the Costume Society), vi, 1972, pp. 36–42.

open shape of black fancy straw, with little jet pompoms to match the trim of the Allison dress and pink clover and ties of pink velvet ribbon under the chin—in short a thoroughly feminine affair.

The excursion to Ely had been one of several weekend sorties into the countryside which in August and early September took the place of the annual holiday. Two of them, to Guildford and to Farnham, combined business with pleasure, as Edward used the opportunity to visit several Surrey professional contacts. A bone-shaking rail journey back from Ely, together with long drives along rough Surrey roads and indigestible hotel food, eventually caused Jeannette enough discomfort to make them abandon such excursions after the first week of September and confine their outings to leisurely walks on the Common, quiet dinners at neighbours' houses, a visit to the Strand Theatre on 1 October, a prize-giving at St Thomas's two days later and, on Saturday 6 October, a series of six calls, all on foot, in the Piccadilly region.

At home there was more than enough to keep Jeannette busy. Although as early as mid-May Edward had gone off 'into some transports' on finding Jeannette buttonholing round a shawl, the preparations for the baby had been slow in starting. For a while they had to compete with the essential alterations to her own wardrobe and with the exceedingly full social schedule. 'There is an immense amount of work in these baby things' she sighed at the end of July on completing the sixth petticoat and starting on the first of the little nightgowns. The advice, which she had in vain sought from her mother, was eventually provided by cousin Alice Scott, by then the mother of eleven children; patterns came from Butterick's; fabrics, ribbons and lace from 'the Stores', Evans' and Munro's. The servants were set to hem diapers (Jeannette's Americanism for nappies). Mrs Marshall's four little nightgowns were retrimmed by Jeannette to her own liking, and she also shortened the six flannel wrappers her mother had made. With the basic wardrobe ready, she settled down to the more entertaining business of the dressy monthly gowns, trimmed with lace and white satin ribbon, and the 'extra-special' robe. There were also the baby's baskets and cot to be ordered from Munro's. This she left till September, perhaps in obedience to the superstition which had expectant parents delay major purchases until the baby was well on the way to be born. The cot with its trimmings, an expensive item, arrived in the fourth week of September. She had it set up on an experimental basis in her room and declared it 'very pretty', with its fancy muslin and valenciennes, all white but for pale blue satin ribbons, its four pairs of sheets, pillowcases, blankets and little down coverlet 'all to match'. It was then stored away in a cupboard.

The nursery itself was of course an afterthought; when the decor of The Limes was being settled in the autumn of 1891, the need for such a room had not occurred to her. Now she fitted it into the larger of the second-floor front spare bedrooms. Equipping it was a matter of one short visit to the Fulham Road. She chose 'bedstead, mattress, bolster, pillow, dressing table, [looking] glass, washstand, fittings, towel rail, 2 chairs & a flap table . . . the whole is under £4!' she exulted. The best linoleum was an extra, as were the blankets, rugs and a small Japanese fire-screen. By 1901 or 1902 when the nursery was photographed along with the rest of the house the screen was still there, but many of the other items, including the lino, had been replaced; the nursery had been promoted to be the child's room, rather than the nurse's.

Eventually, all these preparations tired her out. On 11 October she felt 'knocked up' on waking, breakfasted in bed and did not come down till just before lunch; later she lay on the sofa in Edward's room and discussed the ever-worrying business of how to handle her mother and sister. She roused herself sufficiently to make a pair of muslin curtains for the china cupboard in the drawing-room, along with some more routine sewing, and then went to bed feeling very tired.

The following morning, 'in consequence of a new symptom', she telegraphed for Nurse Workman who arrived at 11 o'clock and was, as usual, unflappable. She approved the arrangements, promised to return the following day and departed, leaving Jeannette to give last-minute instructions to the servants. 'I feel now I have done my best, & must trust to Providence.' Later in the day a telegram went to Mrs Workman to say that Jeannette was still all right. In the evening she wrote to her mother, as Ellen and Ada were due back at Belle Vue that week; 'told her all the arrangements officially, & also that I shd. be glad to see her here, but cannot go there. I feel now very insecure about getting up another day.'

Nevertheless, the next morning she was still up and about, 'notwith-standing rather a set out in the night'. Nurse Workman came to lunch and advised sending for Dr Jeaffreson, who in turn advised that she should now come into residence and assured the Seatons that he himself would be available at any time, though he did not think he would be 'wanted so promptly'. 'I think he will' was Jeannette's own view; that evening, after dispatching another note to Mrs Marshall, she noted: 'I still feel quite well, but am getting quite a figure agn! I am regarded in the light of a phenomenon by Nurse & E. <u>Glückauf</u>.'

The night brought more 'discomfort' and subdued her spirits. She breakfasted in her dressing-gown and by 10.30 had to go upstairs and to lie down. Again a telegram went to Dr Jeaffreson and was followed by another, more pressing one. He came around 11.30, was very kind, promised her chloroform, and then went off for his bag, to return at 2 o'clock.

Her later recollection of the events of that day, 14 October, was rather hazy. By the time doctor returned she had been 'in the direst agony' for quite some time:

To squeeze some one's hand was my only comfort, and that ceased to be one. E. was in a great way, and did all he could, showing the greatest sympathy and feeling. He said he never saw anyone suffer as I did, and Nurse said it was 'very sharp'. When Dr. J. arrived I was begging for the chloroform, and really it was like heaven when I felt myself sinking away with a curious singing in the ears. I knew nothing more till I came to, and heard a baby squalling from somewhere or other, and saw Dr. J. washing his hands, and asking what I shd. like. He suggested tea, wh. I took. He went down to refresh, and came up agn. later. Nurse told me that I had a 'beautiful little girl' (adjective politeness merely!), & when she was washed I was given a tiny, blue, cold little scrap to warm up. The poor mite was no beauty then! E. came up, & kissed me, and looked immensely relieved. He had been walking up & down the dining-room in great anxiety. Had sent messages to M. & A.E. [Aunt Eliza] I have not a clear recollection of the rest of the day (baby was born soon after 4 in the afternoon), but took a little nasty gruel, and some bread & milk or something of the sort. Dr. J. came agn. at 10, and told me he was sure I was an 'old hand'. Thankful it was over. E. wanted to sit up, but it was not necessary. Nurse did, & he left his door open, so as to be within call in a moment if wanted. I scarcely slept a wink. Chloroform and excitement I suppose. Cd. not wonder at it.

'I am a mass of aches from head to foot, and feel as though every muscle is strained. I literally cannot move a bit' Jeannette complained on the day after the delivery. 'Nose even bruised by the inhaler. Poor baby still very plain, and very cold. Nurse says being premature.' For the next few days Jeannette continued to complain of discomfort. 'I suffer considerably but must make the best of it' she wrote on 17 October. *The Times* announcement of her safe delivery appeared that morning and congratulatory cards and letters began to flow in. The baby was thin, she stated on the 18th. 'I am nursing her. Had some discomfort about it at first.'

The breast-feeding lasted for just over three weeks. On the evening of 3 November Jeannette, depressed and more than usually anxious about relations with her mother, broke down when Edward came in to say goodnight. As so often, her depression coincided with his, or perhaps triggered it off. 'I did my best to comfort him, & he lay down outside the bed for a little. He does not like the upstairs room. I am sorry he shd. be so bothered.' Next morning the baby had a stomach upset which Nurse Workman attributed to Jeannette's 'worry'; Jeannette herself laid the blame squarely on the anxieties over the Cheyne Walk business. 'It is too bad of M. & A.' A few days later, after a day of miscellaneous strains, which had included a visit from Ada, she was very sick during the night. 'Worry stopped my digestion' she explained, and went on: 'I am sorry to say I cannot go on nursing the baby, so began weaning. Troublesome.' She expanded about the pain and faintness the weaning was causing her; fomentations were applied, and on 11 November she declared herself to be 'out of the wood'.

To explain what had happened to bring matters to crisis-point, it is necessary to go back to a scene, on the day of Jeannette's confinement, which has some of the elements of burlesque. At some point between 11 and 11.30 that morning, a few minutes before Dr Jeaffreson's first visit, Mrs Marshall and Ada walked into the bedroom in which Jeannette lay in the throes of the first stage of labour. 'Singularly inconvenient time for a visit' she was to comment as soon as she found strength to recount the events of that day: 'I managed to bear my sufferings pretty well before them, but was very thankful when they left. M. brought me some sweet little spoons, but I scarcely knew how to thank her or look at them. A. was only in the room about a minute, M. about 10. She was agitated, but made a remark to Nurse about not wishing to see E. wh. showed that she felt the same!'

In response to Edward's message announcing the birth of her grandchild, Mrs Marshall on 15 October sent a note 'to say she cannot come for a day or two. Felt it much, but tried to make the best of it. Had to tell Nurse something. She is very indignant.' It was little consolation that neighbours and Edward's family enquired after the health of mother and child. When Jack Buchanan, Edward's nephew, came over to ask after her, Jeannette noted that her husband's relatives were much kinder than her own; but when Alice, Jack's mother, called to bring her good wishes and stayed to tea with her brother, Jeannette complained that she could hear her sister-in-law's voice, resounding from the floor below, 'like a coffee mill'.

Two days after the delivery she scribbled a pencilled note, urging her mother to come. A similar note went off to Ada on the following day, and on Tuesday, 18 October, Ada paid a first call, staying about twenty minutes. 'She was so stiff & cold (probably feeling awkward) that I was glad when she went, & had a weep while Nurse saw her out.' After this first visit, Ada came like clockwork, on several successive Tuesdays, and was a little more amiable. On the second visit she presented Jeannette with a pretty little turquoise and gold brooch from Florence. But this visit was no more a success than the previous one: 'I get quite into a fever at the idea of her coming, & am in a perspiration with the effort of keeping up conversation on indifferent subjects . . . Evidently M. thinks I am lying here for the sake of it, but I really could not sit up. A. is very unsympathetic.'

The date was 25 October and Jeannette had been in bed for eleven days. Dr Jeaffreson, who called twice a day, was pleased with his patient's progress. Mercifully, she wrote, he had not kept her on slops; there was clearly nothing wrong with her appetite. But it was not until the twelfth day after the delivery that she recorded his advice to get out of bed and on to the sofa 'for a little change'.

A fortnight after she had taken to her bed she at last let the nurse dress her, lying down, in her dressing-gown, '& then the sofa was put by the bed, & I slid onto it'. Cook then pushed the sofa nearer to the windows, and there Jeannette lay until after tea and supper Edward carried her back to bed. 'Still I am getting better, & Baby improves' she wrote that day. It took her another three days to graduate to an armchair ('Feel as weak as a cat'), and then three more days passed before she moved into the drawing-room, on the same floor. At last, twenty days after the confinement, Edward 'very carefully' helped her down to lunch in the dining-room. In another few days she felt sufficiently strong to come down to breakfast, and when eventually she allowed her husband to take her out for a drive in a hired carriage on two successive fine afternoons, 13 and 14 November, her recovery was complete.

There is nothing to indicate that, beyond a pronounced and extended bout of after-pains and the lassitude induced by a short, sharp labour, there was anything unusual about Jeannette's physical condition in the month after the delivery. The weakness she complained of may have been the effect rather than the cause of what kept her so long in bed. If Ada on her second Tuesday visit had implied that Ellen, and indeed herself, suspected Jeannette of shamming weakness, they were almost certainly putting an unkind construction on her inability to return to a normal pattern. Nurse Workman, whose acquaintance with Marshallic vagaries dated from many years back, and Dr Jeaffreson (who, judging by Jeannette's descriptions of his visits, knew how to handle a wrought-up patient), may have recognized that Jeannette's inability to resume everyday activities was a paralysis of will bordering on hysteria. Every day in the safe fastness of her bedroom delayed the confrontation with her mother and Ada. It needed the doctor's gentle urging (backed presumably by the efforts of Nurse Workman and, of course, of Edward himself) to make her move to other parts of the house, let alone leave the safety of The Limes.[4]

By the time of Ada's fourth Tuesday visit, Jeannette had for several days taken her meals downstairs. To the worry of this visit she attributed the episode of sickness which in turn precipitated the weaning.

Suddenly it seemed as if the bonds of indecision had been removed, allowing the processes of normal life to take over again. Three days after the weaning the nurse and her small charge moved to the second-floor nursery and Edward came down to what was now the parental bedroom, 'from the spare-room, wh. he has taken an intense dislike to'. By 15 November, a Tuesday, Jeannette's impatience with her sister's visits was allowed free rein: 'A came, & I had a "turn-up". Cannot go on in this unsatisfactory way. She went into hysterics wh. startled E. She is so excitable & queer that it is impossible to argue with her.' On the following Tuesday there was a fresh scene: 'E. at home, so I suggested her going in, & making it up. She behaved absurdly, so stiff & riling, & then went into hysterics agn. He was shocked. She _is_ strange. Brought me a comical hood, knitted. Hopeless affair!'

Jeannette's ambiguous style left it uncertain whether the last remark of that passage related to the hood itself or the entire future of her relationship with her mother and sister. Both she and Edward were in fact still prepared to try and mend things. When Mrs Marshall did not

[4] It could perhaps be argued that Jeannette was giving herself airs, usurping the pattern prevalent among ladies of fashion now that women were no longer having to make sure of using to the full the short months of freedom from pregnancy. Ettie Grenfell who gave birth to her first-born, Julian, in 1888, after a labour of six hours and an uneventful delivery, was allowed no visitors other than her husband and her closest family for a fortnight 'as was the custom'. She went downstairs three weeks after the delivery, and for a drive a week later. See Nicholas Mosley, _Julian Grenfell, His life and the times of his death_ (New York, 1976), p. 12.

respond to a note from Edward suggesting they would both call, Jeannette decided to beard the opponents at Cheyne Walk all by herself. She called at Belle Vue within forty-eight hours of Ada's last visit to The Limes and 'had tea & talk with M & A. They were lugubrious, blamed me for weaning the baby, (when it is their fault), & were very affectionate. Altogether they made me miserable, & are so fundamentally wrong in their ideas, that arguing is of no use.'

This aborted attempt at peacemaking was the last meeting with her mother and Ada for a long time to come. Perhaps to avoid another confrontation with Ada, Edward and Jeannette, having entrusted the baby to Mrs Workman, decided to spend a long recuperative weekend at Eastbourne, from which they did not return until late afternoon on Tuesday, 29 November. Meanwhile Edward had yet again written to Mrs Marshall to say that, 'if agreeable', he would call on her on their return from the seaside. Ellen's 'very disagreeable' reply ('It is very foolish of her, but she does not want to make it up, I suppose') precipitated a plan to spend Christmas out of London and accordingly a booking was made at the Eversfield Hotel in Hastings. Next, Seaton burned more bridges by his attempt at argument by correspondence: 'E. is preparing a long letter to M., setting forth our view of the case.' 'Very worrying' noted Jeannette and herself dropped a few lines to her mother to prepare her for Edward's letter, which after modifications went off on Tuesday, 6 December.

To this letter, too, he received no reply. It may have crossed in the post with another one, also dated 6 December, in which Ellen informed Jeannette of the death of Uncle Edwin Williams, and expressed 'rather more pacific feelings'. It was the second death which had hit Ellen's family in the first week of December: Jeannette had only just heard from Aunt Eliza that her epileptic cousin Edward Startin had jumped overboard from the ship which was bringing him back from South Africa, and drowned almost within sight of the English coast.

This time it was Jeannette who responded to her mother's letter in a manner which, if her own account is to be credited, can only be described as brusque and under the circumstances, unkind: 'Clinched the matter by replying instantly, & told her we were going away for Xmas.' And this piece of discourtesy marked, for the time being, a stalemate in the quarrel.

One of the immediate effects of the estrangement was, of course, that Mrs Marshall had still not seen her grandchild; Jeannette, in the remaining weeks of 1892, never once referred to this circumstance. In bizarre adherence to convention, among the few Christmas presents she sent out that year before going to Hastings were a gilt and green glass gum-bottle for her mother and a silvered velvet brush for Ada. She herself received on 21 December a pair of blue vases from her sister, and a muffin dish from her mother. She did not record whether in thanking them for these presents she had reported that the muffin dish had been smashed in the post.

Another discordant aspect of the whole business was that in the anxious weeks during the autumn of 1892 Jeannette repeatedly referred to her mother and Ada, by a spoonerism which she attributed to Edward, as the Wayne Chalkers.

In 1891 it had taken Jeannette some courage to bring herself to call her fiancé by his first name. She now experienced similar inhibitions with regard to her child. In the early weeks she wrote of the new member of the family as 'the baby', and once or twice referred to her by the sexless pronoun, 'it'. Then, four weeks after her birth, the little girl appeared set to shed her anonymity: 'We settled Baby's names, after much "woffling". I suggested Rosalind as being pretty & uncommon, and we both like Mary, wh. is a Seaton name. So those are to be her appellations.' However, the christening was postponed until the New Year and in the meantime Jeannette continued to write of 'the baby', or at best 'Baby'. In a show of affection after the return from Eastbourne she was called 'my "duckums" ', and again, after a stomach upset, 'my duckie'; but never 'Rosalind' or 'my daughter' or 'our child'. Never once did Jeannette in the 1892 diary write of any resemblance of Rosalind to herself or to Edward or to other members of the family; never once was there evidence of the relationship between mother and child giving rise to hitherto unknown feelings of tenderness and protectiveness. Pride there was in plenty: as Rosalind changed from a thin, dark-complexioned 'scrap' with a funny little face, whose crying and grunting disturbed Jeannette, to a nice little thing with eyes that 'are getting bigger and darker every day', she could be shown off to friends and relatives who admired and praised the baby, just as six months previously they had admired and praised Jeannette's taste in interior decoration. When the child was carried downstairs to be shown off to visitors it was almost as if the mother too met her for the first time; Jeannette's descriptions of Rosalind's progress coincided with such special occasions. 'Her little wig is a trifle ruddy, but she has a dear little face, and a lovely skin. I think she is very well made too, and her ears, hands & feet are nice, so we must be thankful.' When this was written, Rosalind was nearly two months old; but that she smiled and cooed and waved her arms and kicked her legs, or appeared to recognize mother or nurse, was not recorded. And never once was there any mention of Edward's encounters with the child whom he had awaited with so much enthusiasm.

Late in November a day was judged fine enough for Rosalind's first outing: 'After lunch, Nurse & I took the baby for its first walk. The outdoor garments are a success.' Jeannette did not record which outfit her daughter had modelled that afternoon. The opulent pelisse of beautifully embroidered China silk which, in a boxful of other elaborate garments, had arrived from the Shanghai in-laws a week earlier, was suited only to special occasions; this time mother and Nurse almost certainly chose the silk-lined cream-coloured fine serge cloak, square-shaped, with yoke, cape and collar, trimmed with valenciennes and cream satin ribbon, and a bonnet to match, all of Jeannette's making. 'We walked to the Pavement & back to Mrs Fletcher's upon whom we called. She & 2 old ladies there, who all worshipped the baby, and said what a pretty child she was. She had a lucky egg given her, & held it tight.' This egg and a silver and coral rattle, a family heirloom brought by Aunt Eliza, were the only toys given to Rosalind in her first ten or eleven weeks.

When on the afternoon of 14 October Nurse Workman brought the tidings of Jeannette's safe delivery down to the kitchen quarters, the three servants, 'immensely relieved', had 'jumped for joy'. Alice Dix, the parlour-maid, had in fact given notice three weeks earlier on the plea of wanting to learn dressmaking and becoming a lady's maid. 'Don't believe she will do for it, but of course she must do as she likes' commented her employer. Finding a new domestic could have been a sore trial to Jeannette just before she was laid up; however, she solved the problem within a matter of hours by promoting the under-maid, with a rise to £16 a year, and requesting the cook to write for her sister, 'a "strapping" young person', to come as replacement for the under-maid. During the visit to Eastbourne Edward and Jeannette made time to buy 'some brooches for our domestics as a reward for their good behaviour while I was laid up'. Nicely set amethysts went to the cook and the newly promoted parlour-maid. The new under-maid was also included in the bounty, though all she got was a 'little mosaic affair'.

To replace the 'monthly' Mrs Workman with a permanent babies' nurse was not as easy. Already during the pregnancy Mrs Workman had performed some of the functions which under more favourable circumstances would have devolved on Jeannette's mother. When in search of concrete information about the processes of pregnancy and childbirth, Jeannette 'very unwisely' consulted a 'Dictionary of Medicine' and got herself thoroughly depressed by what she found in it, it was Mrs Workman who dispelled her fears and answered the multitude of questions, too private—or too revealing of ignorance—to be asked of Edward. And it was Mrs Workman who supervised the practical arrangements for the delivery and after the birth provided an appreciative commentary on the qualities and virtues of the child. Before she left Jeannette had her down to sit with her and talk during a whole afternoon: 'I do not like her going, & she can't bear it. She wd. have liked to stay!' She was paid £20 (twice the usual fee, and £5 more than had been agreed when she was first asked to attend Jeannette; but then she had stayed six weeks instead of the usual four), and left on 2 December 'all but crying, & I felt like it too!'

The first aspect of the highly recommended Nurse Walker who replaced her was not altogether encouraging: 'She looks 55, calls herself 35, is hard featured, & has an odd lingo, but seems pleasant.' After she had been up to the nursery '& made friends with Nurse No. 2', Jeannette admitted to being rather worried though Nurse Walker seemed careful and appeared to be fond of the baby. She was not entirely reassured when Mrs Workman on a visit to The Limes professed some anxiety about the child who, as it happened, developed a touch of diarrhoea within nine days of the Walker takeover. But when Mrs Workman returned a few days before Christmas, she declared the little girl to be thriving, and Jeannette now felt that the nursery once again was in reliable hands. Accordingly, on the 23rd Edward and she left to spend six days at Hastings.

The smoothly working household staff was no doubt one of the reasons why Jeannette felt entitled to leave her two-months old baby over Christmas in charge of an untried nurse, a risky business without the fall-back of a grandmother or an aunt to supervise the arrangement. But Hastings was only just over sixty miles away, and telegrams, though not as quick as a telephone call, took as little as an hour or two to reach their destination. So to be away on the south coast was perhaps not as risky as going out for the evening leaving a baby-sitter in sole charge.

The Seatons had sufficient reason to feel they needed a change. To the anxieties of the family rows on Jeannette's side were added Edward's troubles, both the Soden affair and the perennial difficulties of a job which depended on the co-operation of local government committees. Then they were hit by a couple of extra blows in quick succession. First, on 15 December, came a 'most startling and dis-agreeable piece of news', that a miniature of Jeannette had been stolen from an exhibition at Newcastle; 'E. said a "d", & so did I inwardly! Such a thing never happened before, wh. is no consolation to us. It is unlucky, and most dreadfully aggravating.' When the very next day a seemingly greater misfortune hit them, Jeannette appeared relatively less upset: 'Cook woke us up with an awful thump at the door at 7.20 o'clk. to tell us burglars had been in the house, & taken her purse & watch from the kitchen! I was so startled that I jumped to the awful conclusion that baby was very ill, perhaps dead, & was relieved for the moment. Went down & saw the dining-room & study in a dreadful litter, & the kitchen the same.' The police inspector who arrived after breakfast 'looked wise & took notes'. 'Have no faith' was Jeannette's comment on his bluster. What had been taken, besides cook's posses-sions (which were valued at £5) were six small silver objects, mostly wedding presents, two greatcoats of Edward's, a set of his false teeth (value £10), a gold pencil-case given to Jeannette by her father, and nearly £4 out of her personal purse (she kept another for household expenses); the loss of money was to her the greatest blow for she was about to purchase Christmas gifts and would now have to trim down her ideas to a much smaller budget. The thieves had come in by a staircase window, facing on to the back garden, and had 'found out all we had out in the silver line'. They had also forced Jeannette's desk in the dining-room, but must then have been disturbed, by Nurse and Rosalind, it was thought, so that they fled without touching anything above the ground floor. There was no hint of a speculation on who the thieves might have been, no suggestion that the theft might have been an inside job or indeed that their late parlour-maid could have been connected with burglars.

The following evening Jeannette and Edward went to the theatre, 'as a treat' after all their troubles. Jeannette for this outing wore her grey brocade 'best' trousseau dress, 'turned in a little' at the seams. She had let it out with Ada's help to fit her figure in the fourth or fifth month of pregnancy. But now she had gone back to her normal dimensions, a fact of which she was not a little proud.

The Hastings holiday was a success. Each day a bulletin from Nurse Walker confirmed that Baby was well. Five of the six days were fine, and after the weeks of being shut in Jeannette enjoyed the long walks, although they made her legs ache. Edward, for his part, was stiff as a result of two swims, on Christmas Eve and on the 27th, despite the cold East wind; for a man who had only ten days earlier caught a cold with attendant aches and pains, consequent to the thieves making off with his winter overcoats, he was proving very hardy. On the penultimate day at the Eversfield they heard that the miniature had been recovered. 'Best piece of news for a long time! The thief sent it back as the authorities were making it very hot for him. My portrait in the papers, duplicated for the police stations: 15000 handbills etc. Really I must be notorious, if not celebrated!'

On Christmas Day, after the 11.15 service at Christchurch ('Very high, & incensed, & candled, & a hesitating parson') and a walk through old Hastings, she had written to Ada, 'to make one more attempt at reconciliation', asking her and Mrs Marshall to dine at The Limes on New Year's Day. 'Very good of us, I think!' The 'disagreeable letter from A. utterly declining to come here', which reached Jeannette on the morning after their return to London, destroyed the good mood buoyed up by the recovery of the miniature. 'E. much put out, & I very wretched. It is downright cruel of them to behave like this.' She was miserably depressed all day, cried a great deal, and summarized it all with the words 'Final Rumpus' at the top of the diary page. But by New Year's Eve she had recovered her composure:

We sat up rather late, & were awake at 12 o'clk, when we wished each other a happy new year. We have had many blessings, but some troubles. Still I think & hope that we may go forward with courage into the new year, and be as happy as we have been in 1892.

These sentences closed the last of Jeannette's daily entries. The few remaining pages of the 1892 volume were devoted to reading lists, lists of letters dispatched and 'Births, Deaths and Marriages' entries for the years 1893–5, after which she discontinued the practice of diary-keeping for good.

In the earliest years of Rosalind's childhood the breach with Cheyne Walk continued relentlessly; to compensate somewhat, there was a *rapprochement* with John, still in Russia, but now on correspondence terms with his elder sister. Tradition has it that he eventually got a chair at St. Petersburg university, but there is no evidence that he ever became anything other than a high-school teacher ('profesiòr' in Russian) or a tutor or secretary. Rumours about his impending marriage to a rich merchant's daughter also reached London, but there is no evidence of that either. When his niece grew out of the nursery years and learned to read, there would be occasional picture postcards addressed to her by the faraway uncle, and one or two books of Russian tales, with exotic pictures of horse-mounted princesses who fought fiery dragons, and Pushkin's learned cat on a golden chain, which walked round and round a legendary oak.

As she remained an only child, Rosalind's nursery was naturally a lonelier place than the annexe across the yard in Savile Row. On the other hand, though there was hardly any contact with her mother's family and the relatives on Edward's side were mostly either too far away or past childbearing age, she grew up less isolated than Jeannette. From the age of three she attended the kindergarten of Elm House, a small school a few hundred steps to the west of The Limes; her first report claimed that she had 'improved greatly . . . through contact with other children'. And when, in 1902 or so, the Seatons moved to Pimlico, the choice of the house, 93 St George's Square, SW, was to some extent dictated by the wish to supply a desirable social setting for Rosalind's secondary education. They decided on Frances Holland School, of which the Graham Terrace section, opened in 1881, was within reasonable distance of their new home. Several friendships Rosalind made at Graham Terrace lasted well into her middle age.

To Jeannette, the move back north of the river meant the resumption of a richer, more sociable existence. Living in Pimlico (and later once more in Chelsea) encouraged her to resume some of the interest in embroidery and other applied arts which had fascinated her in her youth. In 1905 and again in 1912 she exhibited examples of her beadwork, in early Art-Deco manner, at the Arts and Crafts Exhibitions which had gradually become the home for a more catholic selection of amateur work than that which had been shown by the post-aesthetic avant-garde of the late 1880s and early 1890s. And, once again, her London extended to the far sides of the Park, to Bayswater, Notting Hill and Kensington; the move to Pimlico had also made the doctors' area between Oxford Street and Regent's Park as accessible as it had been from Cheyne Walk. Only Holloway was excluded once and for all when Aunt Eliza died in 1904 in the house at 76 Parkhurst Road, to which she had moved in 1886.

The turn of the century saw the peak of Seaton's professional activity. In 1908 the St Thomas's lectures were discontinued. Two years later he retired (or was made to retire) from the Surrey position on grounds of impaired health. As pensions had not yet been introduced in the local government sector, the Surrey authorities appointed him to the almost entirely honorary post of consulting MOH, at a salary of £300 a year. Even though their earlier foresight rewarded them with a supplement of some £250 a year in interest,[1] the Seatons now had to make do with only about half of their earlier income. Cuts had to be made. One obvious economy was to move to a more modest home. Accordingly, in 1911 they exchanged the house in St George's Square for a smaller one, 14 Walpole Street, in Chelsea. Before long, they received another financial blow: in the summer of 1914, the Surrey consultancy was withdrawn.

Edward survived this setback by only a few months. On 20 February 1915 he died of influenza with bronchial complications, in Walpole Street, not far from 77 Sloane Street, where he had been born some sixty-seven years earlier.

The trauma of Edward's death deepened the financial worries which the loss of the consultancy had brought about. The constant preoccupation with money, the struggle to maintain standards on a dwindled income and (until 1921) in the face of rising costs, were a strong undertow in the first ten years of Rosalind's diaries, the entire run of which extended, in five five-yearly volumes, from the second week of May 1916 until the end of 1940. Jeannette had periods of insouciance

---

[1] At 5 per cent on savings of £300 a year for eighteen years.

when she showed little concern over their tenuous financial situation. By contrast, Rosalind, eager to exploit the new freedom which had come to young women with the onset of the First World War, felt the shortage of funds as a grievous constraint.

For a year or two after her father's death she carried on as if cash were no issue; her several attempts at voluntary war work smacked of the frivolity of the cossetted only child. Then the zeppelin raids of the summer and autumn of 1917 proved too much for Jeannette's nerves (Rosalind alleged that they were the direct cause of her mother's heart attack in September of that year), and mother and daughter decided to evacuate to Oxford. In the new setting Rosalind settled to a paid job in a matter of two or three months. Her clerical work at the School of Rural Economy carried a salary which grew from £125 to £150 a year, and gave her a permanent appetite for earning.

The return to London proved expensive, as their house in Walpole Street had been given up in early 1918 after a bomb on the neighbouring Royal Hospital had broken the drawing-room windows. And so in March 1919 Jeannette applied to Ellen for a little assistance to help with the expenses of their move to 29 Oakley Street. Relations with Cheyne Walk had been slightly patched up at some point before the beginning of Rosalind's diaries in the spring of 1916. At roughly monthly intervals Jeannette, often accompanied by Rosalind, would visit Cheyne Walk; Ada, too, would occasionally come to Walpole Street. Christmas and birthday gifts were exchanged and in October 1917 Mrs Marshall sent Jeannette a cheque to help meet the cost of dilapidations at Walpole Street. But in 1918 there appear to have been only three or four occasions on which Jeannette travelled from Oxford to see her mother and sister, the last of which was in July. And eight months later, in response to Jeannette's 'most carefully expressed' letter, 'making a most reasonable claim for a little assistance', came not a cheque from Mrs Marshall but an unpleasant letter from Ada. Jeannette chose this occasion to enlighten her daughter about the background of the 1892 quarrel; her vindication of her own and Edward's positions must have been effective, for it caused Rosalind to vituperate: 'It isn't comfy to feel one has criminals as relations and that is what those two women are.' A further letter from Ada, trying to justify her position, did not improve matters.

Then, on 5 April 1919, Ada wrote to say that their mother, now aged nearly eight-eight, had that morning died. On the next day Jeannette, without Rosalind, went over to Cheyne Walk. What passed between the sisters on that occasion was certainly not amicable nor conciliatory. On 8 April Jeannette sent Ada a message to say she would not attend the funeral, and once again all direct contact ceased. Ellen's will drawn up in March 1893, at the height of her quarrel with Jeannette and Edward, had never been revoked. And so Ada got her mother's entire estate, including all that had under Ellen's marriage settlement been vested in her husband for the duration of his lifetime, and to which all three surviving Marshall children, Jeannette, Ada and John, might have been thought to have equal rights.

Nevertheless, on her mother's death Jeannette came into the legacy left to her under her father's will and that, with Rosalind's increasing earnings, meant that from about 1920 the cloud of pecuniary embarrassment lifted somewhat from mother and daughter. On returning to Chelsea Rosalind had decided to exploit the skills acquired before the war at art school and the taste and dexterity she shared with her mother and other Marshalls. She painted lampshades, designed clothes and drew pierrots and colombines on menu and Christmas cards; she also decorated sets of nursery furniture, a well-paid job which on occasion brought her up to £12 10s. a week plus expenses. Gradually the first commissions, crumbs which came to her by way of encouragement from practising artists and art-loving friends, grew into a useful freelance business.

Her clients were the fashionable young, whose style she soon adopted. It was important to her career to be seen around, at the cocktail parties frequented by the smart set, in the right restaurants and night clubs, and to watch polo at Hurlingham and tennis at Wimbledon. She stayed out late several times a week dining and dancing, in the West End rather than at private parties. Dancing had been important in Jeannette's youth, in part because the parties and balls at which one danced were also the occasion for meeting the crowds of young men out of which one's eventual marriage partner might emerge. For Rosalind, as for other girls of her stamp, dancing not only represented the opportunity to be in the company of men, but was an avocation of singular attraction, part sport, part frenzy, to which they devoted the bulk of their leisure hours. She went through phases in the 1920s when each day's record contained some reference to dancing. There were impromptu dances to a gramophone at a friend's house and riotous dancing till five in the morning at the Chelsea Arts Ball; there were dancing lessons to learn the 'blues' in 1923 and the 'Charleston' in 1927. She danced at the fancy dress balls which were the rage in 1923; at *thés dansants* whenever her work allowed it; at the Hammersmith 'Palais de Dance', although she thought it 'pretty low etc.', in 1919, and at the new Mayfair Hotel in 1927. She fussed about finding men to accompany her to parties and agreed to dance with partners to whom she had not been introduced. She danced within eight weeks of her grandmother's death and nine days after the death of her uncle. She raved about 'two perfect American dancers' whom she had seen in a West End night club in 1923, Fred Astaire and his sister Adele.

She also occasionally smoked and rode pillion on a motorbike; she used slang and wrote 'h–ll' and 'd—d' in the diary (in 1892, it will be remembered, her mother admitted to having uttered an inward 'd' when under extreme stress). For Jeannette's 'feeling as queer as Dick's hatband' Rosalind substituted feeling 'dicky', or 'seedy', or 'puce', especially after 'beastly' or 'filthy' meals out; she knew 'awful' friends and 'horrible' girls, and she 'roared with laughter'. Many of the people she came across were 'rather comm', or 'not quite quite', or 'hidge'. 'What a beastly place the world has become since the War' she complained in 1919; the people in the Park were now 'ghastly'. 'How times have changed' she sighed in 1921, aged twenty-nine.

There is no evidence that she was much more relaxed about sexual matters than Jeannette had been at a comparable age. Jeannette had objected to the nudes at the Royal Academy; Rosalind, after a visit to the London Zoo, noted that the uninhibited behaviour of the monkeys on Monkey Hill gave her the 'creeps'. The crowd she moved in may have embraced a few of the fashionable dogmas of sexual freedom; the nearest evidence of it in the diaries was some plan of a mixed tour of the Pyrenees, which never materialized. She flirted assiduously and somewhat indiscriminately, as her mother too had done in her twenties and early thirties, and, unlike her mother, had many opportunities for tête-à-tête encounters with the men who interested her. Such occasions, on which she found herself alone in the presence of a man who attracted and amused her, and whom she sought to attract and entertain, occurred in all sorts of places and at all times of the day and the night, in art studios and night clubs, on the river and going home by taxi after a ball, in the motor cars which took her for a spin in the country or on a visit to a friend's weekend cottage. That all this engendered opportunities for sexual activity is certain, but no sign of it appeared in her jottings, except perhaps that she occasionally noted the date when her menstruation started. However, the fact that her periods were irregular was a sufficient reason to mark their onset, which she did by an asterisk or by some coy euphemism such as 'pain in front', 'not feeling too energetic', or 'un peu souffrante' in her diary. In her thirties, the condition became so marked as to require treatment. When she chose as her physician a woman, Dr Benham, Rosalind was probably motivated by modesty rather than by any feminist predilection.

There was another, major, difference between her life in her young womanhood and that of her mother. Unlike Jeannette who had had no regular companion within her own age group, with the exception of Ada, Rosalind spent her days, at work and play, in the company of other young people. Frances Holland and then art school had resulted in lasting friendships, some of which later helped to shape her adult life. Several of her friends married early and now had homes of their own. A few owned weekend cottages. With the advent of the motor car, the habit of spending one or two nights a week out of town had spread even to the young and relatively impecunious. Rosalind frequently went to stay with friends in the country, in houses with no servants and no ceremonial, where cats and dogs were admitted to the living room (in Jeannette's homes the cat had been a mouser and kept to the kitchen quarters), and young mothers nursed and played with their first babies without the help of professional nannies.

Such intimate contact with her contemporaries brought occasional insights into other people's lives which would have been foreign to Jeannette. 'Ba confessed she had no use for religion' Rosalind wrote in 1922 of her closest friend, Barbara Sichel, whom she had known ever since they had been schoolgirls together at Frances Holland; '. . . neither, really & truly I believe, has Frances Temple. No one has in these days.' Mrs Temple had, as Frances Anson, also been one of Rosalind's earliest friends. A few months before Rosalind's reflections William Temple, her husband, had been promoted to the bishopric of Manchester; in time he would become Archbishop of Canterbury.

Ba Sichel and Rosalind met several times a week, either at the studio to which they both had access for their art-work (Ba too went in for applied art), or over lunch or tea. The young men who took them out by and large belonged to the same set, so that they would form a foursome to dine and dance in town. On occasion Ba and Rosalind also holidayed together, with or without Rosalind's mother or Ba's sister, Helen, though Ba, Rosalind complained, was by no means an ideal travelling companion. The Seatons, mother and daughter, had resumed continental travel in 1920, when Mrs Marshall's death had removed some of the restraints on their budget. Together, they covered some of the ground familiar to Jeannette since the 1870s and '80s—Pontresina, the Italian Riviera, the Auvergne; to these they added in August 1926 a trip to the Vosges. But Jeannette was no longer the intrepid traveller who ran up and down alpine mountain-sides. Already in 1920 Rosalind observed that the high Pontresina altitudes caused her mother breathing difficulties, though she was still game for strenuous long walks. So Rosalind's most ambitious, 1922, jaunt was made without her mother. With one of her women friends she toured northern Italy, sightseeing in Venice, Padua, Verona and Milan, as well as spending some time at the Italian Lakes and in Switzerland. Back in London, she exulted that the entire three weeks' trip had cost just over £40.

It was the venturesome Ba who in 1927 organized a spring holiday in Suffolk. She and Rosalind stayed for a week in a fisherman's cottage at Kessingland near Lowestoft in primitive conditions with no water laid on in the house. They ate freshly caught fish and heated kettles for the bath and for washing-up, and froze and got drenched walking in the face of easterly gales—a whole world away from the comfortable Malvern hotel where Rosalind and Jeannette would spend a fortnight later that year.

'Mother, I know, thinks I am "fast" ' she wrote at the age of twenty-nine. Her habits had become those of a young woman of means who thought little of the cost of the weekly visit to the hairdresser or of hailing a taxi when late for an appointment. Her taste in clothes ran to the expensive, and she had neither the training nor the time to make her own. In consequence, she was often acutely anxious about money and complained that her mother persisted in letting financial matters slide. It was not until 1927 that both Rosalind's and Jeannette's money troubles ended. On 3 November 1927 Rupert Leslie, the son of well-to-do parents and himself a regular army officer with a promising future, asked Rosalind to marry him. She was thirty-five, only a year younger than her mother had been at the time of Seaton's proposal. Her answer was 'a very good equivalent of "Yes" instead of my usual "No"!!' Reporting it in the diary, she added: 'The darling', which was how she referred to Jeannette when she did not call her Mum, 'seemed not unpleased, I'm thankful to say.'

It was in fact at least the third time that Rosalind's affections had been seriously committed and therefore not the puzzling, obstacle-ridden novelty the five months' engagement had been to her mother thirty-six years previously. Even the 'business' talk at which Captain Leslie told his prospective mother-in-law of his financial position, and Jeannette in return revealed her own and Rosalind's precarious situation, passed off 'v. amicably'. 'Mum is such a darling to leave us to ourselves so obligingly' wrote Rosalind; her mood during the fourteen weeks' engagement was buoyant, at times 'absurdly happy'. Even an inopportune attack of mumps did not depress her.

The wedding took place on 9 February 1928. Her cousin George Buchanan gave Rosalind away. This time too, as in 1892, the bride omitted to describe the ceremony.

The wedding was no sooner over than Jeannette, as her mother before her, started to bemoan her lot, which was indeed not enviable. She had suffered a number of minor mishaps in the previous three years, having become rather accident-prone. She found it increasingly difficult to cope with the servants. In short, at seventy-two, Jeannette was beginning to show her age. Moreover, it must have been clear to her that nothing could replace her daughter's companionship: she would be left behind, while the new bride adjusted to married life in army postings sufficiently distant from London to make each of her visits to Chelsea into an event.

The gap left by Rosalind's defection could certainly not be filled by Ada, with whom Jeannette had had no contact for some three years. The last time the sisters had seen one another was at John's funeral, in early 1925. John had returned to London in 1904 or so, having been 'invited' to leave St Petersburg after the outbreak of the Russo-Japanese War on the suspicion of being a foreign spy, and had settled to a bachelor existence in Bloomsbury. He lived in rooms in Guilford Street and spent most of his waking hours in the Reading Room of the British Museum on various literary and philological pursuits, all connected with Russia. The fruits of his researches, published over the years, were a few articles on topographic and literary themes, and a successful primer, *Russian Self-Taught*, which went into many editions; the last one appeared in 1957 and cost 3s 6d.

Since their mother's death in 1919 and the subsequent rupture of relations between his sisters, he was a relatively regular visitor at Oakley Street. Rosalind found him seedy, prosy and generally boring.

He filled the drawing-room with smoke, she complained, and brought her his tax returns to wrestle with. 'Mother loathed him' she claimed on an occasion when he had exasperated her particularly. Then, in the winter of 1924–5, when John was sixty-seven, there was a gap of some three or four months without news of him in the diary; eventually, on 5 February 1925 Ada's message broke the silence:

Uncle John met with an accident in the fog in Middle Temple Lane on Jan. 11, the day after his return from Spain, broke his leg, was taken to Barts where he died as a result of the accident & complications at 7 o'c this morning. Oh! how wretched & bitter we feel that we were never told & could not go to see him & do what we could. What a <u>wicked</u> woman my Aunt is. Poor man—his whole life & death have been a pathetic tragedy. He was always kind to me.

The funeral took place on 9 February at the Golders Green Crematorium. Jeannette and Rosalind went there by tube and found a peculiar gathering: besides Ada, flanked by her two domestics, there was Mr Large, the lawyer called in to deal with John's affairs, and three strangers—a 'full fledged black' and two other men—who had come to pay their last respects to John at 'a strange cold little service'.

The meeting between the sisters which, at the insistence of Mr Large, took place after the funeral was not satisfactory. John had died intestate, and Ada had been given letters of administration for his estate which amounted to a little over £3,000. The cash she probably divided with Jeannette; John's own drawings and water-colours she must have appropriated, for they eventually reappeared as legacies in her own will.

Before Rosalind had time to regain her breath after the return from the four weeks' honeymoon which had taken the Leslies as far as Majorca, she was forced to decide on her immediate priorities. Habit (and a raging cold) won, and after one night with Rupert at his parents' home in Bolton Gardens, she transferred to Oakley Street. The choice was sufficiently bizarre to make her rethink where her allegiance now lay. 'It really isn't right' she ventured after one night under Jeannette's roof, and on the third day she moved back to Bolton Gardens. Variations of this sequence were repeated several times in the early months of her marriage, with several homes, Oakley Street, Bolton Gardens and the ever-changing houses on the periphery of Rupert's army postings constantly in play.

Rosalind's and Rupert's only child, Caroline, was born at Oakley

Street on 30 April 1929. 'Darling baby ... Absurdly like Rupert ... perfectly healthy & very bobbish, thank God' wrote Rosalind. Some months later she noted that her mother was 'so pleased with Caroline'. But Jeannette, aged nearly seventy-four when her grandchild was born, was in fact too old to enjoy her new role, and her increasing infirmity caused new problems for Caroline's nomad parents. Within two years of the child's birth the Oakley Street home had to be closed down. Jeannette moved in with Rosalind and Rupert, and her last years were spent in the relative discomfort of camp-following. She died on 20 May 1935, two months short of her eightieth birthday, and was buried next to her husband in Brookfield Cemetery, Woking. Rosalind was her only heir.

Ada, still Jeannette's shadow, died a year and a half after her sister, in December 1936. An attempt at reconciliation in 1930 had failed and the sisters had until the very last continued on their separate ways. Rosalind was not mentioned in her aunt's will. It may have been this omission that gave rise to the tenacious family myth that Ada's estate had been willed to the Battersea Dogs' Home. In reality, the bulk of Ada's considerable estate was left to University College Hospital, to be applied, in the name of John Marshall FRS, to a purpose connected with the advancement of surgery. By a coincidence, the legacy amounted to about £30,000, the same as the heiress Elizabeth Walton had fed into the coffers of the Williams family a hundred and twenty years earlier. Lesser sums went to Epsom College, also in memory of her father, and to establish a musical scholarship for the blind, named after the blind Aunt Eliza Williams. There were some further small legacies, including £100 for Ada's grandniece Caroline, whom she had most probably never met. Caroline also got a pearl necklace (which had been a gift to Ada from her parents) and a 'bracelet composed of family miniatures'; this, a present in the mid-1860s from a grateful patient, shows all six Savile Row Marshalls, parents and four children—tiny tinted photographic likenesses of a united household.

THE SEATONS

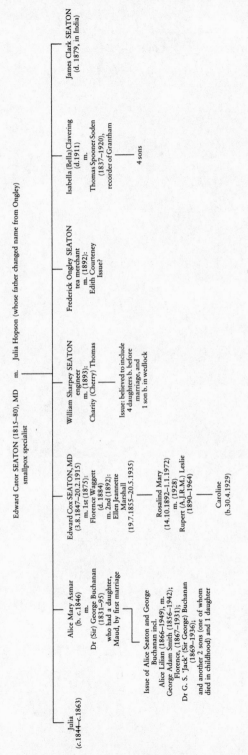

Edward Cator SEATON (1815–80), MD m. Julia Hopson (whose father changed name from Ongley)
smallpox specialist

Julia
(c.1844–c.1863)

Alice Mary Asmar
(b. c.1846)
m.
Dr (Sir) George Buchanan
(1831–95)
who had a daughter,
Maud, by first marriage

Issue of Alice Seaton and George
Buchanan incl.
Alice Lilian (1866–1949), m.
George Adam Smith (1856–1942);
Florence, (1867–1931);
Dr G. S. 'Jack' (Sir George) Buchanan
(1869–1936);
and another 2 sons (one of whom
died in childhood) and 1 daughter

Edward Cox SEATON, MD
(3.8.1847–20.2.1915)
m.1st (1875):
Florence Waggett
(d. 1884)
m.2nd (1892):
Ellen Jeannette
Marshall
(19.7.1855–20.5.1935)

Rosalind Mary
(14.10.1892–1.1.1972)
m. (1928)
Rupert (A.J.R.M.) Leslie
(1890–1964)

Caroline
(b.30.4.1929)

William Sharpey SEATON
engineer
m. (1893):
Charity (Cherry) Thomas

Issue: believed to include
4 daughters b. before
marriage, and
1 son b. in wedlock

Frederick Ongley SEATON
tea merchant
m. (1892):
Edith Courteney
Issue?

Isabella (Bella) Clavering
(d.1911)
m.
Thomas Spooner Soden
(1837–1920),
recorder of Grantham

4 sons

James Clark SEATON
(d. 1879, in India)

INDEX

Cambridgeshire Militia, 42–3, 60

Campbell, Lord Colin, youngest son of the 8th Duke of Argyll, 43

Canut, Monsieur, Léon, and May, 18. *See also*: Noël, Mme

Carriages and other horse-drawn vehicles; their coachmen, 24, 29, 46–9, 82–3, 123, 135, 147, 149, 173, 177, 181, 185, 201, 207–9, 230. *See also*: London—transport and traffic problems

Carter, Hilary Bonham, d. 1866, first cousin of Florence Nightingale; member of LSA, 19

Cartwright, Hamilton, dentist, 102, 107

Cassal, Mr, student at University College, London, 67

Cassavetti, Euphrosyne, born Ionides, mother of Mary Zambaco, 110

Casson, Mr, beadle at University College, London, 66–7

Castañeda, John, *c.* 1834–1900, surgeon; friend and assistant of JM, 26–7, 127

Catalani, Signor, musician acquaintance of the Marshalls, 88

Cemeteries, graves, 6, 29, 82, 247

Challice, John, 1815–63, physician, Liberal politician, MOH Bermondsey, tract-writer for LSA, 20

Chaperones, chaperoning, 42, 51, 77, 105, 109–10, 167, 189, 197–200, 203; post-1914, 242, 245

Chapman, Canon, 204

Charities, charity performances, do-gooding, 69–70, 121, 134–5, 145, 247. *See also*: Bazaars; Ladies' Sanitary Association

Chartist riots (1848), 4

Chelsea, 174, 180–1, 184, 195, 208–9, 216, 239, 245. *See also*: Belle Vue House

Chessar, Jane Agnes, 1835–80, educationist, on staff of Home and Colonial School, on London School Board for Marylebone, 1873, 15–16, 20, 75

Children, childhood, 7–9, 10, 18, 20, 30–1, 91, 130, 149, 153, 226, 246–7

Christian, Prince of Schleswig Holstein, husband of Queen Victoria's daughter Helena, 149

Christmas, 34–5, 38, 182, 197, 199, 202, 232–3, 235–7

Churches and other places of worship, 6,

35–7, 40, 135, 148–50, 158, 176, 181, 195, 204, 218, 219, 237

Clapham, J. H., 143

Clapham, South London, 47, 195, 207–9, 216, 218, 224, 234

Clark, Andrew (Sir), 1826–93, physician; president of RCP, 186

Class, social strata, v, 41, 156, 160. *See also*: Status

Clergy, clergymen, 34, 59, 75, 153, 237

Clough, Anne Jemima, 1820–92, educationist; first principal of Newnham College, Cambridge; trained at the Home and Colonial School, 15

Clubs, clubland, 24, 43, 50, 55–7, 147–9, 172

Cluff, James Stanton, 138

Coates, Mr, William Marshall's clerk at Ely, 185

Cobden-Sanderson, Thomas James, 1840–1922, bookbinder, printer; pioneer of Arts and Crafts, 164

Cockct, Mrs, dressmaker, 29–30

Colloms, Brenda, 20

Collyer, Kate Winifred, later Mrs Benjamin Walker, *fl.* 1891–1914, miniaturist, and her work, 225, 236–7

Colvin, Sidney (Sir), 1845–1927, art and literary critic, 126

Concerts, concert-going, 43, 47, 116, 119, 152, 161, 218. *See also*: Music

Condolences, 30–1, 34, 47, 90–1, 112, 192

Cornforth, Fanny (professional name of Sarah Cox), later Mrs Timothy Hughes, later Mrs John Schott; D. G. Rossetti's model and mistress, 112

Coronio, Aglaia, born Ionides, and family, 110, 118–19

Correspondence, telegrams, 18–19, 31, 57, 82, 89–93, 95–6, 99, 110, 111, 112–16, 124, 126, 140, 158, 168–71, 184–5, 188–92, 196, 203–4, 211–12, 216, 218, 220, 222–3, 227–30, 232–3, 236–7, 238, 240–1. *See also*: Condolences; Etiquette

Costume, clothes, fashion, 13, 27, 33, 36, 38–9, 48–9, 51, 53, 61–3, 71, 73, 88, 98, 107, 136, 141, 146, 148–52, 161–2, 164, 175, 186, 195–6, 198, 203–4, 214, 216–17, 236–7, 241, 244; aesthetic, artistic, 117–21, 146; babies', children's, 18, 21, 26, 211,